Examining Patients

Examining Patients
An introduction to clinical medicine

SECOND EDITION

Edited by
Peter J. Toghill MD, FRCP
Consultant Physician, University Hospital, Queen's Medical Centre, Nottingham.

Edward Arnold
A member of the Hodder Headline Group
LONDON BOSTON MELBOURNE AUCKLAND

First published in Great Britain 1990, second edition 1995, by
Edward Arnold, a division of Hodder Headline PLC,
338 Euston Road, London NW1 3BH

Distributed in the USA by
Routledge, Chapman and Hall, Inc.
29 West 35th Street, New York, NY 10001

British Library Cataloguing in Publication Data
A catalogue record for this book is available from the British Library

ISBN 0 340 589663 (Hb)

1 2 3 4 5   95 96 97 98 99

Typeset in 9/11pt Palatino by
Setrite Typesetters, Hong Kong
Printed and bound by Dah Hua Printing Press Co., Ltd. Hong Kong

Preface to the First Edition

Sir William Osler encouraged students of medicine to 'Learn to see, learn to hear, learn to feel, learn to smell and to know that by practice alone you can become expert.' What he said still applies. We need to listen to our patients to understand their symptoms and we need to observe them with our critical senses to elicit physical signs. These are skills that every doctor can achieve, but they require strenuous effort.

My reasons for editing a new book on symptoms and signs are twofold. Firstly, time has moved on and the patterns of disease are changing. In the western world we are faced with an ageing population for which special skills are required to assess physical and mental health. Life support systems and organ transplantation demand accurate evaluation of the signs of brain death. Readily available air transport has brought the diseases of the tropics into the developed world. New illnesses such as the immuno-deficiency syndromes have appeared bringing with them new, subtle and previously unfamiliar physical signs. Secondly, there is a risk that the new technology such as CT scanning and echocardiography will seduce doctors and medical students away from the art of clinical examination. Let us hope that these new machines will bolster the art rather than undermine it. We can now demonstrate better how physical signs arise and what they actually mean.

This book is meant primarily for medical students in their clinical years but we hope it will be used by general practitioners and postgraduates as a basis for their everyday work. Once the basic grammar of the language of medicine has been learned the vocabulary can be added by everyday experience. We have used the earlier chapters, dealing with the examination of the major systems, as a framework on which to build descriptions of more specialized topics. In this way as well as being a textbook of symptoms and signs it serves as an introduction to clinical medicine in the widest sense. Obviously in a book of this kind it is impossible to be entirely comprehensive but we have deliberately included some rarities that demonstrate instructive features.

The contributors are mainly from the Nottingham Medical School which was established in 1970 as the first new medical school in the United Kingdom in the 20th century. They have based their chapters on experience gained in a large and busy district general hospital at the hub of England.

Nottingham is not the best place to study tropical disease so I have recruited Professor Gordon Cook's enormous experience to help with the chapter on tropical diseases. At present the consequences of infection with the human immunodeficiency virus are only just reaching the English Midlands and Ian Weller, from the Middlesex Hospital, London, has dealt with this topic.

Though based on medicine as seen in the United Kingdom this book is intended for worldwide use since the correct clinical interpretation of physical signs is necessary for all. We have to bear in mind that much of the world's population does not have immediate access to simple X-rays let alone MRI scanning. There is no excuse for inadequate clinical examination either in centres of excellence or in hospitals with limited technical and financial resources.

Peter Toghill

Nottingham, 1989

Preface to the Second Edition

Examining Patients was first published in 1990 and its wide acceptance by medical students, in the UK and overseas, has encouraged production of a second edition for publication in 1994. In this age of rapidly advancing technology I hope that its direct, personal, hands-on approach to patients will demonstrate how much can be achieved by skilled history-taking and clinical examination. Not every patient needs a battery of blood tests or expensive imaging!

Colour has been added to this second edition to present clinical photographs more realistically and also to enhance the clarity of the many tables that appear throughout the book. Important information has been coded as follows: green for causes of clinical conditions; yellow for checklists of important points to bear in mind or act on; purple for diagnostic features. *Examining Patients* was never intended as a comprehensive textbook but its purpose as a learning manual for those early days on the wards is maintained. I hope that general practitioners and postgraduate students will continue to find it useful in their day-to-day work.

I am grateful to my colleagues for revising their sections and for contributing new ideas. Professor Peter Rubin has added a new chapter on physical signs in pregnancy — a topic not previously dealt with in other books on medical physical signs. With our multiracial society new problems are being encountered in haematology and Dr Jalihal from Baroda has expanded the chapter on 'Anaemia, blood diseases and enlarged glands'. Critics of undergraduate and postgraduate training in the UK complain that we often teach about diseases that have no relevance to everyday life. I do not think this is necessarily true but I have added (not as a sop to the critics I hasten to say) a new chapter dealing with 'Black-outs, collapses and shock', problems which frequently confront medical students and young doctors in Accident and Emergency departments. In response to requests from new clinical students we have added a glossary of medical terms.

Sadly, Professor Tony Mitchell died in 1991, shortly after the first edition was published. He was the mentor and inspiration for many of us here in Nottingham and as a tribute to his memory I have left his chapter on 'History taking' untouched. It cannot be improved upon.

The patient–doctor relationship is crucial to the successful conduct of clinical medicine. This is established by taking a history and examining the patient yourself. I hope that this book ensures that this is learned properly at the start so that it can become a skill honed to perfection by a lifetime of practice.

Peter Toghill

Nottingham, 1993

Acknowledgements

I am grateful to the contributors and to other colleagues who have helped in the production of this second edition. As before the majority of the illustrations have been prepared by the Audio-Visual Department of the Queen's Medical Centre, Nottingham and I owe much to the skill of Geoff Gilbert, who has taken many of the photographs, and Lyndon Cochrane who has prepared the diagrams. Churchill Livingstone, Edinburgh, have kindly allowed us to reproduce some ECGs from Professor Hampton's book and Fig. 17.12 is reproduced by permission of HMSO. My sincere thanks go to all the patients who have allowed themselves to be photographed for educational purposes; no book on physical signs could be produced without such illustrations.

The editorial staff of Edward Arnold have been most supportive and it was their encouragement which stimulated the production of this second edition. My secretary Elizabeth Myers has helped with the typing and the book has been wordprocessed by Pauline Morrell. Our medical students in Nottingham have reviewed many chapters and have offered constructive and, often, pungent criticism.

Geoffrey Walker, a former colleague, valued friend and travelling companion for many years, has spent long hours reading and revising the script. I am particularly grateful to him for taking on this onerous task and completing it so efficiently. I have been fortunate in having the constant support and encouragement of my wife Rosemary who has, over these last few months, not only organized my activities, but read this new edition and prepared the glossary.

Contents

xii *Contents*

Contributors

B. R. Allen FRCP
Consultant Dermatologist, University Hospital, Nottingham

S. P. Allison MD, FRCP
Consultant Physician, University Hospital, Nottingham

T. H. D. Arie FRCP, FRCPsych
Professor of Health Care of the Elderly, University of Nottingham

N. J. Barton FRCS
Consultant Orthopaedic Surgeon, University Hospital, Nottingham and Harlow Wood Hospital, Mansfield, Notts

M. J. Bendall MD, FRCP
Senior Lecturer and Consultant Physician, Department of Health Care of the Elderly, University Hospital, Nottingham

C. J. Bignell FRCP
Consultant in Genitourinary Medicine, Nottingham City Hospital

R. Cantwell MB, MRCPsych
Lecturer in Psychiatry, Medical School, University of Nottingham

G. C. Cook MD, DSc, FRCP, FRACP
Professor of Medicine, London School of Hygiene and Tropical Medicine; Honorary Consultant Physician, Hospital for Tropical Diseases, London

I. W. Fellows DM, MRCP
Consultant Physician, Norfolk and Norwich Hospital

N. R. Galloway MD FRCS
Consultant Ophthalmic Surgeon, University Hospital, Nottingham

K. P. Gibbin MA, FRCS
Consultant Otolaryngologist, University Hospital, Nottingham

R. B. Godwin-Austen MD, FRCP
Consultant Neurologist, University Hospital, Nottingham, Derbyshire Royal Infirmary and Pilgrim Hospital, Boston

J. R. Hampton DM, DPhil, FRCP
Professor of Cardiology, University of Nottingham and Consultant Physician, University Hospital, Nottingham

S. S. Jalihal MD, MRCPath
Consultant Haematologist, Scunthorpe General Hospital, South Humberside

I. D. A. Johnston MD, FRCP
Consultant Physician, University Hospital, Nottingham

the late **J. R. A. Mitchell** MD, DPhil, FRCP
formerly Professor of Medicine, University of Nottingham and Consultant Physician, University Hospital, Nottingham

Margaret Oates DPM, FRCPsych
Senior Lecturer in Psychiatry, University of Nottingham and Honorary Consultant Psychiatrist, University Hospital and Mapperley Hospital, Nottingham

P. C. Rubin DM, FRCP
Professor of Therapeutics, University of Nottingham and Consultant Physician, University Hospital, Nottingham

R. B. Tattersall MD, FRCP
Professor of Diabetes and Consultant Physician, University Hospital, Nottingham

P. J. Toghill MD, FRCP
Director of Continuing Medical Education, Royal College of Physicians, London and Emeritus Consultant Physician, University Hospital, Nottingham

1
History-taking

J. R. A. Mitchell

Definitions
Why bother?
The contribution of the history
Why we do it
How to do it
What have you achieved?
References and further reading

We must teach the student how to collect the facts

(Pickering 1958)

Sir George Pickering believed that a well-taken history was a record of the patient's experiences, not only of the current illness for which help was being sought, but of his life, work, family situation and previous health. Properly presented, this history would then allow any subsequent reader or listener to feel that they had lived through and shared those experiences. Pickering also recognized that in addition to the cold facts which the history-taker is trying to elicit, a patient is continually offering valuable clues to his attitudes, knowledge and beliefs about his health by the manner in which he provides the information and by the opinions and fears which colour the story he is telling. His own teacher, Wilfred Trotter, has emphasized the importance of this additional information when he observed 'Disease often tells its secrets in a casual parenthesis'. Before we describe how to elicit both the facts and these nuances, we need to clarify some of the terms we are going to use.

Definitions

Symptoms

These are the things which patients have either noticed for themselves or will recollect when appropriate questions are put to them. Some symptoms also have an externally observable element which can be subsequently shared with the interrogator. They can thus form part of the physical signs of that illness (a swollen leg; a weak arm; a lump in the breast; a skin rash) but many symptoms cannot be cross-checked in this way (chest pain; headache; a numb arm; pins and needles in the feet). Many important diseases have no observable abnormalities whatsoever, so their recognition will depend entirely on the skill and accuracy with which the patient's experiences are elicited and recorded. For example, the common and troublesome condition of migraine has no abnormalities which can be detected by an outside observer, so the correct labelling of the visual disturbances, headaches and vomiting hinges on the patient's story. Similarly, in the effort-related chest pain we call angina pectoris, the pattern of pain may be all that we have to rely on when we have to decide whether to embark on invasive high-technology tests.

The physical signs of the illness

The recognition of these will be covered in subsequent chapters. They are those things which the examining doctor finds. They may, as outlined above, overlap with the patient's symptoms, but more often provide additional information about them. For example, if you find that the legs are swollen, this may merely confirm what the patient has told you, but if you also find an irregular pulse, an enlarged heart and an elevated jugular venous pressure, you are now beginning to point your finger at the heart as the likely culprit.

Finally, when the symptoms and signs have been elicited, the doctor may need to seek help in reaching a working label for the problem by embarking on a series of investigations such as blood tests, x-rays, electrical recordings or isotope imaging.

Why bother?

A particular assembly of body size, shape, facial features, hair and eye colouring enables you to differentiate between students in your year so that you can predict their responses to particular situations and can modify your own actions accordingly. So too will the symptoms, signs and investigative findings enable you to recognize an illness and apply to it a working label or diagnosis. Remember that the name of the illness is of little interest to the patient, except as a topic of social conversation, for what he wants to know is what the label will do to his life: 'Will I die?'; 'Can I return to work?'; 'Will I be disabled?'; 'Can I marry and have children?'. This requires us to judge the future course of the patient's illness and thereby to offer him a prognosis. A working label enables us to consult colleagues, books and scientific journals to determine, from past experience, how the illness is likely to behave. We can then decide whether treatment is necessary or of proven effectiveness, so that a balance-sheet of benefit and harm can be drawn up and the patient can share with us the decisions about what needs to be done.

The contribution of the history

Where patients cannot provide a record of their experiences (for example, because speech has been lost after a stroke; inability to speak the same language as the doctor; infancy; disturbances of consciousness) the attending doctor has to rely on evidence provided by relatives, bystanders or neighbours, and ambulance personnel, so must begin his search for a diagnosis under the same difficulties as our veterinary colleagues. Additionally, in medical and surgical emergencies, the manifest need for life-saving action will temporarily take precedence over the step-by-step recording of the history, so that the attending doctor will recognize hypoglycaemia and correct it before asking the patient about the causes of death of his grandparents, or will correct life-threatening asthmatic airways obstruction before quizzing the patient about his pets and hobbies.

Nevertheless, the majority of patients who you will be asked to see in your early days in clinical medicine will be out-patients or ward admissions who will not, at that time, be desperately ill. In such circumstances, we did a study to assess the relative contributions of history-taking, of physical examination and of investigation by taking a series of patients who we saw in a general medical out-patient clinic. We asked the doctors involved to write down their working diagnoses after reading the referring general practitioner's letter, after taking the history, after examining the patient and after all the tests had been completed. These step-by-step interim diagnoses were then compared with the eventual diagnosis which was reached after a further period of out-patient follow-up. Table 1.1 shows the results and indicates that the most crucial step in reaching a final diagnosis which differed from that already reached by the referring general practitioner was history-taking, the subsequent examination and investigation producing a much lower yield. Thus, in a medical out-patient clinic, if you have 30 minutes to offer a new patient, I would suggest that 15 minutes for the history, 10 minutes for examination and for planning any tests needed and 5 minutes for telling the patient what it all means and what is to happen next would be a sensible time-allocation.

Table 1.1. How we reach a diagnosis in new medical outpatients

	%
Referring GP's diagnosis unchanged	44
Diagnosis changed after history	41
Diagnosis changed after examination	7
Diagnosis changed after tests	8

Why we do it

Before sitting down to talk to your first-ever patient, remind yourself what you are trying to do:

1. To establish the facts about the illness by recording the patient's experiences. You may well be offered the patient's own diagnosis, or another physician's, such as 'indigestion', 'anaemia' or 'arthritis' but remember that behind each label lies a set of symptoms and it is these you must now ferret out.
2. To establish the patient's attitudes to his illness by watching for non-verbal clues and by listening for the hopes and fears with which he clothes his narrative.
3. To establish the doctor's attitude to the patient and his illness. The commonest complaint about doctors is that they neither seem to have the time nor the inclination to listen and the patient who sees the doctor reaching for a prescription pad for a psychotropic drug before he has told his full story must fear that the bulb in the dashboard warning light is being removed as a quicker and cleaner alternative to lifting the bonnet to check the oil-level. A patient of mine said 'I knew he must be an important specialist because he wouldn't let me talk to him' while a colleague commented 'Usually I talk to my patients, but if I have time, I listen to them too'.

How to do it

The skills required are shown in Table 1.2, so let us examine these attributes in more detail:

Understanding Patients will often offer a symptom which may be crystal-clear to them, but which requires immediate probing so that the body-system most likely to be responsible can be identified. 'Dizziness' is a good example, for to one person it could be the sense of rotation and nausea that we all experience after a fairground ride but which in disease terms points to problems in the ear or its neurological connections. Alternatively, to the next patient, 'dizziness' can imply a sense of faintness or lightheadedness which may lead us towards the circulation as a likely explanation (blood-loss, fluid depletion, heart-valve disease or heart-rhythm disturbances, for example). An early interruption (see below), to say 'People can have different sorts of dizziness so let's find out exactly what sort yours is'

Table 1.2. Skills needed for history-taking

The ability to:
Understand and be understood
Obtain relevant information
Interview logically
Interrupt when necessary without inhibiting patient's willingness to talk
Look for non-verbal clues
Establish a good relationship with patient
Be able to summarize the information for succinct presentation on ward round or telephone

will lead you towards a clearer description of the symptoms. You will meet many such situations ('palpitations'; 'black-outs'; 'indigestion' and 'arthritis' for example) and in all of them you need gently to edge the patient away from his label and to uncover his actual experiences.

As well as your ability to understand what the patient is telling you, you must be sure that he understands what you are talking about. Cross-cultural language problems should be self-evident and must be got around by using relatives as interpreters, by mime, by drawing or sometimes (see below) by recourse to four-letter words as opposed to the polite circumlocutions of everyday speech. Even where no language problems appear to exist, the most basic bodily functions may have no counterpart in the patient's polite vocabulary and furthermore, the impolite words vary enormously from one part of a country to another. You need to know what women in your current locality call their periods and it is pointless to ask about eructation, expectoration and passing flatus, when words like 'belch/burp', 'spit' and 'fart', would bring a 'Now I know what you mean, doctor' smile to the patient's face. Reflect with your class-mates on the wide range of words that you used at school to describe the genitalia and do not hesitate to use them instead of penis, testicles and vulva. Never assume that your patients understand their own anatomy, so words like 'stomach', 'kidney' and 'hip' should prompt a gentle interruption to say 'Show me exactly where you mean'.

Essential information can often only be identified retrospectively, so when in doubt, listen patiently while you are told about Auntie Flo's wedding or what they had for breakfast on Easter Monday five years ago. If such a diversionary loop seems likely to lose you and the patient, then play your interruption card.

Interview logically according to the schema outlined

in Table 1.3, but if facts are offered out of sequence, store them in your memory, to avoid asking about them later and hinting to the patient that you weren't really listening. For example, a man may say, in explaining the onset of his own illness 'It began the day we buried the wife' so if, in its logical place, you then say 'And is your wife in good health' you will slip down a notch in the patient's eyes.

Table 1.3. Usual schema for case-history
Name, age and occupation Presenting complaint (PC) History of presenting complaint (HPC) System review (SR) Previous medical history (PMH) Family history (FH) Social and occupational history (SH) Drug history including adverse reactions

Interruptions should be kept to a minimum, but if you do not understand the patient or if he is embarking on a major diversionary loop, then you must say 'Let's try and get that clearer in my mind; tell me exactly . . .'.

Watch as well as listen; it is therefore sensible to jot down rough notes as the patient talks. You can then maintain eye-contact with them and they will not be inhibited by an 'As I was proceeding along the High Street . . .' verbatim-transcription approach of the comic policeman. A fair-copy can then be made later for the records and this gives you the chance to organize times and events in your mind for ward-rounds or case-presentations.

Relationships If you have shown the patient that you are interested and that what you have been doing is 'not merely resigned listening or even politely waiting until you can interrupt' then you have taken the most essential step in patient-care.

The ability to summarize is only attained by practice but the framework described here will help you to acquire an invaluable skill which will stand you in good stead in every branch of medical practice, so good history-taking forms a life-time bonus.

How to begin

The first step to getting an effective working relationship with your patient is to secure an accurate mutual introduction. From the ward-records, the notes or the bed-foot charts you will already know the patient's name, so having checked that its prefix is right (especially Mrs vs Miss vs Ms), I suggest that you approach the patient with an interrogative lift to your voice ('Miss Smith?'), then tell her who you are and check her age and current job. A good phrase is 'I am Miss White, a student doctor, and I have been asked by Dr Brown to help to look after you. Can I sit down and talk to you?'

The presenting complaint (PC)

Many beginnings are counter-productive: 'What are you complaining of?' sounds as though you have already labelled the patient as a whinger; 'What brought you to hospital?' invites the response 'An ambulance'; while 'What is wrong with you?' could provoke 'That's what you're supposed to be finding out'. I think that 'How can we help you?' or 'What is it that you want us to put right?' can get the interview off on a reasonable footing. Try to pin down the symptoms in one or two words, putting down what the patient says, rather than your technical translation of it (black stools rather than melaena; breathlessness and not dyspnoea; swollen legs rather than dependent oedema). If the patient can only offer you a label at this stage, then put it down as 'indigestion' to indicate that clarification will follow in the next section. If the approximate duration of the symptoms has already emerged, you can now take your virgin sheet of paper, write down the date and time of your interview and then begin with:

PC Ankle swelling for 6 months
    Breathlessness for 1 month
    Chest pain for 1 day

The history of the presenting complaint (HPC)

You can then say 'Let's go back to the beginning; tell me how it all started?' or 'When were you last completely well?'. The latter may take you back to their earliest recollections of any illness, so you will immediately be tangling with the patient's previous medical history. If appropriate, you can interrupt them and guide them to their immediate problems, but if in doubt, note it all down chronologically and edit it later. Take them step by step through the evolution of their story, dating critical events as clearly as you can. If the patient sought medical advice, had tests or was admitted to hospital, get as many details as you can, for how a patient was handled can give invaluable guidance as to the thoughts of the attending doctors. Bring the history right up to the time of your interview, including any current treatment plus the details of how the patient arrived in front of you (general practitioner referral; self-referral via Casualty; referral from work). Finally, it is illuminating at this stage to ask the patient what they think the illness is and whether they regard it as of serious significance.

Since patients often wish to please a helpful doctor and will therefore say 'Yes' to what barristers would call leading questions, throughout this section it is vital to cast your queries in an open form, rather than putting them in a way which itself suggests an acceptable answer. Thus, to the patient who says 'My motions were a funny colour' you should say 'What colour?' rather than saying 'Black?'.

For each of the common symptom-complexes you will soon realize what information you need to elicit and Table 1.4 illustrates this in respect of pain. Many diseases identify themselves by their pain-patterns so that when you ask your patient to show you where his pain is and he places his hand (not a fingertip, since referred pain from deep viscera is never that well-localized) on his epigastrium and he then tells you that over the long term he has a few bad weeks, followed by months of freedom, your index of suspicion of peptic ulceration is already high. If he then tells you that hunger, as at night, is associated with his pain and that food, antacids such as 'Rennies', 'Settlers' or 'Milk of Magnesia' from his local chemist and making himself sick will all promptly relieve the pain, then you are looking at a patient with a peptic ulcer, no matter how many negative barium meals he has had.

Table 1.4. Information to be elicited with respect to pain
If pain is a feature then record:
Site — show me; does it spread anywhere?
Character — what is it like?
Timing — long-term over whole span of illness and in detail when it is there.
Things that change it — what makes it better/what makes it worse?

The system review (SR)

Because patients may not remember everything that has happened to them, or may consider that what they do remember is irrelevant or too trivial to mention, it is permissible to jog their memory with some structured questions and a suggested sequence is shown in Table 1.5. If any system is the prime

Table 1.5. Schema for reviewing systems
General well being — weight; appetite; fever; appearance; sleep; mood.
Cardiovascular and respiratory — exercise tolerance for simple, everyday things like a flight of stairs or mowing the lawn; chest pain; 'palpitations'; leg swelling; cough; sputum.
Alimentary — belly pain; nausea or vomiting; bowel habits and nature of stools.
Genitourinary — frequency of micturition by day and by night; incontinence; pain; frequency and duration of periods; sexual activity.
Nervous — headache; vision and hearing; weakness or disturbed sensation.
Locomotor — joint pain, stiffness or swelling.

suspect from your previous history-taking, then the sub-headings will need to be expanded or if mental illness is deemed to play a part, then you will need to frame additional questions in this area. Remember that one definition of a good psychiatrist is the doctor who takes the proper history first time round. Again, remember not tacitly to accept labels, for the patient's use of them may differ from yours; for example, is 'diarrhoea' one very loose stool each day or six well formed ones?

Previous medical history (PMH)

Some of this may already have emerged during your discussion of the presenting illness, but if not, you should ask 'Have you had any illnesses that kept you off school or work at any time in your life? Have you been admitted to hospital or been seen in an out-patient clinic?'. If such events do emerge, try to work out what might have been going on by recording what the attending doctors did. For example, a 'heart attack' which kept a patient in hospital for only two days sounds of different magnitude to the next patient's who remembers being in a coronary-care unit for five days, during which he had a 'wire into his heart' for pacing, a 'tube into his heart from the groin' which was obviously a cardiac catheter, who was off work for six months and who is now on the waiting-list for coronary bypass surgery. Obtaining clear information about major past illnesses, including the addresses at which the patient was living at the time and the hospitals involved, will enable you to summon up the actual hospital records, to make comparisons of results possible, such as changes in the electrocardiographic patterns, and to avoid duplicating previously-done tests.

Family history (FH)

So often, one is told during a case-presentation that there is 'No relevant family history'. This is arrant nonsense, because even though there may be no similar illnesses in the family, the number, relationships and health of the people who may be asked to care for the patient when your episode is completed will be crucial to your management. Similarly, even for diseases that do not have a major heredofamilial basis, their presence in the family will condition the patient's approach to his own symptoms. Thus, if a patient's father and brother both died of lung cancer at the age of 55, your patient who is now that age himself will be more anxious about his chest pain and cough than you are. A few diseases are of course of genetic origin (haemophilia; abnormal haemoglobins as in thalassaemia and sickle-cell disease; Huntington's chorea with its progression to dementia). Where such a possibility exists, you must enquire about the patient's offspring, parents, uncles and aunts, and about grandparents too. Conversely, an 84-year-old woman with a heart attack cannot possibly be carrying dominant nasty genes, or she would not have survived, so here you are more interested in the role of the family as potential carers. You need to know the state of health of the spouse, children, nephews and nieces, and in particular, whether the old lady, who now seems so charming, has so wrecked their lives in the past that they will not be prepared to disturb their current peaceful state by offering to look after her. 'Family history — nil' is therefore, a foolish misunderstanding of the relevance of the whole family, past and present, to the patient's fears and hopes and to the provision that will need to be made for after-care. Such elements are always present, whereas a direct genetic contribution to the illness in front of you is much rarer.

Social history (SH)

The depth to which you explore this area may be conditioned by the earlier part of your history, by the time available and by the patient's willingness and ability to tell you about himself. At the very least, you must establish where the patient was born, and then for immigrants, find out the date of their move and any other countries they have visited *en route*. The rise in foreign travel makes it vital to quiz patients about their holidays and, if tropical countries were involved, to find out what precautions they took against malaria and what immunizations they received before setting off.

You then need to find out where and how the patient lives (house or bungalow; owned or rented; toilet and bathing facilities; proximity of shops; role of neighbours and of any Social Services support). Tactful exploration of income and commitments can follow, together with details of the educational background. You must then enquire, in all cases, about the occupational history, because some jobs can cause disease (exposure to asbestos, to dyestuffs and to cotton dust for example). All diseases will influence the ability of the patient to return to work in some way and some disease—job combinations will preclude a return to that occupation (a heart attack in a heavy goods vehicle driver or epilepsy in a pilot). Distant jobs may cast long shadows, so the man who is now an 'engineering foreman' may have served his apprenticeship as a boiler-maker in the Clyde shipyards and therefore had heavy asbestos exposure. Where relevant, ask about all previous work and do not be fobbed off with vague titles for jobs; remember that 'Engineer' can cover anything from the man who cleans textile machinery to the man who designed the Humber Bridge and 'civil servant' can range from a secretary to a Driving Test examiner to the Secretary to the Cabinet. Always remember to say 'But tell me exactly what you do?'.

Finally, personal habits must be probed. It is well known that patients will tailor their responses to such questions according to their perception of the questioner's likely attitudes. Even the order of asking such questions can be critical, for with self-completed questionnaires it has been shown that asking about smoking first and cough later will elicit a higher and more truthful answer about cigarette consumption than asking about cough first and smoking second, for in the latter situation the respondent clearly perceives that he might be blamed for his own ill health if he answers truthfully. If you approach patients with a disapproving tone in respect of sexual, smoking and drinking habits, they will deny or underplay them. If I am talking to an ex-Merchant Navy seaman, who then became a regular soldier and who currently runs a public house, I would never believe any vows of temperance offered in response to a question such as 'You don't drink do you?' Instead, I would say 'I bet you've been a bit of a lad; what could you put away when you were on good boozing form — 20 pints of beer a night/a bottle of whisky a day?' An auction for the true level of consumption can then follow and you will be much nearer the truth. You must similarly probe, as though encouraging patients to boast about it, the precise details of their sexual life, without appearing censorious or moralistic (which sex? how many partners? which orifices and how? what precautions against infection have been taken?). To lower the emotional tone before you leave the patient or begin your examination, you could then ask about other leisure activities, hobbies and those often forgotten members of asthmatic or itchy households, their domestic pets.

Ensure that if they have not cropped up before and been woven into the fabric of your chronological account, you make a final check on all medications currently being taken by the patient, including any 'bought over the counter', and enquire whether any of them or drugs taken in the past have produced adverse reactions.

What have you achieved?

If you have shown the patient that you care about his illness and have shared it with him by listening carefully to his story, you have laid the foundations for a good consultation today and for a lifetime of effective medical practice in the future. Moreover, when you go on to say 'Thank you for telling me about yourself; now I would like to examine you' the patient will say 'Of course, doctor' and you can begin to marshal the skills to be described by my colleagues in the next chapters.

References and further reading

Hampton JR, Harrison MJG, Mitchell JRA, Pritchard JA, Seymour C. Relative contributions of history-taking, physical examination and laboratory investigations to diagnosis and management of medical out-patients. *British Medical Journal*. 1975; **2**: 486−9.

Pickering GW. Medicine's challenge to the educator. *British Medical Journal*. 1958; **2**: 1117−21.

Trotter WR. *Collected papers*. London: Oxford University Press, 1941.

2

First impressions

P. J. Toghill

What can be learned from the patient's appearance?
Spot diagnoses
Does the patient look ill?
Facial appearances
Shape and size
Mobility and posture
Your patient's perception of the problem
References and further reading

What can be learned from the patient's appearance?

You must, of course, listen carefully to what your patient says. In all probability he or she is telling you his or her diagnosis. But first impressions are important whether your patient is at home, in out-patients or in a hospital bed. That first glance may short-cut much interrogation and direct questioning along worthwhile channels. In those first few seconds of contact you may:

- make a spot diagnosis
- confirm that your patient is seriously ill
- note facial appearances and stigmata
- assess body shape and size
- look at mobility and posture
- get a feel of your patient's perception of the problem.

How much these first impressions may fit or conflict with your patient's complaints will be learned as the history unfolds.

Spot diagnoses

Some diseases are instantly diagnosable. The big

head of Paget's disease, the rash of ophthalmic herpes zoster and the puckered mouth of scleroderma can be diagnosed at a glance (Figs 2.1–2.3) as can the shuffling gait of Parkinson's disease or the stiff, awkward movements of ankylosing spondylitis. In some diseases a new observer may have advantages. The slow and almost imperceptible change in appearance in myxoedema may be unrecognized by a conscientious general practitioner seeing the patient regularly for a succession of seemingly unconnected trivial complaints; a new doctor immediately recognizing the condition may be astonished by the lack of clinical acumen of the earlier medical attendant.

Local knowledge is important. Appearances familiar to doctors in the tropics may perplex those working in the western world. Cutaneous leishmaniasis in a Saudi visitor might flummox a casualty officer in a UK hospital yet would be quickly recognized in Riyadh. The medical registrar in Hong Kong quickly looks for the nasopharyngeal tumour in his patient with cranial nerve lesions; his counterpart in the UK may not think of that diagnosis when examining a Chinese restaurateur.

Does the patient look ill?

This is a question that every doctor asks himself,

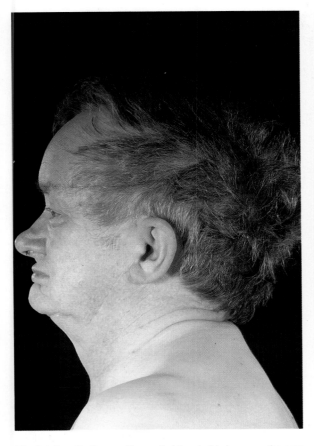

Fig. 2.1 Paget's disease. The vault of the skull bulges over the eyes and ears. A common complaint is that the patient has to buy hats of a larger size.

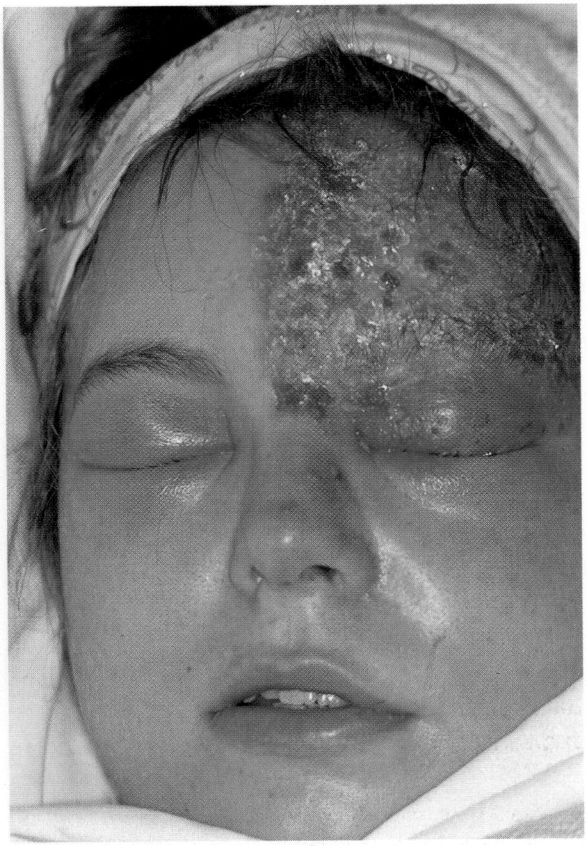

Fig. 2.2 Ophthalmic herpes zoster. The vesicles are limited strictly to the ophthalmic division of the Vth cranial nerve though the opposite side of the face may be swollen during the acute phase of the illness.

either consciously or unconsciously on seeing his patient for the first time. Experience is essential; frequently it is impossible to define specifically why a patient 'looks ill'. Relatives or friends may draw attention to deteriorating health unnoticed by professional health workers.

A common feature of illness is, of course, loss of weight and this needs to be assessed with care. The wasted patient with gaping collar, baggy trousers and tightened belt does not have to confirm his weight loss with documented serial recordings. His skin will be too big for him and will hang in redundant folds over his limbs and trunk. The patient's demeanour may give clues as to the cause of his weight loss. The inexorable morale-sapping progress of disseminated cancer may be suspected at first sight. The perky bird-like features of the schoolgirl with anorexia nervosa may provide early clues as

may the restlessness of the thin thyrotoxic. Patterns of wasting differ with particular diseases and not all are characterized by thin bellies; the protuberant abdomen and leg oedema of the Somali famine victim provides an unhappy reminder of yet another type of cachexia. Conversely some patients may claim to have lost much weight — and even produce supportive documentary evidence; yet their well-being, rounded faces and well-fitting suits and dresses refute this!

Anaemia is another pointer to organic disease but may at times be surprisingly difficult to detect clinically. A haemoglobin level of 7.0 g/dl may be unsuspected in a sunburnt young woman; by contrast a frail, pallid, elderly lady confidently diagnosed as being anaemic will be shown by the laboratory to have a normal haemoglobin. Weather-beaten skin often disguises anaemia in an out-of-doors worker,

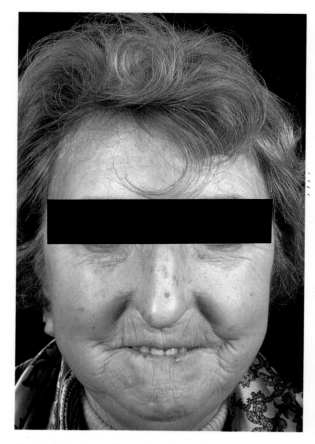

Fig. 2.3 Scleroderma. The puckered mouth is a characteristic feature. Note also the telangiectatic spots on the cheeks and nose.

Facial appearances

Much can be learned from your patient's facial appearance and this may allow a 'spot diagnosis' to be made. Once seen in real life and committed to memory these are often easy to recognize. Unfortunately many of the so-called 'classical' appearances of disease portrayed in some textbooks are so gross that the student or young doctor fails to diagnose the early case. Acromegaly is such an example (see Fig. 12.13). Do not fall into the sin of diagnostic greed in expecting every criterion to be fulfilled before daring to identify a syndrome. Many of these 'spot diagnoses' are dealt with elsewhere and include the endocrinological syndromes of Addison's disease, thyrotoxicosis and hypopituitarism, the chromosomal aberrations of Turner's and Down's syndromes and the skeletal defects of Paget's disease and achondroplasia. Occasionally it may be possible to diagnose systemic disease from a facial rash as with

whereas the pale skin of the tenement dweller may falsely suggest it; a glance at the nail beds and fingers may be more helpful. The traditional inspection of the conjunctiva may be misleading, particularly in those with 'rheumy' eyes. The only infallible guide to anaemia is the measurement of the haemoglobin level. In the haemolytic anaemias such as hereditary spherocytosis, pallor may be tinged with mild jaundice, due to the associated unconjugated hyper-bilirubinaemia. The combined effect is of a characteristic lemon-yellow tinge to the pale skin and white sclerae.

The cause of the increased skin pigmentation of chronic debilitating illness or neoplastic disease is poorly understood but is mainly due to increased deposition of melanin. When this is combined with anaemia the complexion in the white-skinned patient takes on a sallow appearance.

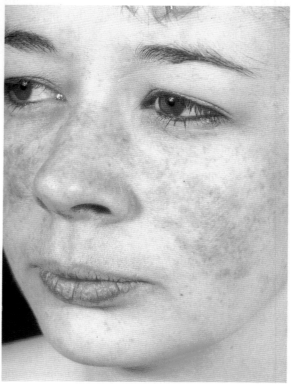

Fig. 2.4 The facial rash of systemic lupus erythematosus (SLE) often described as having a bats-wing or butterfly distribution.

the butterfly rash of systemic lupus erythematosus (SLE) (Fig. 2.4).

What is often more difficult is the recognition of those subtle facial alterations, that hint of personality change, addictions or undisclosed fears. For various reasons your patient may wish to be economical with the truth!

In the western world problems of alcohol loom large. Many alcoholics make no attempt to conceal their addiction which reveals itself in their plethoric facies, glowing rhinophymic noses and an all pervading aroma of alcohol. Others are reluctant to admit to drinking even when questioned directly. Here the whiff of alcohol in the breath in the early morning, the sweating palms and fine tremor may offer some clues. We are all aware of the plethoric facies and suffused conjuctivae of the alcoholic but it is only in recent years that attention has been drawn to the Cushingoid appearance which develops in some of them. The round red face, truncal obesity and slim limbs show superficial similarities to Cushing's syndrome. The distinction may be further blurred by an associated hypertension, now a recognized feature of alcoholism.

The smoker smells of his or her habit and will quickly show you nicotine-stained fingers. Look critically and you will soon learn to identify the 'smoker's face' (Fig. 2.5). Skin wrinkling is unquestionably increased in heavy smokers, producing premature ageing. Its cause is uncertain. Similar skin wrinkling is, of course, seen in chronic excessive exposure to the sun.

A glance at your patient's eyes may show a corneal arcus which is a normal phenomenon associated with ageing but its presence in younger patients particularly those under the age of 50 may point to

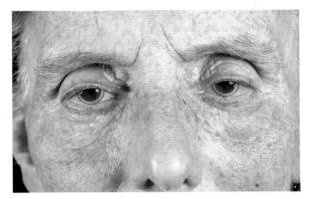

Fig. 2.6 Corneal arcus and xanthelasmata. This combination is strongly suggestive of the patient having hyperlipidaemia and full investigation is mandatory.

an underlying hyperlipidaemia. The combination of a corneal arcus with xanthelasmata (Fig. 2.6) is strongly suggestive of hyperlipidaemia. Look at the ear-lobes; wrinkling of the ear-lobes progressing to deep clefting of the lobe (Fig. 2.7) is strongly correlated with coronary artery disease.

Look for the signs of self-inflicted trauma and disease in the young. Whilst tattoos do not necessarily indicate carriage of hepatitis B, they may be reminders of military service in older men and markers of certain lifestyles in the younger age groups. Red sores round the nose and lips may indicate solvent abuse and round scars on the skin (skin popping) and track marks on the veins are the insignia of the intravenous drug addict. Whilst the young man with expensive after-shave, short hair cut, ear-rings and moustache may well be homosexual, it is important to remember that many homosexuals do not parade their sexual preferences. It is in this last group that the possibility of HIV infection may be overlooked.

The patient's face may betray psychiatric disease. Depression is probably the easiest to identify; the withdrawn, expressionless, retarded patient with advanced disease is quickly identified but milder depression may be difficult to distinguish from simple unhappiness. At the other extreme the hypomanic patient may demonstrate few obvious facial stigmata but the constant flow of conversation and disarmingly frank comments may all alert the doctor.

Red faces deserve attention. A strikingly red face with peripheral cyanosis of the ear lobes and nose tip should always suggest polycythaemia, particularly if there is an associated conjunctival suffusion. Alcoholics often have red faces but rhinophyma (see

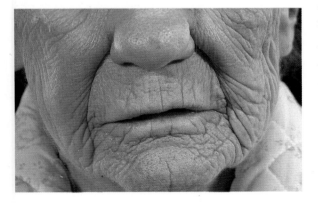

Fig. 2.5 The smoker's face. Premature wrinkling of the skin is a common finding.

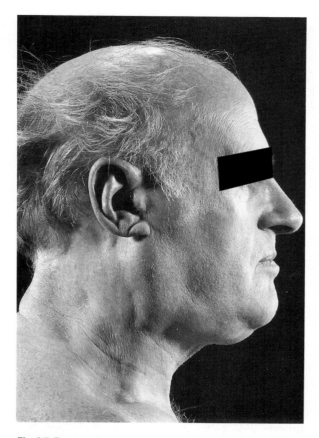

Fig. 2.7 Deep ear-lobe creases: a physical sign linked with coronary artery disease.

Fig. 23.10) is by no means always due to alcohol. Those working in the open air commonly have red faces with telangiectasia of the cheeks and foreheads. A diffuse telangiectatic mat over the cheeks may be seen in patients with cirrhosis and this may be similar to the malar flush of mitral stenosis (see Fig. 16.1) so beloved by the physicians of years gone by. The origin of the malar flush remains uncertain. Gross and bizarre telangiectasia of the face and con-junctivae is a unique and characteristic feature of the rare disease ataxia telangiectasia. Episodic hot flushing or erythema of the face is a common meno-pausal symptom, curiously often less evident to the observer than to the sufferer. A much rarer cause of episodic flushing is that seen in the carcinoid syndrome.

Note must be taken of facial skin colour but this, in white people, is influenced by sun and wind exposure. We must expect considerable variation in the light-skinned races without necessarily impugning disease influences. Some increased pig-mentation of the cheeks and forehead (chloasma) occurs during and fades after pregnancy (see Fig. 11.1). The most gross hypermelanotic pigmen-tation in disease is seen with Addison's disease and with Nelson's syndrome in association with extremely high levels of adrenocorticotrophic hor-mone. The pigmentation of haemochromatosis is characteristically slaty grey. The chronic adminis-tration of some drugs such as busulphan may darken the skin.

Patchy loss of pigmentation of the face may be due to vitiligo, a curious disorder linked with other autoimmune disorders such as Addison's disease, pernicious anaemia and thyrotoxicosis. However, the commonest cause of patchy depigmentation of the skin is following inflammatory skin eruptions. Lack of pigmentation of skin, hair and uveal tract is seen in oculocutaneous albinism.

Shape and size

Loss of weight

This has already been considered as a feature of organic disease. Some of the commoner causes of loss of weight in the various age groups are shown in Table 2.1.

Table 2.1. Loss of weight in youth and middle and old age

Age group	Loss of weight
Young	Malnutrition*
	Diabetes
	Malabsorption
	Tuberculosis*
	Anorexia nervosa
	AIDS
	Chronic infections*
Middle age	Malignancy
	Diabetes
	Thyrotoxicosis
	Malabsorption
	Cardiac cachexia
	Chronic hypoxia
Old age	As in middle age
	Malnutrition and neglect
	Senile cachexia

* Particularly in the tropics.

In the undeveloped countries malnutrition is a common cause of wasting and loss of weight in the young whereas in the western world this is most unusual. Patterns of disease are altering and in the western world tuberculosis has become a rare cause of weight loss in the young, though it is still common in undeveloped countries (Fig. 2.8). The growing menace of human immunodeficiency virus (HIV) infection in Central Africa and parts of the USA brings it to the fore as a more frequent cause of weight loss in young adults.

The syndrome of anorexia nervosa is often diagnosable at first sight. The young girl with gross wasting of limbs and trunk is little distressed by her cachectic appearance even to the extent of denying it entirely. Her face is often bright and alert and the skin of the back and shoulders may be covered in soft downy lanugo hair. The growth of this hair is not confined to anorexics and may be seen in other wasting diseases of the young such as Crohn's disease. In anorexia nervosa the size of the breasts may be preserved contrasting starkly with the loss of fat elsewhere.

In the Western World chronic inflammatory bowel disease and malabsorption are common causes of loss of weight and wasting. In both Crohn's disease and in ulcerative colitis the appearances may be complicated by long-term, high-dosage steroid therapy and surgery (Figs 2.9 and 2.10). Whereas previously Crohn's disease was regarded as rare in Indians and Africans it is now commonly seen in first- and second-generation immigrants to developed countries.

As suggested earlier the weight loss of malignancy can be suspected straight away by the associated pallor, pigmentation and weakness. The degree of

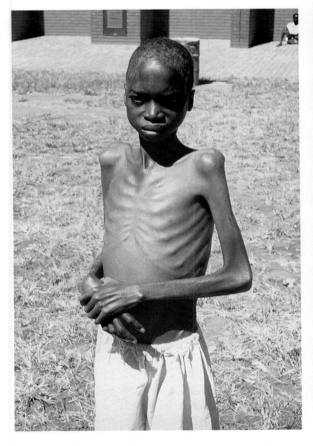

Fig. 2.8 Secondary malnutrition in a Zambian boy suffering from extrapulmonary tuberculosis.

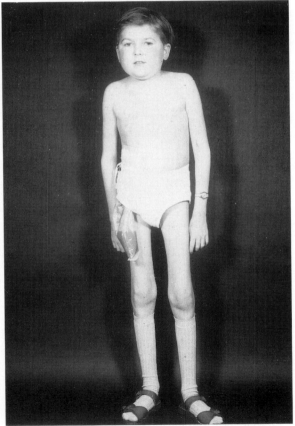

Fig. 2.9 Wasting in ulcerative colitis. This boy had recently had a total proctocolectomy following failed long-term therapy with steroids. His round 'moon-face' contrasts starkly with wasted limbs.

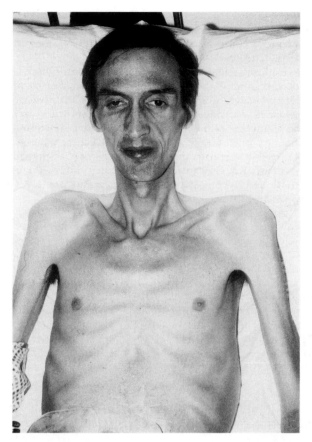

Fig. 2.10 Wasting in Crohn's disease. Abdominal scars and ileostomy bag show the evidence of previous surgery.

weight loss may be disguised by associated ascites and leg oedema; consequently the patient with malignancy may present with wasting of his face, shoulders and neck and swelling of the lower half of the body.

Severe weight loss may be a feature of the last two or three years of life in old age. We can now regard senile cachexia as a specific syndrome. Weight loss may be quite dramatic in those with emphysema or chronic obstructive airways disease in middle age and may give rise to perplexing diagnostic problems.

Obesity

Everyone can recognize a fat person though the definition of the word raises problems. The Framingham study clearly showed that a 20 per cent excess over ideal weight impairs general health and this excess has often been used to define obesity. By this definition up to one-third of the male and more than a third of the female population of the USA are obese.

Obesity may be more accurately quantified in terms of body mass index (BMI) derived from Quetelet's formula (W/H^2 where W is weight (kg) and H is height (m)). Using this method the obese have been divided into three grades: I (BMI 25–29.9) II (BMI 30–39.9) and III (BMI >40). Grade I obesity, using this definition, affects 30 per cent of the adult population of the United Kingdom. Body fatness is a characteristic that is strongly genetically determined though environmental factors may override this, particularly in the younger age groups. In general, heavy babies become plump adolescents and they in turn grow into fat adults. Just looking at fat families confirms that the distribution of fat is genetically determined although in men obesity tends to be more generalized whereas in women fat is deposited over the trunk and buttocks.

Not uncommonly painful fatty deposits develop over the limbs, and to a lesser extent on the trunk, in middle-aged people; this condition has been termed Dercum's disease. Occasionally diffuse lipomata accumulate round the neck and in front of the ears; this bull-necked appearance is called the Madelung collar.

The principal causes of secondary obesity are well known though relatively uncommon (Table 2.2). In fact myxoedema, so often considered, is infrequently associated with significant weight gain. Long and continued high-dosage steroid therapy is a much more frequent cause of obesity than Cushing's syndrome though in both there is a contrast of truncal obesity with slim limbs.

Table 2.2. Causes of secondary obesity

Hypothyroidism
Cushing's syndrome
Hypothalamic disorders
Drugs (steroids and anabolic agents)

Although unrelated to obesity the syndromes of 'body building' must be briefly considered here. Amongst those are the athletes, the weight-lifters, shot-putters and wrestlers who may use anabolic steroids to boost the development of muscles which are hypertrophied by exercise.

Tallness

As with obesity, tallness is mainly genetically determined; however, the effect of beneficial factors, particularly diet, is well demonstrated by the increase in average height of men and women in previously underdeveloped areas. This is particularly noticeable in South East Asia, China and Japan.

Nevertheless there are rare syndromes that need to be recognized. The gigantism/acromegaly syndrome is described in more detail elsewhere but sometimes young patients do present because of unusual tallness (Fig. 2.11).

Klinefelter's syndrome is a congenital chromosomal abnormality with an additional female chromosome so that instead of being a normal XY male, the patient is XXY. These sterile men are unusually tall with young-looking faces, a female distribution of body fat and gynaecomastia. The external genitalia are small with small testes. The tallness of these patients is due to an increased lower body segment, i.e. from ground to pubis.

Another rare, but important cause of tallness is Marfan's syndrome, a disorder of dominant inheritance with defective collagen cross-linking as a possible but unproven cause. The prevalence may be between 1 in 50 000 and 1 in 10 000 persons. The associated abnormalities include long, spidery fingers (arachnodactyly), dislocated lens, high arched palate and pectus excavatum. The major threats to life are dissection or rupture of the aorta.

Shortness

As with tallness, most short people are so because of genetic and racial influences. Nevertheless it is of critical importance to remain alert to the many causes of short stature; in some children and a few adults an underlying disorder such as coeliac disease may require therapy. The patterns of dwarfism vary throughout the world but Table 2.3 lists some of the commoner conditions which you should quickly consider when you see a very short person.

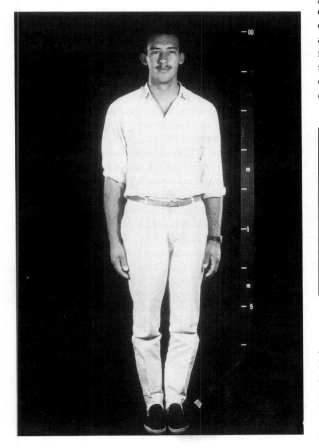

Fig. 2.11 The gigantism/acromegaly syndrome. This young man was brought to hospital by his wife who commented on his heavy facial features and excessive height (204 cm).

Table 2.3. Causes of short stature

Constitutional
Emotional deprivation
Achondroplasia
Down's syndrome
Turner's syndrome
Rickets (dietary and renal)
Coeliac disease
Cretinism
Pituitary syndromes
Severe malnutrition

Of these syndromes one of the commonest is achondroplasia which is seen as the circus dwarf. Here the arms and legs are very short, the head appears large, and the bridge of the nose depressed (Fig. 2.12). Apart from the mechanical problems of the very short stature, general health is not impaired.

Down's syndrome due to trisomy of chromosome 21 is well known and is usually quickly recognized even by lay persons. Babies and young children with Down's syndrome are of normal size but their subsequent growth slows and adult patients with Down's

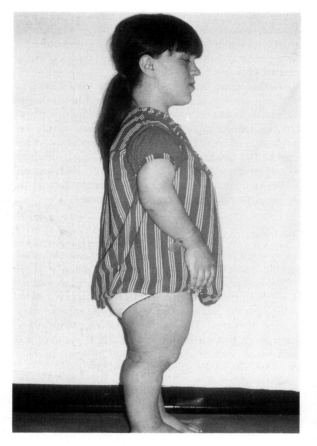

Fig. 2.12 Achondroplasia.

syndrome are rarely taller than 10-year-old children. The characteristic features include 'Mongoloid facies' with prominent medial epicanthic folds to the eyes, a flattened bridge to the nose, gaping mouth and broad, fissured tongue (Fig. 2.13(a)). The hands are broad with a single transverse skin crease and incurved little fingers. Many patients with Down's syndrome are now surviving into middle age when the facial appearances may be less characteristic (Fig. 2.13(b)).

Adult girls with Turner's syndrome (Fig. 2.14) rarely exceed 150 cm in height. In this syndrome of XO karyotype the subjects have a somewhat masculine shape with wide shoulders and, characteristically, a webbed neck, a low hair-line and an increased carrying angle.

Mobility and posture

An essential part of the formal examination of the musculoskeletal and nervous system is to watch your patient walk, stand, turn and sit down. If he is mobile, by the time he reaches you, this part of your assessment will have been performed. He will have shown if he has stiff, fixed and painful joints, and he will have shown if he has involuntary movements and if he can maintain his posture.

Your patient's perception of the problem

Why do patients visit doctors? Most do so because they are ill or because they have symptoms, lumps, rashes and swellings for which they require explanations. But these are not the only reasons. Some come because they need confirmation or certification that they are well. Others come for 'second opinions' — confirmation or otherwise of what has already been decided by other doctors. Some come for personal advice about their business, family or love lives; they are using their doctors as priests, lawyers or friendly neighbours. Usually the reason for the consultation is clear; occasionally the introductory symptoms or signs may be used as an excuse to lead on to a more serious worry. The 'by the way doctor' throw-away line at the end of the interview may reveal the critical problem, concealed and delayed by embarrassment, shyness or abject terror. It is for the doctor to latch on to the significance of the particular remark, hint or gesture. Do not miss the 'red flag' symptom; all too often it may pass unnoticed and unexplored.

Accompanying spouses, relatives or friends may give you further clues about your patient's perceptions about his disease. The presence of companions often has covert significance that requires careful and perhaps sensitive appraisal. Watch for those non-verbal clues! A husband may be brought reluctantly to the doctor's surgery by his wife who is quite properly concerned about his deteriorating health. Despite the husband's resentment she must be given an opportunity to talk confidentially. Alternatively, an over-protective mother may seek to dominate a consultation about her son's trivial health problems. A doctor must know when a 'one-to-one' consultation is needed.

However, there are often times when the evidence of witnesses — be they wives, workmates or strangers — is essential. A few minutes spent ques-

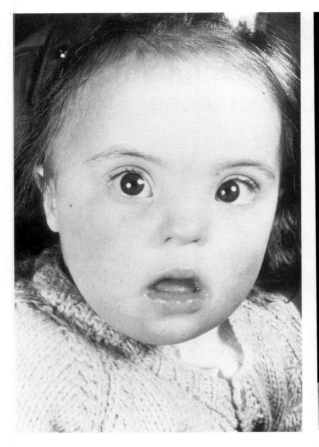

Fig. 2.13(a) Down's syndrome in childhood.

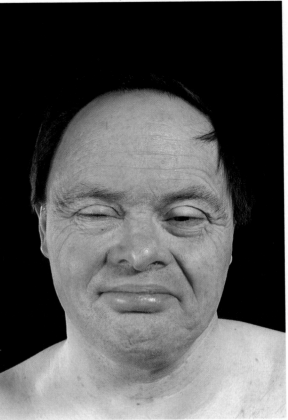

Fig. 2.13(b) Down's syndrome in a 51-year-old man.

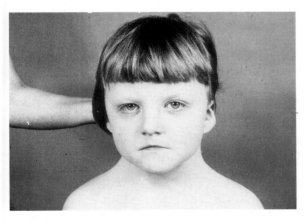

Fig. 2.14 Turner's syndrome. Note the webbing of the neck.

tioning someone who actually saw a 'funny turn' may be of more value than the cost of a CT scan, EEG and 24-hour tape combined. Information of this kind is priceless — disregard it at your peril!

References and further reading

Bates BA. *A guide to physical examination*, 4th edn. Philadelphia: Lippincott, 1987.

Browse N. General and facial appearances. In *An introduction to the symptoms and signs of surgical disease*, 2nd edn. London: Edward Arnold, 1991, 202–9.

3

The symptoms and signs of cardiovascular disease

J. R. Hampton

> Symptoms
> The physical examination
> References and further reading

Symptoms

Disease of the cardiovascular system causes five main symptoms: pain in the chest, breathlessness, ankle swelling, palpitations, and dizziness or black-outs. All of these can occur with disease of other systems, and they also occur in healthy people. A carefully taken history is often the best way of deciding whether the symptoms are significant, and whether they are due to some non-cardiovascular disease.

Chest pain

The important cardiovascular causes of chest pain are cardiac ischaemia (lack of oxygen supply to the heart muscle), pericarditis and dissecting aneurysm. Cardiac ischaemia may be related to exercise when it causes the pain called angina; it may be reversible but not closely related to exercise when it is sometimes called 'unstable' angina, and it may be persistent when blockage of a coronary artery causes myocardial infarction. The important non-cardiovascular causes of chest pain are those that arise in the pleura, the oesophagus and the chest wall.

Cardiac ischaemia

Ischaemic pain is felt in the front and the centre of the chest. It is usually described as 'tight', 'pressing', or 'crushing'. It frequently radiates (spreads) to the left arm and less frequently to the right arm and to

the back; sometimes it radiates to the neck, jaw and teeth and although this is less common it is virtually diagnostic of cardiac ischaemia.

Angina occurs at times when heart work is increased so that there is a greater demand for oxygen by the heart muscle. Thus angina characteristically develops with exertion and it is relieved by rest; it seldom lasts more than 15 minutes. It is often induced by emotional stress and by sexual intercourse. It is worse in cold and windy weather and during exercise after a meal. It is often associated with breathlessness due to temporary left ventricular dysfunction; in patients with mild heart failure angina often occurs when they lie down at night. It is relieved within seconds or occasionally minutes by glyceryl trinitrate and the response to this can be used as a diagnostic test. When a patient says that trinitrate takes more than 10 minutes to work, the pain is probably not angina. If chest pain is thought to be ischaemic bear in mind risk-factors and family history (Table 3.1).

Table 3.1. Important points to think about if chest pain sounds ischaemic

Prolonged pain suggests myocardial infarction
Smoking history
Other risk-factors such as hypertension, diabetes or hyperlipidaemia
Symptoms suggesting anaemia
Symptoms suggesting heart failure
Family history of myocardial ischaemic disease

'Unstable' angina is a term used in several different ways. By some definitions it includes newly developed angina, or angina that is increasing in severity and frequency. Other definitions use the term to mean angina occurring at rest, the pain being relieved by glyceryl trinitrate. The term 'crescendo angina' is sometimes used to describe worsening angina that may come on at rest, is recurrent and forces the patient to take frequent glyceryl trinitrate tablets.

Angina is most commonly confused with non-specific chest pain. This is very common in young and middle-aged men. This pain may have a similar distribution to angina, affecting the central chest and left arm, but it is unpredictable. It is not closely related to exertion but it may develop at the end of a busy day. It is not associated immediately with emotion, but it is more common at times of emotional stress. It is never induced by intercourse. Although patients may claim relief from nitrates, the effect is very slow.

Myocardial infarction (death, or necrosis, of heart muscle) occurs when occlusion of a coronary artery causes irreversible ischemia. Coronary artery occlusion is usually due to thrombosis on top of a pre-existing atheromatous plaque, but this can only be inferred from the patient's symptoms and signs and from the results of investigations. Coronary artery occlusion can also cause sudden death, so the term 'heart attack' is usually used to encompass both myocardial infarction and sudden death.

Pain due to a heart attack is similar in nature to angina but it usually lasts for several hours and a diagnosis of infarction is unlikely if the pain settles within 30 minutes. Pain lasting longer than 48 hours is unlikely to be due to infarction, though when pericarditis complicates infarction then the pain may persist for several days. The pain of a myocardial infarction is usually, though not necessarily, suf-ficiently severe to make the patient sweat, and the pain is often accompanied by vomiting. Glyceryl trinitrate is ineffective and powerful analgesics such as morphine are needed for pain relief.

Pericarditis

Pericarditis causes a pain with a distribution similar to ischaemia, but it is often made worse by breathing and it is markedly affected by posture. It is usually worst lying flat and is relieved by sitting up and leaning forward.

Dissecting aneurysm

Dissection of the aorta causes severe central chest pain that is often described by the patient as 'tearing'. It typically radiates through to the back. It is often sudden in onset and it is frequently accompanied by dizziness or transient loss of consciousness.

The causes of chest pain, other than that due to cardiac ischaemia, are shown in Table 3.2.

Breathlessness

Breathlessness is very difficult to define. It may result from cardiac or respiratory disease, or from anaemia but most commonly it is due to obesity and a lack of physical fitness (Table 3.3). Whatever the cause it is usually first noticed on exertion, though with increasing disease it may occur at rest. The identification of the system responsible for breathlessness depends on associated symptoms and on the physical examination.

Breathlessness may result simply from anxiety: a patient who 'feels the need to take occasional deep breaths' seldom has a physical problem. Over-breathing due to fright or anxiety can be recognized because

Table 3.2. Other causes of chest pain (excluding cardiac ischaemia). The associated physical signs are discussed later

Cause of pain	Physical signs
Aortic dissection	Unequal arm pulses, aortic regurgitation, pericardial friction rub
Pericarditis	Pericardial friction rub, venous and arterial paradox with tamponade
Pleuritic pain	Unequal chest movements, pleural rub
Pneumothorax	Hyper-resonance, reduced breath sounds
Oesophagitis	Usually none
Oesophageal rupture	Signs of pain, shock, pleural effusion (usually on left)
Nerve root pain	Spinal pain, neurological abnormalities
Bone and muscular pain	Local tenderness

Table 3.3. The main causes of breathlessness

Obesity
Lack of physical fitness
Anaemia
Heart failure
Respiratory disorders
Pulmonary embolism

it causes paraesthesiae (pins and needles) around the mouth and in the fingers.

Cough and wheeze characteristically accompany breathlessness due to respiratory disease (see Chapter 4), but in fact also occur with cardiac disease and hence the old terms 'bronchial asthma' and 'cardiac asthma'. When the left ventricle becomes inefficient due to any heart disease, the pressure in the left atrium rises; this increases the pressure in the pulmonary veins and capillaries and the lungs become stiff. Compression of bronchi may cause a wheeze, and this becomes worse as left atrial pressure rises. Initially the patient may have a dry cough, but when the left atrial (and therefore pulmonary capillary) pressure exceeds the oncotic (osmotic) pressure of the plasma, fluid will leak into the alveoli and 'pulmonary oedema' is then said to be present. The patient then begins to cough up frothy sputum which may be pink, or sometimes stained with blood.

The frothy sputum coughed up because of pulmonary oedema must be differentiated from the thick, sticky, yellow or green sputum that is produced by patients with chronic bronchitis, chest infections or bronchiectasis.

With a rise in the left atrial pressure and increasing stiffness of the lungs, the patient becomes breathless on lying flat. This is called orthopnoea. This results from two circulatory changes: first, on lying flat approximately half a litre of blood that is pooled in the leg veins whilst standing is returned to the effective circulation, thus increasing the work of the heart. Second, in the upright position hydrostatic pressure helps drain the upper lung zones into the left atrium so that respiration can continue in the upper zones even though the lower parts of the lung are congested. This hydrostatic effect is lost when the patient lies flat, the whole of the lung then being affected by the raised left atrial pressure.

The typical symptoms of a patient with poor left ventricular function are therefore breathlessness on mild exertion and a need to sleep propped up. The patient may wake during the night extremely breathless, wheezing and coughing up pink, frothy sputum. He feels the need to get out of bed and walk about

and often opens the bedroom window to 'get more air'. Such attacks are called 'paroxysmal nocturnal dyspnoea' or 'cardiac asthma'.

It is important to remember that orthopnoea is also a symptom of patients with chronic airways disease. Their breathing movements are largely diaphragmatic and they have to sit upright to give the diaphragm the greatest possible movements.

Ankle swelling

Ankle swelling may be due to cardiac disease, to venous or lymphatic obstruction in the legs, or to a low plasma albumin which may be the result of liver, kidney or gut disease. When fluid collects between the cells in the loose tissues of the ankles and feet 'oedema' is said to be present and this is one of the features of heart failure. Oedema accumulates when the venous pressure plus the hydrostatic pressure of the upright posture exceeds the oncotic pressure of the plasma. The problem is exacerbated by a sequence of physiological processes that lead to salt, and so to water, retention. If the patient is lying in bed the oedema collects over the sacrum rather than in the ankles.

Ankle oedema due to heart failure, unlike that resulting from unilateral venous obstruction, is symmetrical. The patient may complain of aching legs but the feet are not actually painful.

Palpitations

'Palpitation' is a term that means different things to different people, but the best definition is an awareness of the heartbeat.

To understand and diagnose the nature of palpitations it is necessary to think in terms of the electrocardiogram (ECG). The word 'rhythm' is usually used to describe the sequence of electrical activation within the heart and its subsequent muscular activity. 'Rhythm' thus applies to the electrocardiogram rather than what the patient feels. Normally the heart is controlled by repeated depolarization of the sinoatrial (SA) node and from there activation spreads through the atria to the atrioventricular (AV) node, down the His bundle and its branches to the ventricle (Figs 3.1 and 3.2). Under these circumstances the heart is said to be in 'sinus rhythm'. The activation sequence can also begin in the atria, in the AV node, or in the ventricles, and the heart is said to be in an atrial, AV nodal (properly called 'junctional', but usually just called 'nodal') and ventricular rhythm. In any of these abnormal rhythms there may be single abnormal beats or there may be a sustained rhythm.

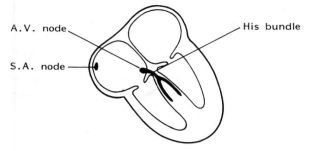

A.V. node

His bundle

S.A. node

Fig. 3.1 The conducting system of the heart.

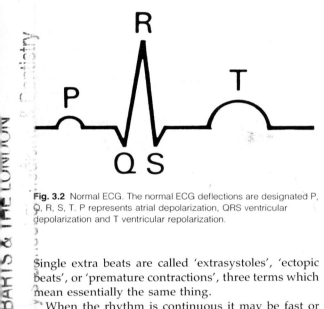

R

P

T

Q S

Fig. 3.2 Normal ECG. The normal ECG deflections are designated P, Q, R, S, T. P represents atrial depolarization, QRS ventricular depolarization and T ventricular repolarization.

Single extra beats are called 'extrasystoles', 'ectopic beats', or 'premature contractions', three terms which mean essentially the same thing.

When the rhythm is continuous it may be fast or slow; fast rhythms are called 'tachycardias' and slow rhythms are called 'bradycardias', but these are relative terms and there is no absolute rate above which 'tachycardia' is present or below which there is a 'bradycardia'. The precise diagnosis of the cause of palpitations depends on recording an ECG while the patient has symptoms. Typically the patient will say that he or she is perfectly well at the time he actually sees a doctor, but even then a carefully-taken history will usually allow you to make a reasonably accurate diagnosis.

Variations in heart rate

Everyone is aware of his or her heart beating rapidly due to extremes of exertion or emotional stimulation and this is entirely normal. The range of the normal heart rate is very wide; in athletes it may be as low as 40/min at rest, and in healthy people extreme exercise

can raise it to 180/min. If the patient can count his heart rate at a time he has palpitations and it is between 50 and 150/min and is regular, it is likely that sinus rhythm is present.

The heart rate is unnaturally increased (and the patient is thus more aware of it) in the presence of anaemia, blood volume loss and hyperthyroidism and these possibilities must be explored in the rest of the history and examination.

Missed and extra beats

Palpitations due to extrasystoles can usually be diagnosed quite easily from the patient's description. The heart 'lurches' or 'jumps out of the chest'. 'Hit one, miss one', 'misses a beat', 'all over the place', are common phrases for a patient to use. The patient is not usually conscious of the early beat but of the long ('compensatory') pause that follows it and the beat that follows this pause. The return of normal sinus rhythm is usually accompanied by a beat that the patient calls 'strong' because the long diastole of the compensatory pause allows the left ventricle to become unusually full and so to expel a large volume.

Extrasystoles can occur at any time, but most often the patient notices them while relaxing, particularly in bed at night.

The distinction between supraventricular and ventricular extrasystoles cannot be made from the history; for this the ECG is essential. However, making the distinction is of little importance to the patient. Supraventricular extrasystoles have no significance at all and, although in large groups of patients those with ventricular extrasystoles are more likely to have heart disease than those without, in the absence of any other evidence of heart disease the excess risk to an individual is not worth bothering about. Reassurance is all that is needed.

Runs of palpitations

'Paroxysmal' in this sense simply means intermittent. At times the patient is aware of a rapid heart beat that is usually regular, although with atrial fibrillation it is irregular (Fig. 3.3). A typical attack of a parox-

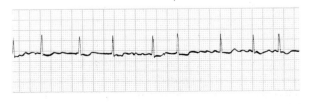

Fig. 3.3 ECG showing atrial fibrillation.

ysmal tachycardia involves a sudden change of cardiac rhythm so the attack begins suddenly. The heart is 'too fast to count'; the rate is usually in the range of 150 to 250/min. The short diastolic period between beats means that the left ventricle is stimulated to contract before it has had time to fill and even at a high heart rate cardiac output falls. Left ventricular failure may develop and as left atrial pressure rises the patient becomes breathless. Reduced cerebral blood flow may cause dizziness and even a loss of consciousness. The short diastole means reduced coronary flow (which is mainly diastolic) and the combination of this and the increased myocardial oxygen demand caused by the tachycardia may precipitate angina even in people with normal coronary arteries. Breathlessness, dizziness, or chest pain associated with a tachycardia is extremely serious, and emergency hospital admission is essential.

A paroxysmal tachycardia will typically stop suddenly and the patient will soon recover completely, but often the patient describes the attack as 'dying away'.

Attacks of a paroxysmal tachycardia are usually unpredictable but in some people they are induced by exercise. They may be stopped by any procedure that reflexly stimulates the vagal nerve. The patient may have noticed that breath-holding, rubbing the eyes or the carotid artery in the neck, or inducing vomiting may stop the attack. If not, he should be told about these things and a definite response will help to make the diagnosis.

Paroxysmal tachycardias have to be distinguished from sinus tachycardia and the most useful features of the history are a sudden onset and sudden cessation and the situations in which the attacks occur. Sinus tachycardia builds up and dies away slowly and occurs during exercise or emotional stress; true paroxysmal tachycardias begin suddenly and unpredictably.

Syncope (see also Chapter 15)

'Syncope' means sudden loss of consciousness with a fairly quick recovery. The most common cause is simple fainting but cardiac arrhythmias, both tachycardias and bradycardias, may be responsible. The ultimate cause of loss of consciousness is a lack of oxygen supply to the brain and this may also cause an epileptic seizure. Seizures, or fits, may thus have either a cardiac or a neurological cause and differentiating the two can be extremely difficult. In general terms it depends on the identification of other symptoms that are more clearly suggestive of disease in

one system or the other, or in detecting physical abnormalities in one system during the examination.

As with palpitations, patients are usually perfectly well at the time they consult a doctor but the history can be extremely helpful.

Simple faints Fainting is due to a combination of vagal nerve over-activity causing marked sinus bradycardia, with peripheral vasodilatation that causes hypotension. Everyone faints at times but some people faint more easily than others. A faint is best identified from the circumstances in which it occurs — in hot and crowded rooms, in church services before breakfast, or in operating theatres. The patient is only unconscious for a short time and recovers on lying (or falling) down. The subject is seldom aware of the bradycardia though witnesses may describe the pulse as slow and may even say that the heart has stopped. There is usually associated sweating and pallor.

'Micturition syncope' is a variation on this theme. The patient gets up at night to urinate; having been asleep in a warm bed his blood pressure is already low and he is vasodilated. Micturition may be associated with vagal activity and bradycardia and the subject faints. Women rarely suffer from this syndrome because they sit down to micturate!

Stokes—Adams attacks When there is complete dissociation between atrial and ventricular conduction (complete or third-degree heart block) the ventricles beat at their own inherent rhythm of 20—40/min (Fig. 3.4). The extreme bradycardia and poor cardiac output lead to heart failure and occasionally the ventricular rate may become so slow that the patient loses consciousness. This may last only for a few seconds but such episodes may be recurrent and they are called 'Stokes—Adams attacks' after the Irish physicians who first described them (see Fig. 15.1).

Aortic stenosis may also be responsible for syncopal attacks occurring with exertion.

The causes of syncope are summarized in Table 3.4.

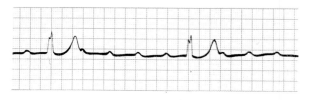

Fig. 3.4 ECG showing complete heart block. Note that the ventricles are beating at their own slow rhythm, quite independent of the atrial activity.

Table 3.4. Causes of syncope

Simple faints
Micturition syncope
Tachy- and bradyarrhythmias
Postural hypotension (see Table 13.4)
Stokes—Adams attacks (see Fig. 15.1)
Aortic stenosis

Other features in the history important in cardiovascular disease

So far we have considered the symptoms that a patient may describe as part of the history when cardiovascular disease is the main problem. The remainder of the history — the 'systems review', the past history, the family history and the social history — are also important not only because they may point to other, unrelated, diseases but because they may give clues to the cause of symptoms.

Systems review

Most cardiovascular diseases do not actually make a patient feel ill in himself and weight gain due to fluid retention is more common than weight loss. However, weight loss is a feature of infective endocarditis (infection on the heart valves) and it is sometimes seen in patients with very severe heart failure ('cardiac cachexia') when the excess fluid has been removed by diuretic treatment.

Patients with heart disease usually sleep normally unless they are wakened by angina or orthopnoea. Their appetite is unimpaired except when heart failure causes liver distention or when they are being treated with too much digoxin.

Some points which may need to be considered in the 'systems review' in a patient with cardiovascular disease are listed in Table 3.5.

Past history

Obviously a past history of myocardial infarction or a stroke will point to cardiovascular disease, but it is

Table 3.5. A check-list for the 'systems review' for a patient with cardiovascular disease

System	What the patient may complain of	Possible cardiovascular interpretation
Respiratory	'Asthma' Wheezing at night	Left ventricular failure
	Coughing up blood	Pulmonary emboli Mitral stenosis
Gastrointestinal	'Heartburn'	Angina
	Vomiting Anorexia Weight loss }	Digoxin toxicity
	Jaundice	Hepatic congestion due to CCF
Nervous	Headache	Severe hypertension Cranial arteritis
	'Strokes'	Cerebral emboli
	Dizzy turns and black-outs	Tachy- and bradyarrhythmias
Renal and urinary	Urinary infections 'Cystitis' }	Chronic pyelonephritis → hypertension
	Haematuria	Renal emboli, endocarditis
Musculoskeletal	'Growing-pains' in childhood	Rheumatic fever → chronic rheumatic heart disease
	'Arthritis'	Aortic incompetence and/or pericarditis due to systemic lupus erythematosus
	Painful back	Aortic incompetence due to ankylosing spondylitis

also important to ask about previous rheumatic fever. This is a disease of children, now rare in the western world but still a problem in developing countries, which is characterized by a prolonged generalized illness with joint pains and sometimes by involuntary movements called chorea ('St Vitus dance'). The late consequences are stenosis or incompetence of the heart valves, so when a patient complains of breathlessness or ankle swelling and admits to rheumatic fever in childhood, rheumatic valvular disease is very likely. The possibility of rheumatic heart disease must be considered in any patient said to have, or found to have, a heart murmur but it is also helpful to find out whether the heart murmur had been mentioned after routine medical examinations in childhood, during pregnancy, in the services, or for employment and insurance.

Family history

Heart attacks sometimes run in families. There is an increased risk if a parent or sibling died of a heart attack before the age of 50; beyond this the family history becomes progressively less important. If there is a very strong history suggesting heart attacks in young relatives the possibility of inherited disorders of lipid metabolism or of hypercoagulable states must be considered.

Social history

Smoking habits are extremely important in any patient suspected of having coronary artery disease and cigarette smoking is the major risk-factor for this. Although the excess risk declines if the individual stops smoking, it does not return to normal levels for 10 years or more.

Alcohol intake is also important, for alcohol poisons the heart muscle and causes 'alcoholic cardiomyopathy'. This is a condition that can cause arrhythmias (hence palpitations) and heart failure. A high alcohol intake may also increase the blood pressure.

There are no occupations, other than those associated with smoking and drinking, that are strongly linked with heart disease, but heart problems prevent patients from following some forms of employment. Thus it is important to know if a patient is an airline pilot, an engine driver, or if he needs to hold a Heavy Goods Vehicle or Public Service Vehicle driving licence: people in any of these categories will lose their livelihood if heart disease is proved. This may colour the history the patient gives and also affects their attitude to their disease.

The physical examination

Examination of the cardiovascular system should be performed in five stages:

- general appearance
- physical signs associated with the arterial circulation
- physical signs in the venous circulation
- physical signs in the lungs as part of the circulation
- physical signs associated with the heart itself

In each stage it is important to think logically and to relate the findings to the anatomy and physiology of the circulation. Although the usual sequence of 'inspection, palpation, percussion, auscultation' should be remembered, these four methods of examination have a different importance in the four stages.

General appearance

The main features that may be apparent from the general appearance of the patient are:

- evidence of generalized disease
- evidence of pain
- evidence of heart failure
- evidence of an impaired regional circulation

Evidence of a generalized disease

During the initial assessment of a patient (inspection) it may be possible to identify at a glance signs or syndromes that might be related to the cardiovascular problem. An example of this might be the diagnosis of thyrotoxicosis in a patient with heart failure. Table 3.6 lists some associations which are also mentioned in other sections of this book.

Other important physical signs which may be noticed during this initial survey include:

Corneal arcus and xanthelasmata As has been explained earlier an arcus is commonly seen in elderly patients (arcus senilis) and is of little significance. However, when it is present in young patients (arcus juvenilis) and is associated with xanthelasmata (see Fig. 2.6) there is a strong possibility of hyperlipidaemia being present.

Xanthomata Tendon xanthomata (Fig.3.5) and nodular xanthomata (see Fig. 18.8) are rare physical signs seen in patients with uncommon forms of familial hyperlipidaemia.

Wrinkled or clefted ear-lobes These are statistically associated with coronary artery disease (see Fig. 2.7).

Table 3.6. 'Spot diagnosis' syndromes that may be associated with cardiovascular disease		
	Syndrome	Cardiovascular disease
Chromosomal	Down's	Septal defects
Endocrine	Thyrotoxicosis	Atrial fibrillation, heart failure
	Myxoedema	Angina, pericardial effusion
	Acromegaly	Enlarged heart
	Addison's	Hypotension
Musculoskeletal	Marfan's	Aortic disease
	Ankylosing spondylitis	Aortic regurgitation
	Rheumatoid arthritis	Pericarditis
	Scleroderma	Cardiomyopathy
Miscellaneous	Paget's	High output heart failure
	Alcoholism	Cardiomyopathy

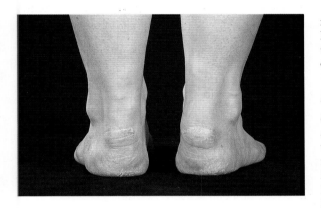

Fig. 3.5 Tendon xanthomata. These lesions, characteristically seen on tendons over extensor surfaces, occur in patients with familial hypercholesterolaemia. They should always be searched for in young patients with cardiovascular disease, particularly if there is a strong family history.

Three important but non-specific signs must always be looked for:

Fever The combination of a raised temperature and a generally ill appearance is a feature of infective endocarditis. A raised temperature also occurs for a day or two after a myocardial infarction or pulmonary embolism.

Clubbing of the fingers Finger-clubbing occurs in a wide variety of diseases including chronic infections, cancer and gut diseases (see Tables 4.7 and 4.8). In the cardiovascular system the two important causes are cyanotic congenital heart disease, which often causes very severe clubbing, and infective endocarditis.

Splinter hemorrhages Linear red or black streaks called 'splinter hemorrhages' under the finger or toe nails are a feature of infective endocarditis (Fig. 3.6). However, they are usually the result of trauma, and they may also result from emboli of non-infective origin.

Pain

Cardiac The pain of myocardial infarction is severe and the patient looks distressed. He may be pale and will often be cold and sweaty. He lies still, but he may vomit (see Table 3.7).

Pericarditis The patient is uncomfortable lying on his back but prefers to sit up and lean forward. Respiration is often painful.

Limb ischaemia With severe ischaemia of the leg the patient may sit with the leg hanging over the side of the bed because raising it makes the pain worse. The leg will be white or sometimes bluish.

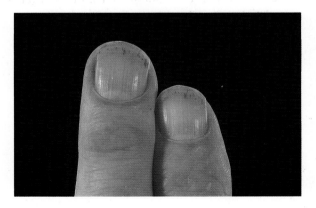

Fig. 3.6 Splinter haemorrhages of the nails.

Table 3.7. Physical signs to look for in patients with possible acute myocardial infarction

Signs of pain (sinus tachycardia; cold, clammy
    periphery)
Sweating
Signs of heart failure
Arrhythmias
Hypotension or hypertension
Pericardial friction rub

Heart failure

Breathlessness   In mild failure the patient may appear normal at rest or on mild exertion; breathlessness will only become apparent on undue exertions such as climbing stairs. Watching the patient undress may reveal just how breathless he really is. In severe failure the patient is breathless at rest and he is unable to lie flat.

Patients with pulmonary oedema may have a cough and a wheeze that can be heard from the end of the bed and may cough up frothy, pink, or even faintly blood-stained sputum.

Cyanosis (see also Chapter 4)   Cyanosis simply means blueness. There are two forms of this, central and peripheral. Central cyanosis occurs when more than 1.5 g of haemoglobin are deoxygenated. It occurs when severe heart failure prevents proper oxygenation of blood in the lungs; when lung disease is severe enough to prevent oxygenation even though the circulation is adequate; when there is a bypass or 'shunt' that allows blood to pass from the venous or 'right' side of the heart to the arterial or 'left' side without passing through the lungs; and when there is an abnormally high haemoglobin (polycythaemia).

Central cyanosis must be distinguished from peripheral cyanosis, which is said to be present when the circulating blood as a whole is adequately oxygenated but a local abnormality of circulation makes one or more of the extremities appear blue. The most common cause of this is cold but peripheral cyanosis also occurs when there is poor and slow bloodflow due to arterial blockage, or when venous return to the heart is obstructed by occlusion of a vein so that the blue colour of the venous blood becomes apparent.

Evidence of local impairment to circulation

Obstruction to arteries, veins, or lymphatics can cause

abnormalities that are immediately apparent on general examination.

In the extreme case, lack of arterial supply to a limb will cause gangrene: the toes or foot (occasionally the hand) appear black and the tissue is obviously dead (see Fig. 12.21). In slightly less severe cases the skin is white or sometimes bluish, the skin is cold to the touch and the patient is unable to move the affected part (Fig. 3.7). In milder cases still the skin will be cool compared with the opposite limb and there may be reduced hair growth.

Acute venous obstruction (see below) is characterized by a swollen, blue and tender leg while lymphatic obstruction causes a swollen leg which is usually a normal colour and is not tender. With lymphatic obstruction the oedema does not easily pit (see Fig. 19.8).

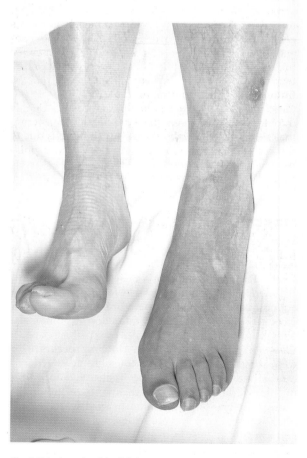

Fig. 3.7 Ischaemia of the left foot.

Examination of the arterial circulation

Presence of pulses

A pulse can be felt whenever an artery is close to the surface of the body; the ease with which a pulse can be detected will obviously depend on how fat the patient is.

The aorta can often be felt in the mid-line of the abdomen in thin people, but not in those who are even moderately obese or who have well-developed muscles in the abdominal wall. If the aorta can be felt very easily the possibility of a bulge or weakness of its wall (an 'aneurysm') must be considered (see Fig. 6.32). The pulses that can most easily be felt are:

Superficial temporals These are branches of the external carotids and they are felt just in front of the upper border of the ear-lobe; they run upwards and medially over the forehead. The importance of these arteries is that they can become involved in a generalized inflammatory condition of arteries called 'giant cell arteritis' or 'temporal arteritis' (Fig. 3.8); this is mainly a disease of old people which causes generalized muscular aches and pains, headaches and sometimes blindness because of involvement of the retinal artery (see Fig. 20.6). In this condition the temporal arteries are thickened, tender and may be thrombosed and therefore not pulsating.

Carotid arteries These can be felt by pressing deeply into the neck between the larynx and the sternomastoid muscle. Usually the pulse felt there is due to the common or external carotid artery, and a pulse may be felt even when the internal carotid is thrombosed. Because the carotid arteries are large they are

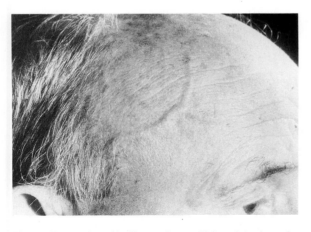

Fig. 3.8 Temporal arteritis. The arteries are thickened, tender and often non-pulsating. Patients complain of soreness of the scalp particularly when brushing the hair.

good for assessing pulse character (see below) but more important is that a narrowing in these arteries may cause turbulent flow which can be detected as a 'bruit'. A bruit is simply a rushing noise in time with the pulse, best heard with the diaphragm of the stethoscope. Bruits are important because they indicate the presence of arterial disease, usually atheroma, which may be responsible for neurological events such as strokes and transient cerebral ischaemic attacks. An arterial bruit must be distinguished from the radiation of the murmur of aortic stenosis which will be described later; simply, if there is a systolic murmur that originates in the aortic valve, it is almost impossible to identify carotid bruits separately.

Brachial arteries Brachial arteries can be felt on the medial side of the upper arm just above the elbow, and just below the elbow on the medial side of the antecubital fossa: this is the pulse usually used for the measurement of blood pressure.

Radial arteries These pulses are felt in the lateral side of the arm, immediately medial to the radius. Although they are the most accessible pulses, the arteries are relatively small and therefore not ideal for assessing pulse character or even heart rate (see below).

Femoral arteries These are felt at the mid-inguinal point (half way between the anterior superior iliac spine and the centre of the symphysis pubis). Their presence or absence is important in two circumstances. First, one of the causes of high blood pressure is a coarctation of the aorta, a condition in which a congenital narrowing of the descending aorta prevents adequate blood supply to the kidneys and the lower half of the body. In this condition the femoral pulses are difficult to feel, are usually delayed compared with the brachial pulses and they may be absent. Secondly, in a patient who might have peripheral vascular disease, one or both may be absent and either may have an audible bruit indicating narrowing of the artery.

Popliteal arteries These arteries are often very difficult to feel. They run behind the knee in the mid-line and can be felt by firm pressure in the upper part of the popliteal fossa; it is necessary to compress the artery against the back of the femur if the pulse is to be felt at all. If the foot pulses are present it is fair to assume that the popliteal artery is patent in that leg even if it cannot be felt.

The foot pulses Two pulses should be palpable in the foot, though if either is symmetrically absent then this may simply represent a normal variant. The dorsalis pedis artery runs on the superficial aspect of the foot in the mid-line and the posterior tibial runs behind and below the medial malleolus. These pulses may be absent if there is narrowing or blockage of one of the more proximal arteries (femoral or popliteal) or may be blocked individually by emboli arising anywhere in the arterial circulation.

The positions of the important pulses are shown in Fig. 3.9.

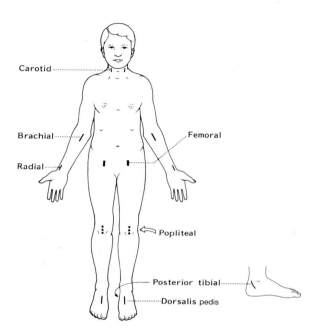

Fig. 3.9 The position of the arterial pulses. Palpation of the leg pulses is of critical importance in patients with peripheral vascular disease. The dorsalis pedis artery can be felt along a line from midway between the malleoli to the proximal part of the first metatarsal space. The posterior tibial artery can be palpated midway between the medial malleolus and the prominence of the heel.

The pulse rate

The pulse rate is usually, but not necessarily, the same as the heart rate. It is best counted against a watch for 30 seconds and the figure doubled to give a rate per minute. When the heart beat is irregular, so that some diastolic periods are shorter than others, the left ventricle will have a variable time to fill so the amount of blood expelled with each beat (the stroke volume) will vary. A small volume may be associated with a low systolic pressure in that beat and the combination may mean that the beat will not cause a palpable pulse in a peripheral artery. Therefore, if the pulse is irregular, it is best to listen with a stethoscope at the cardiac apex and to record the 'apex rate'.

There is a wide range of the normal heart rate. In the new born the rate may be over 150/min, but it slows in the first year or two. Athletes may have a heart rate as low as 40/min and in young people physical or marked emotional stress can increase the heart rate to nearly 200/min. The maximum heart rate becomes less with increasing age and as a simple guide the maximum predicted rate is 220 minus the patient's age in years. The common causes of sinus brady- and tachycardia are shown in Tables 3.8 and 3.9.

Heart rates between 50 and 150/min are most likely to represent a normal heart rhythm, but there can be exceptions and these will be discussed later.

Table 3.8. Causes of sinus bradycardia	
Physiological	Trained athletes
	Sleep
Pathological	Myxoedema
	Drugs (e.g. β-blockers)
	Vasovagal attacks
	Hypothermia
	Raised intracranial pressure

Table 3.9. Causes of sinus tachycardia	
Physiological	Exercise
	Emotion
Pathological	Fever
	Thyrotoxicosis
	Shock
	Blood loss
	Cardiac and/or respiratory failure
	Drugs (e.g. aminophyllin)

The pulse rhythm

The word 'rhythm' is used in different ways. As applied to the pulse it simply means whether it feels regular or not. As discussed previously, the word 'rhythm' properly applies to the electrical pattern of stimulation of the heart that is reflected by the electrocardiogram (ECG).

The normal heart beat is initiated by depolarization of the sinoatrial node in the right atrium. Contraction of the atrium cannot be detected by palpation; the arterial pulses are caused by contraction of the left ventricle. The depolarization of the sinoatrial node is affected by the vagus nerve, an increase in vagal activity slowing the frequency of depolarization. Vagal activity is affected by respiration so the heart may speed up and slow down with each breath. This is obvious in young people but it becomes less with increasing age; the effect of the vagus is absent in people with abnormalities in the autonomic nervous system, as may occur in diabetes.

Although a regular pulse in the range 50–150/min is likely to represent sinus rhythm, there are other regular rhythms with this rate. For example, atrial flutter with two-to-one block can give a pulse rate of 150/min: here the atria are being stimulated to contract at 300/min but only alternate beats are conducted to the ventricles, so the ventricular rate is half that of the atrial rate. With four-to-one block the ventricular rate is a quarter of the atrial rate (Fig. 3.10). Occasionally, ventricular tachycardia (a rhythm in which the

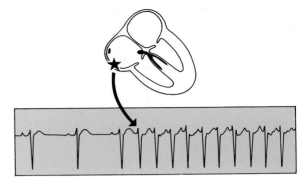

Fig. 3.11 ECG showing supraventricular tachycardia.

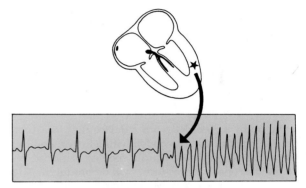

Fig. 3.12 ECG showing ventricular tachycardia.

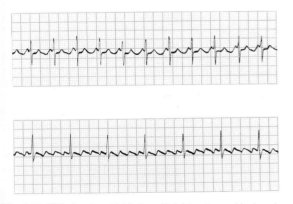

Fig. 3.10 ECG showing atrial flutter with (a) two-to-one block and (b) four-to-one block.

heart rate is controlled from an abnormal or ectopic focus in the ventricles) causes a regular heart rate in the range 100–150/min. More often, ventricular tachycardia produces a heart rate of about 200/min, but supraventricular tachycardias (most due to a focus around the atrioventricular node) lead to a similar heart rate and these rhythms can only be distinguished with an ECG (Figs 3.11 and 3.12).

Irregular heart rhythms are either due to extrasystoles or to atrial fibrillation. In extrasystoles the heart is occasionally stimulated by an ectopic focus which can be either in the ventricles or around the AV node; usually there are several normal beats and then an early one, which is followed by a 'compensatory' pause. The origin of these abnormal beats can only be determined with an ECG (Fig. 3.13).

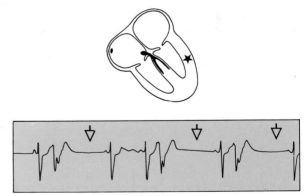

Fig. 3.13 ECG showing extrasystoles. The arrows indicate compensatory pause.

In atrial fibrillation the heart is totally irregular (Fig. 3.3). Unless the patient is treated with digoxin the ventricular rate is usually rapid and may be as fast as 200/min.

Table 3.10. Physical signs that may be associated with 'palpitations'

Rhythm responsible for palpitations	Physical signs to look for
Sinus tachycardia (see also Table 3.9)	Anxiety Thyrotoxicosis Heart or respiratory failure Signs of anaemia or blood volume loss
Extrasystoles	Usually no physical signs other than the irregular pulse, though there may be other evidence of heart disease
Paroxysmal tachycardia (either supraventricular or ventricular)	Signs associated with ischaemic heart disease Signs suggesting rheumatic heart disease Thyrotoxicosisis Enlarged heart suggesting cardiomyopathy
Atrial fibrillation	Rheumatic heart disease, especially mitral stenosis Thyrotoxicosis Evidence of alcoholism Evidence of recent myocardial infarction

Some important points about palpitations are summarized in Table 3.10.

The pulse character

If the pulse is recorded with a device that measures the rise and fall that can be felt with a finger, and the rise and fall is displayed on a moving paper or on an oscilloscope, a 'wave-form' will be produced. The shape of this wave-form is what is meant by 'pulse character'.

The wave-form of the normal pulse is made up by a rapid up-stroke, a very brief plateau and a less steep down-stroke (Fig. 3.14). The down-stroke is interrupted by a 'dicrotic notch' which coincides with closure of the aortic valve, but the notch can seldom be appreciated clinically.

In aortic valve stenosis the up-stroke of the pulse is slowed and the plateau prolonged; the 'plateau pulse'

is characteristic of significant aortic stenosis, but it does take quite a lot of practice to detect this with confidence (Fig. 3.15).

The normal blood pressure (BP) in an artery reaches a peak of about 120 mmHg and a minimum of about 80 mmHg (see below). The pulse pressure is therefore 120 − 80 = 40 mmHg, and it is this difference that can be felt in the pulse. It is not possible to judge any absolute figure, but a narrow pulse pressure (say, 110 − 90 = 20 mmHg) is typical of a 'plateau pulse'.

If the pulse pressure is wide the down-stroke of the wave-form is steep and the pulse seems to drop rapidly. This is described as a 'collapsing pulse'. In aortic valve incompetence, the diastolic arterial pressure begins to approach the diastolic pressure in the left ventricle, which is usually only 5−10 mmHg. A typical blood pressure in a patient with a collapsing pulse of aortic incompetence might therefore be 150/50, the pulse pressure thus being 100 mmHg.

A similar pulse pressure is present when the systolic pressure is high but the diastolic pressure is

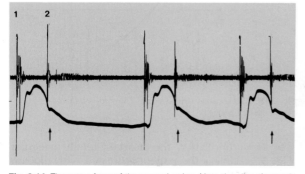

Fig. 3.14 The wave form of the normal pulse. Note the dicrotic notch (arrowed) and the phonocardiogram tracing above.

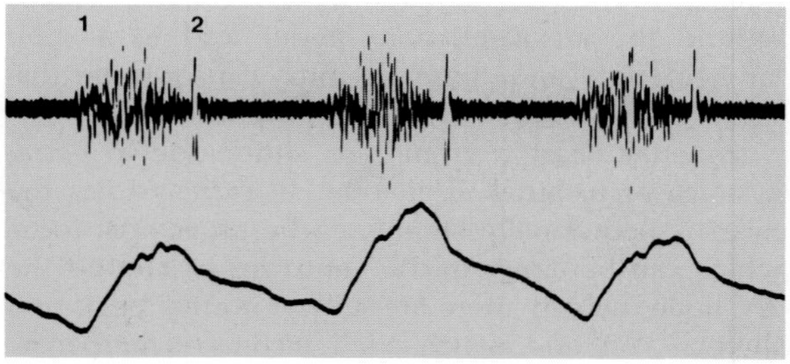

Fig. 3.15 The pulse form in aortic stenosis (the plateau pulse). The phonocardiogram is shown above.

normal — this is characteristic of old people who have rigid arteries so the BP might be 190/90 and the pulse pressure would again be 100 mmHg. This sort of pulse can be very difficult to distinguish from the collapsing pulse of aortic incompetence.

The term 'volume' is sometimes applied to the pulse and to some people means much the same thing as pulse character. A peripheral pulse cannot have a 'volume' so the term is meaningless and should not be used.

The blood pressure

The pressure of the blood within an artery cannot be assessed simply by feeling the pulse. Blood pressure is measured with a sphygmomanometer with which a variable pressure is applied to the upper arm to find out how much pressure is needed to impair blood flow.

Fat arms take more compressing than thin ones, so a record made in a fat arm may give a spuriously high value for the blood pressure. Therefore the size of the cuff should be appropriate to the patient and the cuff width should be about 40 per cent of the arm's circumference. In practice, standard cuffs are used in adults but the possibility of a falsely high result in fat people must be kept in mind.

To measure the blood pressure:

- Place the cuff fairly tightly round the upper arm
- Ensure that the brachial artery is at the same level as the heart
- Find the brachial pulse by palpation at the elbow
- Inflate the cuff until the brachial pulse can no longer be felt
- Place the diaphragm of the stethoscope over the position of the brachial pulse
- Reduce the pressure in the cuff slowly, by not more than 2 mm per heart beat. The pressure in which the pulse can first be heard is the systolic pressure, the highest pressure generated by the heart
- Continue to reduce pressure slowly. The intensity of the pulse sound will increase and then change character, becoming 'muffled'. Reducing the pressure by a few more mm of mercury will lead to the pulse sound becoming inaudible

There has in the past been a disagreement as to whether the point of muffling or of disappearance of the sound should be taken as the diastolic pressure (the minimum pressure in the artery when the aortic valve is closed and the left ventricle is relaxing). It is now generally accepted that the point of disappear-

ance is closer to the true diastolic pressure and furthermore it is the more reproduceable of the two measurements. The point of disappearance should therefore be recorded as diastolic pressure.

The different sounds heard during the measurement of blood pressure were first described by Karotkoff, who thought there were five different sounds. The first was the appearance of a pulse sound, the fourth was the point of muffling and the fifth was the disappearance of the sound. The second and third sounds related to intensity and character of the pulse sound and these are now only of historic interest.

Hypertension

When the blood pressure is high look for evidence that it has caused damage to 'target organs' (Fig. 3.16):

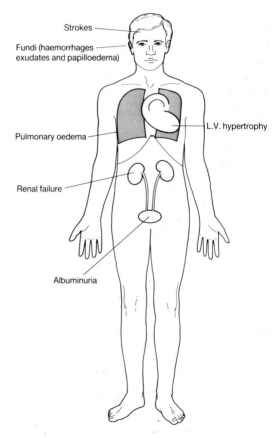

Fig. 3.16 Sites of damage to target organs in hypertension.

- fundi (see Fig. 22.11)
- the heart
- the brain
- the kidneys

Remember that a primary cause of high blood pressure will only be found in 5 per cent of cases, but nevertheless it is important to consider:

- coarctation of the aorta (delayed or absent femoral pulses, collateral pulses over the scapulae)
- Cushing's disease (truncal obesity; muscular wasting; round, red face) (see Fig. 12.14)
- kidney disease (enlarged polycystic kidneys, any signs of renal disease)
- phaeochromocytoma, a rare tumour secreting catecholamines (story of 'funny attacks'; during attack marked sinus tachycardia, cold, clammy skin, left ventricular failure)

Examination of the venous circulation

The features of the venous circulation that are important in the clinical examination are: (a) the peripheral veins themselves; (b) the jugular venous pulse; (c) the size of the liver, for this becomes enlarged as the venous pressure rises; (d) the presence of peripheral oedema.

As with the examination of the arterial part of the circulation, it is best to think of the venous features as a set and group these physical findings together.

The peripheral veins

Superficial peripheral veins can usually be seen in the hands and feet. In the legs, superficial veins may be unusually prominent, tortuous and enlarged and they are then called 'varicose'. These abnormal veins may become thrombosed due to inflammation and this is called 'superficial phlebitis': the affected vein can be seen as a red cord under the skin, which is tender to touch. Phlebitis is usually associated with peripheral swelling, or oedema (fluid collecting in the interstitial tissues). Varicose veins can bleed into the skin and can ulcerate; patients who have had varicose veins for years may have a brownish discoloration of the skin due to repeated bleeding.

The deep veins to the legs are situated within the main muscle mass and therefore cannot be seen or felt. They can become thrombosed at times when the blood is hypercoagulable and the patient is immobile, typically after surgical operations, childbirth and after trauma when the leg is immobilized in plaster. The physical signs of a deep vein thrombosis (or DVT) are

extremely unreliable and are neither sensitive nor specific. There may be no abnormal physical signs at all and the supposedly classical abnormalities may be present without thrombosis.

However, for what they are worth the signs are:
Swelling of the leg Symmetrical swelling of both legs is likely to be due to heart failure or a low plasma albumin level, but when the legs are a different size a DVT becomes more likely. The circumference of the thigh and calf should be measured with a tape-measure, at a defined distance above and below a fixed point such as the anterior tibial tubercle.
Pain When the muscle mass containing the affected vein is squeezed the patient complains of unusual pain. In the presence of a venous thrombosis of the calf, sharp dorsiflexion of the foot will be painful (Homan's sign).
Warmth A leg in which there is a DVT is warmer to touch than the normal leg. This is because the returning venous blood is diverted through the superficial veins which become more prominent.
Discoloration A leg with a DVT is usually bluish in colour, though when the thrombosis is very severe marked swelling may prevent arterial flow into the leg and this causes the 'white leg of pregnancy' which is, in fact, very rarely seen.

Although deep venous thrombosis usually affects the legs, the major veins of the arms can also be thrombosed, particularly after trauma or when invaded by a tumour in the axilla or mediastinum.

The jugular venous pulse

The jugular veins show a pulsation which is important for two reasons. First, its position reflects the pressure within the right atrium. Secondly, the wave form of the pulsation helps in the diagnosis of a variety of quite different conditions. The abbreviation 'JVP' is sometimes used to mean 'jugular venous pulse' and sometimes to mean 'jugular venous pressure'.

Because there is no valve between the jugular veins and the right atrium, the veins in the neck act as a manometer: the height of the column of blood above the heart measures right atrial pressure. The pulsation in the jugular vein reflects pressure changes in the right atrium.

There are two jugular veins on either side of the neck, internal and external. The external vein is easier to see: it runs from the mid-point of the clavicle upwards to cross the sternomastoid muscle obliquely. Although easily seen when distended it may give a false idea of the right atrial pressure because blood flow in the vein may be obstructed as the vein passes through the fascia under the clavicle and for this reason the internal jugular vein should be identified whenever possible. The internal vein runs deeply from the sternoclavicular joint upwards and laterally to the angle of the jaw, thus passing underneath the external jugular vein (Fig. 3.17).

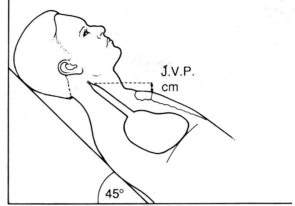

Fig. 3.18 The height of the jugular venous pulse.

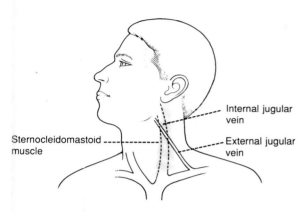

Fig. 3.17 The position of the internal and external jugular pulses.

The jugular veins can be identified more easily by asking the patient to perform a Valsalva manoeuvre, which is forced expiration against a closed glottis (tell the patient to 'strain as if having your bowels open'). The increased intrathoracic pressure raises right atrial pressure and the jugular veins become distended.

The jugular venous pressure

The measurement of any pressure requires a reference point and in the case of the jugular venous pressure this should properly be taken as the centre of the right atrium. The right atrium cannot, of course, be approached directly by clinical examination but its centre lies 5 cm vertically below the manubriosternal angle whatever position the subject is in (Fig. 3.18). The right atrial pressure can therefore be measured (in cm of blood) by adding 5 cm to the vertical height above the manubriosternal angle to which the jugular veins are distended. The normal right atrial pressure is 5 or 6 cm of blood so this is usually discounted and the jugular venous pressure is measured using the manubriosternal angle as the reference point.

It is essential to appreciate the importance of measuring the vertical height of the jugular venous

pressure above the manubriosternal angle. In a normal subject the right atrial pressure is such that the jugular veins are not distended at all on sitting upright, but on lying down the veins may be filled for the whole of their length. On the other hand, in a patient with severe heart failure the right atrial pressure may be so high that the jugular veins are distended up to the angle of the jaw or above even when the patient sits upright. There is therefore no set position for the patient in which the venous pressure should be measured: the patient should simply be asked to recline at whatever angle makes the top of the column of blood in the jugular veins most obvious.

Jugular venous pulsation

The jugular venous pulsation essentially reflects the sequence of pressure changes within the right atrium, but the wave form of the venous pulse is complicated by transmission of a pulse from the carotid artery that runs adjacent to the internal jugular vein. The venous pulse therefore has three components which are called 'a', 'c' and 'v' (Fig. 3.19).

The 'a' wave is due to atrial contraction: it is accentuated when right atrial pressure is high as in pulmonary hypertension and it is lost when atrial activity is disorganized by atrial fibrillation.

The 'c' wave is transmitted from the carotid artery.

The 'v' wave occurs while the tricuspid valve is shut and is therefore associated with atrial filling. It may in part be caused by upward doming of the valve as the right ventricle contracts. When the tricuspid valve

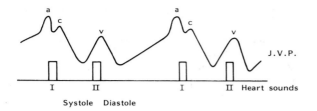

Systole   Diastole

Fig. 3.19 The components of the jugular venous pulse.

is incompetent, the blood flow due to right ventricular systole is partly ejected back into the right atrium and the 'v' wave is accentuated. Because the mechanism of the 'v' wave is different under these circumstances it is sometimes called a 'systolic wave'.

The trough between the 'a' and 'c' waves is called the 'x' descent, and that between the 'c' and the 'v' is the 'y' descent.

The pulsation in the jugular vein can most easily be appreciated at the top of the distended part of the vein. As with the measurement of the jugular venous pressure, it is important to place the patient in whatever position makes this most obvious; examination can be markedly helped by arranging a tangential light to fall across the neck. The pulsation in the jugular vein can easily be confused with carotid artery pulsation because the internal jugular vein and the carotid artery are adjacent. The arterial and venous pulsations can be distinguished in the following ways:

- an arterial pulsation can be felt. A venous pulsation is usually impalpable, although with tricuspid regurgitation it may be possible to feel the systolic wave in the jugular vein (see below)
- gentle pressure just above the clavicle will obliterate a venous pulsation and the vein will fill above the point of pressure. An arterial pulsation will not be affected
- the pulsation in the jugular vein is best seen at the limit of venous distention, so its position in the neck will change when the patient sits up or lies down
- deep inspiration reduces intrathoracic and therefore right atrial and jugular venous pressures. The position of the venous pulsation therefore moves downwards in the neck on inspiration and upwards on expiration. The position of an arterial pulse is unaffected
- there are no valves between the superior vena cava, the right atrium, the inferior vena cava and the hepatic veins. Thus if pressure is applied over the liver just below the ribs, blood will be

expressed from the liver and the right atrial pressure will rise with a consequent rise of the jugular venous pressure and pulsation. This is called the 'hepatojugular reflux'
- the pulse wave-form in the carotid artery is a simple 'up and down', but that of the jugular venous pulse is more complex. Even though it can be difficult to identify the individual component of the venous wave-form, it is usually quite easy to see as a rapid oscillation at the top of the venous column

Conditions that can be diagnosed from the jugular venous pulse

Heart failure   If the jugular venous pressure is greater than 6 or 7 cm above the middle of the right atrium, i.e. more than 2 or 3 cm above the manubriosternal angle, the filling pressure of the right atrium is abnormal and 'heart failure' is present. When making this diagnosis it is important to ensure that the jugular veins are pulsating and that the height of the jugular venous pressure is affected by position and expiration; if this is not so the distension of the jugular veins may not reflect right atrial pressure and may be due to obstruction to venous return by a mediastinal tumour, such as lung cancer.

Tricuspid regurgitation   A prominent 'v' wave which collapses due to a deep 'y' descent indicates tricuspid incompetence. The downward equivalent of the systolic wave in the jugular veins is a similar pressure wave in the inferior vena cava and hepatic veins, so causing distention and pulsation of the liver.

Heart block   In complete heart block the atria contract independently of the ventricles, so the 'a' waves in the jugular venous pulse are not regularly followed by 'c' or 'v' waves. At times the right atrium will by chance contract against a closed tricuspid valve; when this happens the whole of the right atrial stroke volume will be expelled up the superior vena cava. This will cause a sudden and marked single pulsation in the neck which is called a 'cannon wave'.

Pulmonary hypertension   High pressure in the pulmonary artery due, perhaps, to recurrent pulmonary emboli, causes a rise in right ventricular pressure and so a rise in right atrial pressure. The 'a' wave is then prominent and can be seen as a regular 'flick' in the jugular pulse. The same appearance is seen when right atrial pressure is high independently of the right ventricular pressure, for example in tricuspid valve stenosis or (very rarely) when the tricuspid valve is occluded by a tumour called a myxoma.

Constrictive pericarditis   The pericardium is usually a

thin structure which has no influence on the performance of the heart. In some chronic diseases, typically tuberculosis but also after viral inflammations of the pericardium or in collagen diseases, the pericardium becomes thickened and stiff. On inspiration the pericardium is pulled down by the diaphragm and the heart is compressed. Instead of the usual fall in venous pressure on inspiration the jugular venous pressure rises and at the same time the reduced inflow to the heart reduces left ventricular output and the systemic pressure falls. These abnormal responses to inspiration are called venous and arterial paradox.

The liver as part of the venous circulation

As we have already seen, a high right atrial pressure for any reason will be reflected by a raised pressure in the superior and inferior vena cavae and so to a high pressure in the hepatic veins and in the liver itself. The liver becomes engorged (congested) with blood and is swollen. The normal liver lies entirely beneath the ribs on the right side and cannot be felt, though in the presence of chest diseases the diaphragm may be pushed down so that the liver edge becomes palpable. If the liver edge can be felt it is therefore necessary to percuss the chest to define the upper margin of the liver; in heart failure this will be in the normal place (see Fig. 6.11). The degree of liver enlargement should be expressed as a number of cm below the right costal margin.

A congested liver is tender and this is one of the characteristic features that separates the hepatic enlargement due to heart failure from that of most primary liver diseases. Congestion of the liver can cause an ache in the upper abdomen and this is particularly common with long-standing tricuspid regurgitation. Prolonged heart failure can be a cause of jaundice and in extreme cases they may be splenic enlargement.

Oedema and the venous circulation

When the pressure in the capillaries exceeds the oncotic (osmotic) pressure of the blood, fluid will leak out of the circulation into the interstitial spaces. This is one of the characteristic features of heart failure, where not only is the right atrial and therefore the venous pressure raised, but a series of physiological changes lead to sodium and therefore to water retention. This extravascular tissue fluid is called 'oedema' and the fluid can collect in various parts of the body. Most commonly it is seen in the soft tissues

around the ankles but the same process leads to fluid in the alveoli of the lungs where it is called 'pulmonary oedema'. Fluid can also collect in potential spaces such as the peritoneum (where the fluid is called ascites), in the pleural cavities (pleural effusions) and in the pericardium (pericardial effusion).

Peripheral oedema

A combination of a raised venous pressure and the hydrostatic pressure due to the height of the heart above the feet, means that in patients with heart failure fluid collects first around the ankles. The ankles are seen to be swollen and on moderately firm pressure an imprint of the fingers is left which gradually fills in. The ankle swelling of heart failure is symmetrical, unlike that resulting from venous obstruction in the leg. When patients lie in bed the most dependent part of the body is the sacrum and buttocks and fluid may collect here as much as round the ankles. However, remember that most patients with ankle swelling do not have heart disease (Table 3.11).

Table 3.11. The main causes of ankle swelling
Immobility (see Fig. 13.3)
Venous insufficiency (varicose veins)
Deep vein thrombosis
Venous obstruction in pelvis or abdomen
Heart failure
Lymphatic obstruction
Low plasma albumin
Idiopathic oedema (mainly in women)

The lungs as part of the circulation

One of the early manifestations of heart failure is a rise in the left atrial pressure. This causes an increase in the pulmonary capillary pressure and so to an engorgement and a stiffening of the lungs. This causes breathlessness and sometimes a soft wheeze can be heard. With increasing left atrial pressure the oncotic pressure of the blood may be exceeded and fluid will then leak into the alveoli themselves. This can be heard as a crackling sound, initially at the lung bases but spreading throughout the lung fields as heart failure increases. These crackles must be differentiated from those due to pneumonia or fibrosing alveolitis; the best way of making this distinction is from the association of other evidence of cardiovascular disease in the history or examination.

The examination of the heart

The position of the heart in the chest (Fig. 3.20)

Knowing the position of the heart, its chambers and its valves within the chest is the key to understanding not only the physical examination of the heart but also the electrocardiogram, the chest x-ray and the echocardiogram. It is therefore worth thinking about basic anatomy before discussing the physical signs in the heart that can be detected on clinical examination.

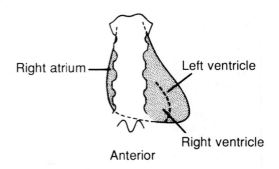

Fig. 3.21 The position of the chambers on the front of the heart.

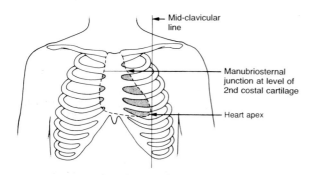

Fig. 3.20 The position of the heart in the chest (anterior view).

Seen from the front, the heart is roughly triangular in shape. The heart lies mainly beneath the sternum, with the base of the triangle just projecting to the right of the sternum and the apex being in the left side of the chest, in a line (the 'mid-clavicular' line) below the mid-point of the clavicle. The cardiac apex is usually in the fifth rib interspace.

The cardiac apex forms the most important single physical sign in the cardiovascular system for its position indicates the size of the heart. The cardiac apex beat is defined clinically as the furthest point out from the mid-line and the furthest point downwards where the heart beat can be felt: this point corresponds accurately to the position of the true cardiac apex. Note that it is not necessarily the same point where the cardiac impulse can most easily be felt: this is sometimes called the 'point of maximum impulse' (or 'PMI') but this is not useful as it does not necessarily identify heart size. The cardiac apex is normally formed by the left ventricle. The right ventricle occupies most of the front of the heart and lies beneath and just to the left of the sternum (Fig. 3.21). Enlargement of the right ventricle therefore brings the heart more into contact with the sternum which can be felt to lift with each heart beat. Right ven-

tricular enlargement also pushes the cardiac apex outwards.

The left ventricle lies to the left of, and behind, the right ventricle. Left ventricular enlargement shifts the cardiac apex outwards and downwards, and causes the apex beat to be easily localized and forceful.

The right atrium forms the right border of the heart as seen from the front, but even when enlarged it seldom projects much to the right of the sternum. The left atrium lies at the back of the heart and does not form part of the cardiac silhouette seen from the front. In the side view it forms the upper part of the posterior heart border and is adjacent to the oesophagus.

Figure 3.22 shows a chest x-ray from the front and the side. The plain x-ray does not allow separation of the different heart chambers nor does it show the valves, but in Fig. 3.23 the position of the chambers is outlined. The position of the valves is most graphically demonstrated by an x-ray of artificial valves (Fig. 3.24) which show the aortic and mitral valves lie close to the middle of the heart, as seen from the front, and both are beneath the sternum. We shall see later that this makes nonsense of the terms 'mitral area' and 'aortic area'.

The position of the ventricles, the left atrium and the aortic and mitral valves are well shown by the echocardiogram. One of the standard views is the 'long axis' which makes a slice of the heart from base to apex. Figure 3.25 shows the right ventricle in front and the left ventricle and left atrium behind. The close proximity of mitral and aortic valves is also obvious. Magnetic resonance imaging (MRI) can also be used to demonstrate the position of the chambers of the heart (Fig. 3.26). The mitral and tricuspid valves are shown clearly in the 'four chamber' echocardiographic view, where the echo probe looks at

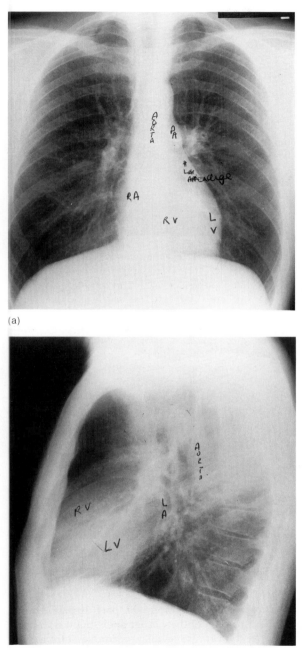

(a)

(b)

Fig. 3.22 Posteroanterior (a) and lateral (b) chest x-rays.

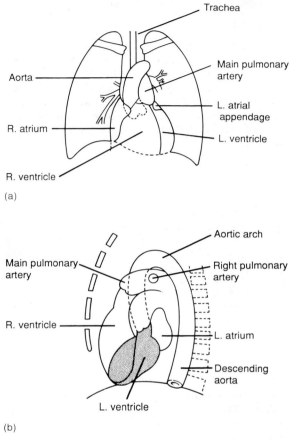

(a)

(b)

Fig. 3.23 Posteroanterior (a) and lateral (b) chest x-rays with chambers outlined.

the heart from the apex (Fig. 3.27). The diagonal position of the septum, with the anterior position of the right ventricle, also explains the positions used for the chest leads of the ECG: leads V_1 and V_2 'look at' the right ventricle, leads V_3 and V_4 'look at' the septum, and leads V_5 and V_6 'look at' the left ventricle (Fig. 3.28).

How to examine the heart

Inspection and percussion   Inspection and percussion of the heart are seldom helpful. Usually the heartbeat cannot be seen and any visible pulsation is probably abnormal. It is very difficult to demonstrate the size of the heart by percussion because of its position behind the sternum and because there is usually lung in front of at least part of it. The only two possible abnormalities are complete absence of cardiac dullness as a result of emphysema of the lungs and increased dullness to percussion to the right of the sternum in the presence of a large pericardial effusion.

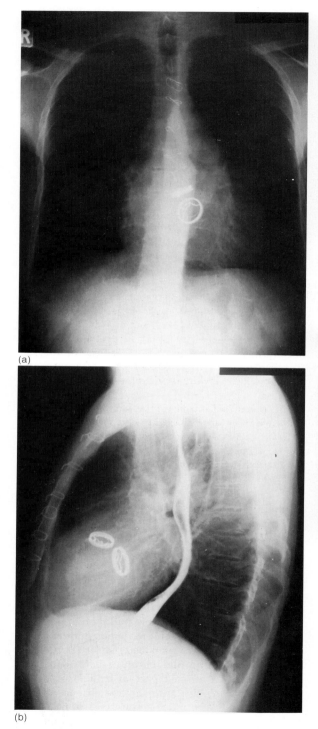

(a)

(b)

Fig. 3.24 The position of the mitral (lower) and aortic (upper) valves demonstrated by an x-ray of artificial valves. Note barium in the oesophagus. Posteroanterior (a) and lateral (b) films.

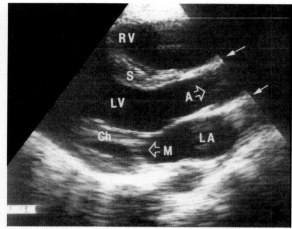

Fig. 3.25 Echocardiogram showing the long axis of the heart. RV and LV = right and left ventricles; S = septum; Ch = chordae. Open arrows indicate aortic (A) and mitral (M) valves. Thin arrows indicate walls of aorta.

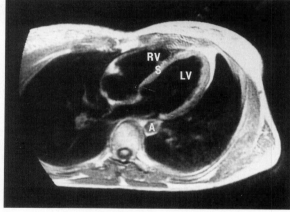

Fig. 3.26 MRI scan of the heart showing the position of the chambers of the heart. Note that the heart is viewed from below. A = aorta.

Palpation   The most important part of palpation is the identification of the cardiac apex, but it is important to feel over the whole precordial impulse for abnormal movements and thrills (palpable murmurs).

If the cardiac apex is difficult to feel the patient should be asked to turn on the left side; this brings the apex more into contact with the chest wall, but the position of the heart does not change. The apex beat may be displaced from its normal position in the fifth rib interspace in the mid-clavicular line by three mechanisms:

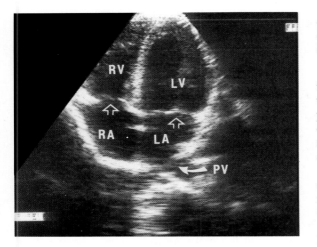

Fig. 3.27 Echocardiogram viewing the heart from the apex. RA and LA = atria; PV = pulmonary veins. Open arrows indicate tricuspid and mitral valves.

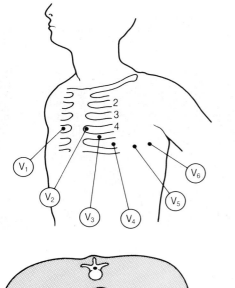

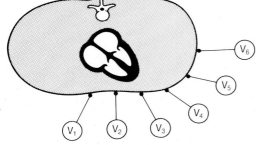

Fig. 3.28 Positions of the ECG chest leads over the heart. Leads V₁ and V₂ 'face' the anterior RV, V₃ and V₄ the septum and V₅ and 6 the LV.

- mediastinal shift
- left ventricular hypertrophy
- right ventricular hypertrophy

Mediastinal shift may occur when it is pulled towards the side of a collapsed or fibrotic lung, or when it is pushed away from the side of a large pleural effusion or a tension pneumothorax. In each case the trachea will deviate from the mid-line in the suprasternal notch and it is important to check this in any patient whose apex beat is displaced.

Rarely the heart may lie on the right side of the chest (dextrocardia) and the apex will then be in the right fifth interspace and the mid-clavicular line but the trachea will be central.

When the apex is displaced by left ventricular hypertrophy (Table 3.12) it shifts downwards and outwards and its position should be described either as being a certain number of cm beyond the mid-clavicular line or it may be related to the anterior axilliary line (a line below the anterior border of the axilla formed by the pectoralis major).

Right ventricular hypertrophy (Table 3.13) also causes an outward shift of the cardiac apex, but the apex beat is usually more diffuse. The important sign is a lifting or heaving motion that can be felt if the flat of the hand is placed on, or just to the left of, the sternum.

The precordial impulse may feel abnormal in the presence of a left ventricular aneurysm; here there may be a diffuse rocking movement between the sternum and the apex.

When the first heart sound is very loud, as in

Table 3.12. The causes of left ventricular hypertrophy
High blood pressure Aortic stenosis Aortic incompetence Mitral incompetence VSD

Table 3.13. The causes of right ventricular hypertrophy
Mitral stenosis Pulmonary stenosis Any congenital heart disease with right-to-left shunt Chronic lung disease Multiple pulmonary emboli

mitral stenosis, it can actually be felt as a sharp 'tap' at the cardiac apex. Any murmur that is loud enough will cause vibrations that can be felt on the chest wall and these are called 'thrills'.

Ausculation

The identification of heart sounds and murmurs with a stethoscope is often thought of as the main art of cardiology, but its importance is over-rated. Identifying the rhythm, the heart size and the presence of heart failure from physical signs are usually much more important.

The heart sounds

There are several noises of short duration that are called 'sounds'. These are associated with the opening and the closing of the valves, but the actual sound is made by sudden changes of velocity in the bloodstream. High-pitched sounds are best heart with the diaphragm of the stethoscope and the low-pitched sounds are best heard with the bell.

The first sound is associated with closure of the mitral and tricuspid valves at the beginning of systole. The mitral and tricuspid components of the first sound can often be heard separately and may be confused with fourth and first sounds.

The second sound is associated with closure of the aortic pulmonary valves and often has two components. In young people the second sound is usually single on expiration, but inspiration delays pulmonary closure as blood is sucked into the chest and the right ventricular output is increased (Fig. 3.29). This doubling of the second sound on inspiration is lost with increasing age. The second sound is widely split with no change of inspiration when excitation of the right ventricle is delayed by block of conduction down the right bundle branch. Such 'fixed splitting'

is characteristic of an atrial septal defect. When excitation of the left ventricle is delayed by left bundle branch block the aortic valve closure will be relatively late compared with that of the pulmonary valve and the pulmonary component of the second sound will precede the aortic components. The second sound will therefore appear double on expiration, but with inspiration the pulmonary component will be delayed so that the two components of the second sound coincide and the sound becomes single. This is called 'reverse splitting'.

The third heart sound is associated with ventricular filling and is heard soon after the second sound (Fig. 3.30). It is dull and low pitched and is nearly always localized to the cardiac apex. A soft third sound may be normal, especially in young people, but in older patients it is usually an indication of heart failure. Most third sounds originate in the left ventricle, but occasionally right ventricular sounds can be identified because they become louder on inspiration.

The fourth heart sound is associated with atrial contraction and therefore occurs at the end of diastole, just before the first sound. When audible it is nearly always pathological and indicates heart failure. Like the third sound, it is low pitched and is localized to the cardiac apex.

In addition to the main heart sounds a variety of sharp, high-pitched clicking noises may sometimes be heard.

Systolic clicks (Fig. 3.31) may be single or multiple. A single early click is characteristic of congenital stenosis of the aortic or pulmonary valve and is probably due to 'doming' of the valve before it opens. Such clicks are followed by an ejection murmur (see below). Late clicks, single or multiple, are often associated with mitral valve prolapse, when one or both cusps of the valve balloon back into the

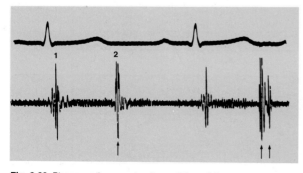

Fig. 3.29 Phonocardiogram showing splitting of the second heart sound on inspiration.

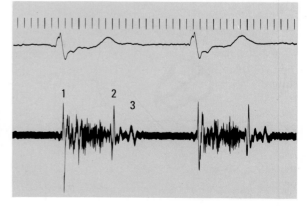

Fig. 3.30 Phonocardiogram showing the third heart sound.

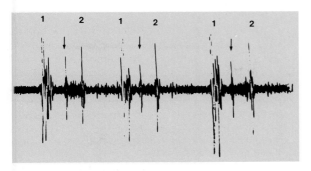

Fig. 3.31 A systolic click (arrowed).

left atrium as the left ventricle contracts. They are usually associated with a systolic murmur due to mitral regurgitation and this murmur is characteristically late in systole.

The 'opening snap' is the classical sharp, high-pitched extra sound of diastole. It indicates mitral stenosis and precedes the characteristic diastolic murmur (see below). Although best heard at the apex it is usually also audible at the left sternal edge and this, together with its high pitch, differentiates it from a third sound. It occurs early in diastole, before the position when a third sound would be heard.

Heart murmurs

A *murmur* is essentially the same thing as a bruit and is due to turbulent bloodflow. Murmurs arise when a valve is thickened and fails to open properly (stenosis) or when it fails to shut properly and leaks (incompetence or regurgitation). Murmurs also occur when an abnormally large amount of blood flows past a normal valve. Murmurs may occur in systole or diastole and identifying these parts of the cardiac cycle is an essential prelude to determining the cause of the murmur.

'Systole' always refers to ventricular systole and is the period between the first and second sounds; its interval is usually shorter than diastole. With increasing heart rate systole and diastole become similar in duration and this can make their differentiation difficult. Systole corresponds to the apical impulse and to the pulse in the carotid artery and it is possible, but extremely difficult, to time systole by feeling the carotid at the same time as listening to the heart. Systolic murmurs are nearly always louder than diastolic murmurs, but the real answer to the problem is that each type of murmur has its own characteristics. With practice these can be recognized without worrying about systole and diastole.

Systolic murmurs occur when the ventricles are contracting: the aortic and pulmonary valves should be fully open and the mitral and tricuspid valves should be completely shut. Failure of the aortic and pulmonary valves to open (valve stenosis) or leakage of the mitral and tricuspid valves (incompetence or regurgitation) therefore causes a systolic murmur.

Diastole occurs when the ventricles are relaxing and blood is flowing into them from the atria. The mitral and tricuspid valves should be fully open and the aortic and pulmonary valves shut. Stenosis of the mitral or the tricuspid valves, and incompetence of the aortic or pulmonary valves, therefore causes a diastolic murmur.

Murmurs also occur when there is an abnormal communication between the heart chambers due to a congenital defect. For example, if there is a ventricular septal defect (VSD) blood will flow across it in systole, when the pressure in the left ventricle is higher than in the right. This bloodflow is turbulent and causes a systolic murmur. With a patent ductus arteriosus blood can flow through the defect in both systole and diastole, leading to a 'continuous' murmur.

Types of murmur When there is resistance to bloodflow, as with valve stenosis, the intensity of the murmur increases to a peak as bloodflow becomes maximal and then decreases. Such murmurs are called 'ejection' in type and a phonocardiogram shows them to be 'diamond' shaped.

Valve incompetence begins the moment the valve should have shut so these murmurs are 'early'; mitral and tricuspid regurgitation tends to persist throughout most of systole and so cause 'pansystolic' murmurs, while aortic and pulmonary incompetence begins early and then decreases, causing a 'decrescendo' murmur.

The position where murmurs are heard Some old books describe 'mitral', 'aortic', 'pulmonary' and 'tricuspid' 'areas', but these are meaningless and inaccurate and should never be used. The heart should be listened to with the diaphragm and the bell in four places: the cardiac apex, the left sternal edge in the second and fifth rib interspaces and the right sternal edge in the second interspace.

The murmurs of mitral stenosis and regurgitation are best heard at the apex. Those of tricuspid stenosis and regurgitation are best heard at the lower left sternal edge and at this point the murmur of a VSD is loudest.

Pulmonary stenosis causes a murmur best heard at the upper left sternal edge. The murmurs of aortic and pulmonary incompetence are best heard somewhere down the left sternal edge.

Some murmurs have characteristic 'radiations': the sound spreads in the direction in which the blood is flowing. Thus the murmur of mitral regurgitation radiates to the axilla and round to the back. That of aortic stenosis radiates to the carotid arteries in the neck. A VSD murmur often radiates up the left sternal edge. The murmur of mitral stenosis and of tricuspid stenosis or incompetence tends to be localized.

The characteristics of individual murmurs

These are summarized in Tables 3.14—3.19 which include characteristic phonocardiograms.

The murmurs of pulmonary stenosis and incompetence are similar to those of aortic stenosis and incompetence but are loudest when the patient breathes in, increasing flow through the right side of

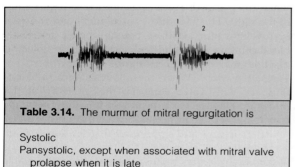

Table 3.14. The murmur of mitral regurgitation is

Systolic
Pansystolic, except when associated with mitral valve
 prolapse when it is late
Best heard at the apex
Found to radiate to the axilla

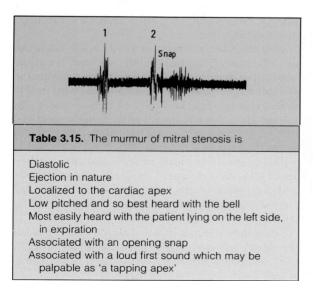

Table 3.15. The murmur of mitral stenosis is

Diastolic
Ejection in nature
Localized to the cardiac apex
Low pitched and so best heard with the bell
Most easily heard with the patient lying on the left side,
 in expiration
Associated with an opening snap
Associated with a loud first sound which may be
 palpable as 'a tapping apex'

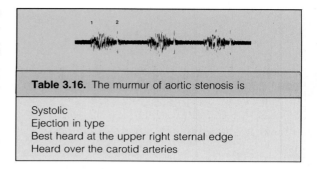

Table 3.16. The murmur of aortic stenosis is

Systolic
Ejection in type
Best heard at the upper right sternal edge
Heard over the carotid arteries

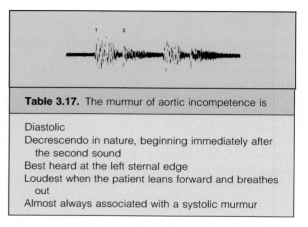

Table 3.17. The murmur of aortic incompetence is

Diastolic
Decrescendo in nature, beginning immediately after
 the second sound
Best heard at the left sternal edge
Loudest when the patient leans forward and breathes
 out
Almost always associated with a systolic murmur

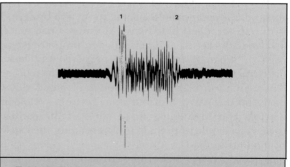

Table 3.18. The murmur of a VSD is

Systolic
Typically pansystolic, but a small VSD may cause an
 ejection-type murmur
Best heard at the lower left sternal edge
Also sometimes heard up the left sternal edge

the heart. Likewise, the murmurs of tricuspid stenosis and incompetence are best heard on inspiration. The murmur of tricuspid incompetence (regurgitation) is hard to differentiate from that of mitral incom-

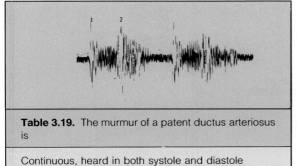

Table 3.19. The murmur of a patent ductus arteriosus is

Continuous, heard in both systole and diastole
Best heard below the left clavicle

petence, but the diagnosis is best made from the jugular venous pulse and from a pulsating liver.

An atrial septal defect seldom causes a murmur itself, but the increased flow through the right side of the heart due to the left-to-right shunt causes a 'flow' or ejection murmur at the pulmonary valve. If there is a large flow through the ASD the increased flow through the tricuspid valve may also cause a flow murmur there, similar to the murmur of tricuspid stenosis.

Other heart murmurs

Heart murmurs do not necessarily indicate intrinsic cardiac disease. Remember that a murmur occurs when a high volume crosses a normal valve as in:

- pregnancy
- anaemia
- thyrotoxicosis
- CO_2 retention
- beri-beri

These conditions may be associated with a sinus tachycardia, a raised jugular venous pressure and mild ankle oedema and are termed 'high output states'.

Many heart murmurs are of no consequence at all and are sometimes simply labelled 'benign'. These can be recognized by the following features:

- no symptoms
- no cardiac enlargement
- always systolic
- usually soft
- usually ejection in quality

These murmurs may be due to minor aortic valve abnormalities, to trivial pulmonary stenosis or to mitral valve prolapse.

The important cardiac abnormalities that are associated with heart murmurs are shown in Table 3.20.

Pericarditis

A wide range of pathological conditions can cause inflammation or irritation of the pericardium producing pericardial friction. In the Western world the commonest cause of pericardial friction is acute myocardial infarction but in undeveloped countries rheumatic fever is still a common cause. Table 3.21 lists the main causes of pericarditis.

Table 3.21. Causes of pericarditis

Pericarditis (viral or bacterial)
Myocardial infarction
Rheumatic fever
Connective tissue diseases
Trauma
Uraemia
Infiltration of pericardium with tumour

Pericardial friction rubs vary from soft shuffling sounds to scratchy noises in time with the cardiac cycle and often influenced by respiration. When a pleural rub is heard in addition the sounds are termed pleuropericardial.

Table 3.20. Cardiac abnormalities associated with heart murmurs

Cardiac pathology	Murmur due to
Rheumatic heart disease	Mitral and aortic stenosis or incompetence; right-sided valves seldom affected
Ischaemic heart disease	Mitral regurgitation or VSD following myocardial infarction
Congenital heart disease	Any abnormal communication between right and left sides of the circulation
Dissecting aneurysm } Collagen disease } Ankylosing spondylitis }	Aortic root dilatation

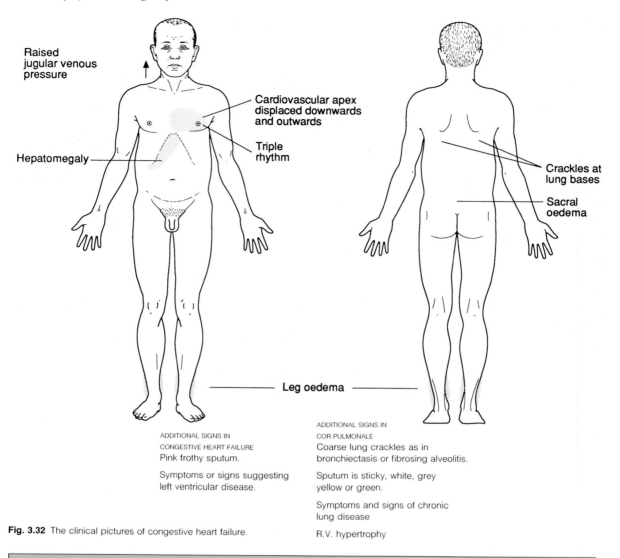

Raised jugular venous pressure

Cardiovascular apex displaced downwards and outwards

Triple rhythm

Hepatomegaly

Crackles at lung bases

Sacral oedema

Leg oedema

ADDITIONAL SIGNS IN
CONGESTIVE HEART FAILURE
Pink frothy sputum.

Symptoms or signs suggesting left ventricular disease.

ADDITIONAL SIGNS IN
COR PULMONALE
Coarse lung crackles as in bronchiectasis or fibrosing alveolitis.

Sputum is sticky, white, grey yellow or green.

Symptoms and signs of chronic lung disease

R.V. hypertrophy

Fig. 3.32 The clinical pictures of congestive heart failure.

Table 3.22. Important causes of left and right heart failure	
Left heart failure	Right heart failure
Ischaemic heart disease	Secondary to left heart disease
	Secondary to lung disease
	Multiple pulmonary emboli (cor pulmonale)
Rheumatic heart disease	Rheumatic tricuspid valve disease (rarely)
Mitral regurgitation	
Aortic stenosis or regurgitation	
Hypertension	
Cardiomyopathy	
Congenital heart disease	Congenital heart disease
VSD	ASD
Patent ductus arteriosus	Any cyanotic heart disease with right-to-left shunt

When fluid is formed within the pericardial sac, as a result of the pericarditis, the two layers of the pericardium separate and the noise disappears.

Effusions in serous cavities

The techniques of identifying pleural effusions and ascites are covered in other chapters. A pericardial effusion may be difficult to detect unless it causes compression of the heart (tamponade) when it will lead to venous and arterial paradox, as described above. Moderate or large pericardial effusions may make the cardiac apex difficult to feel and they muffle the heart sounds. In extreme cases it may be possible to detect an increase in the area of cardiac dullness, particularly to the right of the sternum.

Pericardial effusions have many causes other than heart failure, the most important being infective, inflammatory due to non-infective conditions such as collagen diseases and malignancy. In heart failure there is no inflammatory component at all but in the other conditions inflammation may cause the presence of a 'friction rub' which is usually best heard just to the left of the sternum as a superficial scratching sound in time with the heart beat and present in both systole and diastole (see below).

Heart failure

If a patient's symptoms and signs suggest the presence of heart failure, it is important to remember that this is a description, not a full diagnosis. Congestive cardiac failure (right heart failure secondary to left heart failure) must be distinguished from cor pulmonale (right heart failure secondary to lung disease). The symptoms and signs in these two conditions can be very similar and the two may coexist. Those features common to both and those which may help to make a clinical distinction are summarized in Fig. 3.32.

Right heart failure is not necessarily always due to lung disease and Table 3.22 compares the possible causes of left and right heart failure.

References and further reading

Hampton JR. *ECG made easy*, 3rd edn. Edinburgh: Churchill Livingstone, 1986.
Marriot HV. *Bedside cardiac diagnosis*. Philadelphia: Lippincott, 1993.
Wolfe JHN. *ABC of vascular diseases*. London: British Medical Association, 1992.

4

The symptoms and signs of respiratory disease

I. D. A. Johnston

The history
The physical examination
References and further reading

Respiratory disease is a common reason for patients seeking medical help and accounts for about a fifth of all consultations in general practice. As with other specialties, the taking of a good history — characterizing each symptom and its relationship to other symptoms — is of key diagnostic importance. The main respiratory symptoms will be covered here and important points in the family and drug histories mentioned. You should also remember that, in respiratory disease, a detailed occupational history may be vital, though only brief guidelines can be given here. Accounts of the examination of the respiratory system have in the past often been unnecessarily complicated with the inclusion of many physical signs of little modern value. This chapter excludes such signs.

The history

There are three main respiratory symptoms: breathlessness, cough and chest pain. They are discussed separately, each section including other related symptoms. Wheeze, for example, almost always occurs with breathlessness and is included with it, while sputum and haemoptysis are included under cough.

Breathlessness /dyspnoea.

Breathlessness is one of the commonest medical complaints and may be thought of as an uncomfortable awareness of the need to breathe. The term

'dyspnoea' is often used interchangeably with 'breathlessness', but the latter is preferable.

The sensation of breathlessness that normal people get on strenuous exertion is probably similar to that experienced by patients on mild exertion or even at rest. Three basic mechanisms can lead to breathlessness (Table 4.1) and may act singly or jointly. Thus in asthma, airflow obstruction increases the work of breathing, hyperinflation reduces muscle function and anxiety increases the neurological drive — the combination of these factors, and others, causing breathlessness. Breathlessness arises when there is an abnormal drive to breathe which does not meet requirements or, alternatively, is in excess of requirements.

Table 4.1. Mechanisms leading to breathlessness

1. Increased work of breathing	
(a) Airways obstruction	e.g. asthma
(b) Stiff lungs	e.g. pulmonary fibrosis
(c) Stiff chest wall	e.g. scoliosis
2. Decreased neuromuscular power	e.g. muscular dystrophies
3. Increased drive to breathe	
(a) Chemical drive	e.g. hypoxia, acidosis
(b) Neurological drive	e.g. from stimulation of lung J-receptors as in pulmonary oedema

To diagnose the cause of breathlessness, you must enquire about the following key points (Table 4.2):

Table 4.2. Key points to establish cause of breathlessness
Is it really breathlessness?
Timescale of onset/duration of symptoms
How severe is the breathlessness?
How variable is it?
Spontaneous
Nocturnal
Postural
Precipitating factors
Treatment (including occupation)
Associated symptoms

Table 4.3. Timing of onset of breathlessness		
Seconds/minutes	LVF	
	Pulmonary embolism	
	Pneumothorax	Asthma
Hours/days	LVF	Allergic alveolitis
	Pneumonia	Pleural effusion
	Asthma	
	Adult respiratory distress syndrome	
Weeks	LVF	Anaemia
	Asthma	Pleural effusion
Months/years	Chronic airflow obstruction	
	Asthma	Pulmonary fibrosis
	Anaemia	

* NB (i) There is much overlap between categories; (ii) many causes of breathlessness are omitted.

Is it really breathlessness?

Make sure you understand exactly what your patient is complaining about. Some patients will talk about being 'short of breath' or 'short of puff' rather than using the word 'breathless'. Occasionally patients may talk about being breathless when they are referring to chest tightness or pain such as angina — the two symptoms may often occur together of course. Patients with pleuritic chest pain frequently complain of breathlessness and the two symptoms may indeed coexist as in pulmonary infarction. Such patients may, however, be referring merely to an inability to take a deep breath due to pain — as with fractured ribs.

Timescale

'How long have you been breathless?' or 'When did your breathing difficulties begin?' are vital questions since the causes of long-standing breathlessness are quite different from those in which breathlessness has only been present for the last day or so (Table 4.3). The timescale of the onset of breathlessness therefore is an important diagnostic feature, though there is a lot of overlap. Left ventricular failure can, for example, present as an acute event or gradually increasing over several weeks. Remember that patients are poor at dating the onset of long-standing breathlessness. You should press them on this point — not uncommonly patients who initially say they have been breathless for a few months will admit to progressively reducing exercise tolerance over several years when questioned closely.

Severity

There are two reasons why it is important to document the severity of breathlessness. First, you need to understand how your patient's life is affected by the breathlessness. Second, you need to be able to assess whether any treatment you give is beneficial. There are several well-tried systems of grading breathlessness on three- or five-point scales. A better approach is to ask some general questions such as 'How far can you walk on the flat without stopping?' or 'Can you get up your stairs at home in one go?' together with more tailor-made questions. Thus, you might ask a housewife whether she can do her cleaning or the retired man whether he can still dig his allotment. All such questions clearly need to be appropriate to the degree of breathlessness. Be careful with patients with multiple pathology; the breathless old lady with the arthritic hip and the breathless man with intermittent claudication may both be limited more by pain in their legs rather than their breathlessness.

Variability

Spontaneous Is the breathlessness fairly constant/slowly progressive as often in chronic airflow obstruction or is it more episodic with day-to-day variation as in asthma?

Nocturnal Breathlessness that wakes the patient at night, usually in the early hours, occurs in two conditions which may sometimes be difficult to distinguish: pulmonary oedema and, probably more commonly, nocturnal asthma. First, pulmonary oedema due to left ventricular failure or, now much less commonly, mitral stenosis, causes 'paroxysmal nocturnal dyspnoea . The patient will give you a history of being woken by breathlessness relieved by sitting up or getting out of bed, manoeuvres which reduce the capillary hydrostatic pressure and thus tend to relieve pulmonary oedema. Secondly, poorly controlled asthmatics frequently wake around 2 or 3 a.m. with breathlessness which is usually associated with cough and wheeze of variable severity. This reflects an exaggeration of the normal circadian variation in airway calibre.

Postural Increased breathlessness on lying flat ('orthopnoea') can occur with almost any cause of the symptom and not just cardiac failure as is often thought. It is, however, a particular feature of bilateral diaphragmatic paralysis.

Precipitating factors Breathlessness that relates to some environmental factor, identifiable or not, is usually due to asthma. Some asthmatics, for example, may become breathless when exposed to cats, or a certain perfume or have seasonal symptoms with their breathlessness confined to the summer months when pollen counts are high. Some allergens cause breathlessness due to an alveolitis rather than asthma, as in farmers or pigeon-breeders who develop symptoms 4–6 hours after exposure. Occupation is particularly important: you must ask all patients with persistent breathlessness how their symptoms relate to their work. Two questions will identify the majority of those with occupational asthma — 'Is your breathing (or wheeze/cough) better at the weekends?' and 'Is it better when you are on holiday?' Finally, while almost all breathlessness is worse during exertion, exercise-induced asthma often occurs after exercise.

Treatment Variability due to treatment may be an important clue. Breathlessness relieved by diuretics is usually due to pulmonary oedema, while marked improvement over a few days with steroids strongly suggests asthma or, less commonly, parenchymal disease such as an allergic alveolitis. Rapid relief with a bronchodilator inhaler supports a diagnosis of asthma.

Associated symptoms

As always, the relationship of a symptom to others may be crucial. Breathlessness in a smoker with haemoptysis and weight loss may well be due to pulmonary collapse or pleural effusion due to cancer while its occurrence with wheeze in a young person is almost always due to asthma. Breathlessness is a common symptom of anxiety, often unrelated to exertion and occurring with a wide spectrum of symptoms such as palpitations, tingling in the arms,

dizziness and chest pains. Patients with these symptoms are frequently hyperventilating and may also complain of 'being unable to take a deep enough breath' or 'having to take a deep breath every so often'.

Wheeze

Many students, and doctors, omit to ask patients about wheeze, thinking that patients will not understand. Likewise, wheezy patients often complain primarily of breathlessness. Nevertheless most patients know what wheeze is and if they look blank you can describe it as a whistling sound on breathing out, or in. Wheeze is important because it indicates airflow obstruction (Table 4.4). Many of the important features of wheeze are similar to those described for breathlessness; thus, wheeze that is variable, either spontaneously or following precipitating factors such as exercise, allergens, occupation, drugs (e.g. beta-blockers, aspirin), or wakes the patient at night, is likely to be due to asthma.

Table 4.4. Causes of persistent wheeze
Asthma
Chronic bronchitis
Emphysema
Major airway obstruction, e.g. due to tumour

Cough

Cough may be a troublesome, sometimes distressing symptom. It is a common feature of many respiratory diseases and is therefore rarely of diagnostic help by itself. Cough involves making a forced expiratory effort against a closed glottis which then suddenly opens resulting in an explosive release of air carrying with it respiratory secretions. The cough reflex is initiated by receptors in the larynx and major airways which are stimulated both by material within the airway lumen (such as sputum, foreign bodies or inhaled irritants) and events in the airway wall (such as the effects of infection or sudden large changes in volume in the thorax).

Points about cough

Many smokers and people living in industrial areas regard a cough as a normal part of life and their response to your question 'Do you have a cough?' may often be 'no' or 'just the usual, y'know'. In this case you need to find out what your patient considers is normal, whether the cough has changed recently and in all cases the following features of the cough.

Duration How long has the cough been present? A regular morning cough for many years productive of a little white sputum is characteristic of chronic bronchitis while a cough of a week or two will most frequently be due to the common cold.

Variability Nocturnal cough may occur in asthma and though often combined with breathlessness and wheeze may be the sole presenting symptom of childhood asthma. Likewise daytime cough is variable in asthma while a persistent cough of a few weeks or months in a smoker should make you think of bronchial carcinoma or chronic bronchitis.

If the cough is episodic ask about precipitating factors. Cough related to meals or lying down may be due to aspiration of oesophageal contents. Is the cough dry or does your patient bring up phlegm (productive), or blood (see below)? A longstanding, highly productive cough is usually due to bronchiectasis. Ask about the possibility of foreign-body inhalation (e.g. peanuts) in children; the inhalation of foreign bodies is often unnoticed. Chronic sinusitis may be associated with cough but coexisting intrathoracic problems need to be excluded first.

Type of cough

If your patient has a cough, you will often hear it during history-taking. You may be able to confirm that it is productive but otherwise the character of the cough is rarely any help in diagnosis. With unilateral vocal-cord paralysis (as in recurrent laryngeal nerve palsy, e.g. due to malignant mediastinal invasion) the cough may be rather prolonged and has been likened to the lowing of cattle (hence 'bovine' cough). Laryngitis, especially in children, leads to a rather harsh 'croupy' cough. A weak cough occurs in bilateral cord palsy, respiratory muscle weakness, severe illness of any cause and when cough causes pain.

Sputum

You should ask 'Do you cough up any phlegm?' rather than asking about 'sputum', a term that means nothing to most patients. If the patient's cough is productive then you need first to know how much is being produced. About 100 ml of secretion is produced each day by the normal respiratory tree and this is usually swallowed. Patients can often give a useful guide to sputum volume in terms of, say, an eggcupful or a cupful a day and such volumes are often found with bronchiectasis, sometimes larger

with a lung abscess. One general point about history-taking here. When you ask about, for example, the amount of phlegm or the number of episodes of chest pain 'in a day', what you usually want to know is what is happening over a 24-hour period, while the patient not infrequently assumes you are talking about the 'daytime' as opposed to the 'night time'. You need to be on the same wavelength as your patient.

What about the colour and consistency? Clear or white, grey in industrial areas, sputum (mucoid) is typical of bronchial mucus gland hypersecretion, as in chronic bronchitis. When the sputum is yellow or green (purulent), often thick, it contains white cells indicating infection, except that in asthma green sputum may represent sputum eosinophilia due to the asthma and not bacterial infection. Coal workers may cough up black sputum (melanoptysis). Asthmatics often have very viscid, stringy sputum ('I can't seem to get it out' is a common comment) and less commonly may cough up small bronchial casts (Curschmann's spirals) which may be brown in bronchopulmonary aspergillosis. Frothy, sometimes pink, sputum is seen in severe acute pulmonary oedema but the very copious watery secretion of alveolar cell carcinoma is extremely rare. Offensively smelling sputum suggests anaerobic infection, as in a lung abscess or an empyema with bronchopleural fistula.

Haemoptysis

Coughing up blood causes patients, and often their doctors, to worry about cancer, though this is the cause in only about 3 per cent of cases. Faced with a patient complaining of coughing up blood, two questions first need to be answered. Is it really haemoptysis? Is the blood really coming from the chest? Haematemesis is usually, though not always, easy to exclude, but bleeding from the nasopharynx may be difficult to distinguish. If there is nose bleeding or the blood just appears in the mouth, then a nasopharyngeal source is more likely; whereas if the blood definitely comes up with a cough or is mixed with, or streaked in, the sputum then the chest is the likely source. Blood from the chest is usually bright red, not brown. How much haemoptysis is there? The volume of blood being coughed up is a guide to the immediate seriousness of the problem and is therefore important in management. There is no cut-off point but haemoptysis of more than 200 ml per 24 h has a high mortality. The cause of haemoptysis (Table 4.5) is found in only about half of those presenting with the symptom. Some clues come from

Table 4.5. Causes of haemoptysis

Common	No cause found
	Acute respiratory infection
	Bronchiectasis
	Lung cancer
	Tuberculosis active/inactive
	Pulmonary infarction
Uncommon	Aspergilloma
	Pulmonary vasculitis
	Chest trauma
	Arteriovenous malformations
	Benign tumours
	Foreign body
	Mitral stenosis
	Clotting disorders

the history and examination. Frank haemoptysis with pleuritic pain, breathlessness and sometimes a pleural rub is seen in pulmonary infarction, or with fever, purulent sputum and signs of consolidation in pneumonia. Recurrent haemoptysis over several years is common in bronchiectasis. In a smoker aged 40 years or more, bronchial carcinoma must always be considered. Haemoptysis should never be ascribed to 'bronchitis' before more serious causes have been excluded, and even if they have, it is better to be honest and say that the cause is unknown.

Chest pain

The lung itself is not supplied with pain fibres so fibrosing lung disease, multiple secondaries and diseases confined to the parenchyma do not cause chest pain. Pleuritic chest pain can, however, be very severe. Typically this is a sharp, stabbing pain worsened by movement such as breathing in or coughing. Your patient may say that 'it catches me

when I breathe'. Pleuritic pain can occur due to inflammation of the pleura (pleurisy) since the parietal pleura is very sensitive, or to musculoskeletal causes. Chest wall pain can closely mimic the pain of pleurisy (Table 4.6). The main diagnostic difficulties revolve around infection versus infarction versus musculoskeletal causes. Fever and purulent sputum indicate infection, breathlessness and haemoptysis support infarction and a history of trauma and pain reproduced by tenderness at the site of the pain favour a musculoskeletal cause. This latter physical sign may also occur in pleurisy, however, and the history is often not so clear cut. Central diaphragmatic pleurisy often causes pain referred to the shoulder since the pain fibres from this part of the diaphragm run with the phrenic nerve (C3,4,5) while pleurisy involving the outer part of the diaphragm causes pain referred to the lower chest and upper abdomen. The extremely severe pleuritic pain of the coxsackie viral disease epidemic myalgia (Bornholm disease or devil's grip) in which the intercostal muscles are extremely tender, is fortunately rare. Pain radiating round from the back due to thoracic spine disease as in vertebral collapse sometimes has a pleuritic quality and may be exacerbated by coughing.

Other respiratory chest pains

Large pleural effusions often cause a dull heaviness and pleural malignancy (especially mesothelioma) may characteristically cause a constant, often severe, pain. Pneumothorax may cause a pleuritic type of pain but patients often describe it as a dragging or drawing sensation. Pain and swelling over the sternocostal junction bears the name Tietze's syndrome but it is far more common to find pain on palpation over the sternocostal junctions without swelling. Tracheitis may cause an uncomfortable

Table 4.6. Causes of pleuritic chest pain

Pleural disease	Infective, e.g. pneumonia	
	Pulmonary infarction (pulmonary embolus)	Common
	Neoplastic, primary or secondary	
	Collagen disease	
	systemic lupus	
	rheumatoid arthritis	Uncommon
	Asbestos-related pleurisy	
Musculoskeletal disease	Rib fracture (trauma, cough or pathological)	Common
	Muscular strain	
	Bornholm disease	Rare
	Herpes zoster (pre-rash)	

central chest ache often described as a 'raw feeling' and occasionally mediastinal or hilar lymphadenopathy, as in sarcoidosis, can cause similar problems. Persistent coughing due to any cause may lead to a soreness in the central chest as well as the possibility of causing rib fracture.

Checklist of other important points in the history

The lung is frequently involved in systemic disease and a full history will be needed. The following are points of particular importance:

Ankle oedema The advent of peripheral oedema in patients with chronic lung disease may signify cor pulmonale (right heart disease secondary to lung disease) and indicates a poor prognosis.

Smoking You should get a broad idea of how much your patient smokes and if he has given up, how long ago that was. Chronic bronchitis and emphysema are very uncommon in the absence of a history of smoking, while wheeze in a lifetime non-smoker is usually asthma. The smoker's increased risk of lung cancer declines with the number of years since stopping smoking.

Occupation In respiratory medicine, a full occupational history is often vital, particularly so when your patient has asthma, pulmonary fibrosis or pleural disease. The list of causes of occupational asthma is growing but some important causes are isocyanates (used in paint spraying), flour and grain, epoxy resins (used in adhesives) or colophony (used in solders). In pulmonary fibrosis or pleural disease you need to enquire about mining and asbestos exposure. You may need to dig deep — that year's exposure to asbestos while making gas masks in the Second World War may not result in mesothelioma for 30–40 years!

Drugs Aspirin and other non-steroidal, anti-inflammatory drugs frequently worsen airflow obstruction. Many drugs cause pulmonary eosinophilia. Nitrofurantoin, amiodarone and busulphan are among many drugs associated with pulmonary fibrosis.

Hobbies Budgerigars and pigeons may cause extrinsic allergic alveolitis.

Sexual history You may need to take a detailed sexual history since the possibility of AIDS must always be considered when there are unexplained respiratory symptoms or chest x-ray abnormalities or evidence of opportunistic infection.

Past medical history In particular, ask about past tuberculosis and its treatment, or contact with the disease.

Family history A family history of cystic fibrosis or of emphysema at a young age (as in α-1-antitrypsin deficiency) are important.

Old x-rays Finally, never forget to ask whether your patient has had previous chest x-rays and if so where. A great deal of time and many investigations may be saved if old x-rays are available for comparison.

The physical examination

Extrathoracic signs

Clubbing

Recognizing clubbing of the fingers is easy when it is gross and all the signs are present (Table 4.7 and Fig. 4.1). Less obvious cases engender time-consuming arguments on ward rounds as to whether clubbing is, or is not, present, though the outcome of the argument rarely affects clinical management. It is best to recognize three categories, i.e. clubbing is either definitely present, definitely absent or possible. The pathogenesis of clubbing remains unknown — certainly there is increased bloodflow through the fingers and a neurogenic component seems likely as vagotomy can abolish clubbing. A large number of conditions are associated with clubbing (Table 4.8) and of the respiratory causes bronchial carcinoma is the commonest. Remember that

Table 4.7. Signs of clubbing

1. Increased sponginess of the nail bed
2. Increase in angle between the nail and nail bed, usually, but not always, to $>180°$
3. Increased curvature of nails in both longitudinal and lateral axes
4. Ends of fingers become bulbous

Table 4.8. Causes of clubbing

Congenital
Bronchial carcinoma
Fibrosing alveolitis, asbestosis
Chronic pulmonary sepsis, e.g. bronchiectasis, cystic fibrosis, lung abscess
Infective endocarditis
Cyanotic congenital heart disease
Ulcerative colitis, Crohn's disease
Cirrhosis of liver
Many other, rare, causes, e.g. pleural neoplasm

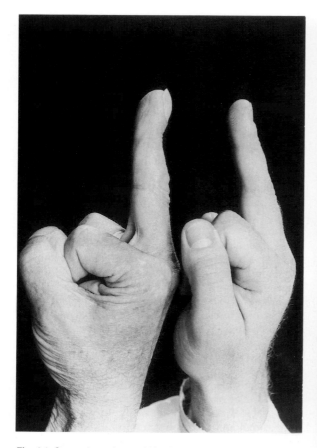

Fig. 4.1 Comparison of normal (right) and clubbed finger (left).

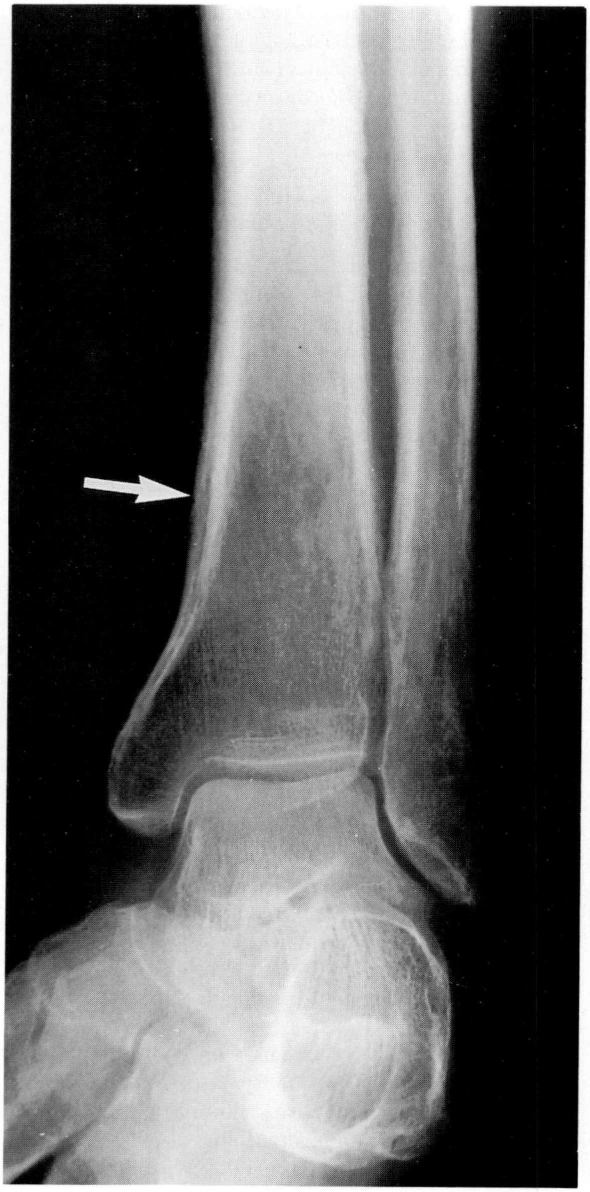

clubbing may be congenital and seems to occur more frequently in black people without any underlying pathology. Patients are often unaware of the changes in their nails, probably because clubbing usually develops slowly. It can also affect the toes.

Hypertrophic pulmonary osteoarthropathy results in pain and sometimes swelling over the ends of the long bones above the wrists and ankles symmetrically. It almost always occurs with clubbing and most cases are associated with a squamous carcinoma of the lung. X-rays show subperiosteal new bone formation on the shafts of the long bones (Fig. 4.2).

Fig. 4.2 Hypertrophic pulmonary osteoarthropathy. Arrow points to subperiosteal new bone formation.

Cyanosis

You should look at the tongue, lips and nails for the blue discoloration of cyanosis. If cyanosis is seen in all these three sites it is termed 'central' (Table 4.9)

and if just seen in the nails, it is 'peripheral'. The ability to recognize cyanosis varies widely among doctors let alone students but cyanosis should be detectable when the arterial oxygen saturation is 80–85 per cent. As an approximate guide only it

Table 4.9. Common causes of central cyanosis	
Acute	Severe pneumonia
	Acute asthma
	Left ventricular failure
	Pulmonary embolus
Chronic	Severe chronic airflow obstruction
	Pulmonary fibrosis
	Right-to-left cardiac shunt

indicates that the blood contains at least 1.5 g/dl of reduced haemoglobin. Cyanosis is easy to detect in polycythaemia but may be absent in anaemia despite severe hypoxaemia. Peripheral cyanosis is usually due to increased oxygen extraction with a slow-moving circulation. It will be seen in cold weather or in Raynaud's phenomenon or peripheral vascular disease.

Superior vena caval obstruction (SVCO)

This condition is most often due to pressure from a bronchial carcinoma or its associated mediastinal glands (Table 4.10). Patients may complain of head-ache and sometimes worsening breathlessness as well as a puffy face, or that their collar feels tight. The resulting signs (Table 4.11 and Fig. 4.3) vary in severity. The dilated veins on the chest wall represent the collateral circulation bypassing the obstructed SVC and returning to the heart usually via the inter-costals and azygos system. The engorged neck veins may be impossible to see if the neck itself is very swollen.

Table 4.10. Causes of superior vena caval obstruction
Bronchial carcinoma — common
Lymphoma — uncommon
Mediastinal fibrosis and other causes — rare

Table 4.11. Signs of superior vena caval obstruction
Dilated veins on anterior chest wall
Engorged, fixed, non-pulsatile jugular veins
Swollen face and neck
Conjunctival oedema

Other signs

The supraclavicular fossae should be closely exam-ined for enlarged glands frequently found in bronchial carcinoma, lymphoma, tuberculosis and sarcoidosis.

Inspection of the chest

Make sure your patient is comfortable, sitting at about 45° and in a good light. A great deal can be gleaned by simple observation of the chest (Table 4.12). Ask yourself whether the chest wall itself is normal, before looking at the pattern of breathing and the movements of the chest.

Table 4.12. Inspection of the chest	
Appearance of the chest wall	
General shape	
Chest deformity	Pectus carinatus
	Pectus excavatus
	Scoliosis
	Kyphosis
	Thoracoplasty
	Chest wall lesions
Breathing	
Rate	
Pattern of breathing	Shallow
	Kussmaul
	Cheyne–Stokes
	Sighing
	Pursed-lip
	Orthopnoea
Chest wall movement	
Expansion	General reduction
	Unilateral reduction
Paradoxical movement	Flail segment
	Intercostal recession
	Indrawing ribs
Abdominal movement	
Use of accessory muscles	

Appearances of the chest wall

Note the general shape of the chest. An increase in the size of the chest in the anteroposterior axis causes patients to look barrel chested. You will see this in patients who have long-standing hyperinflation of their lungs, as in emphysema, and sometimes when there is distortion of the chest due to kyphosis (see below). You will see various deformities of

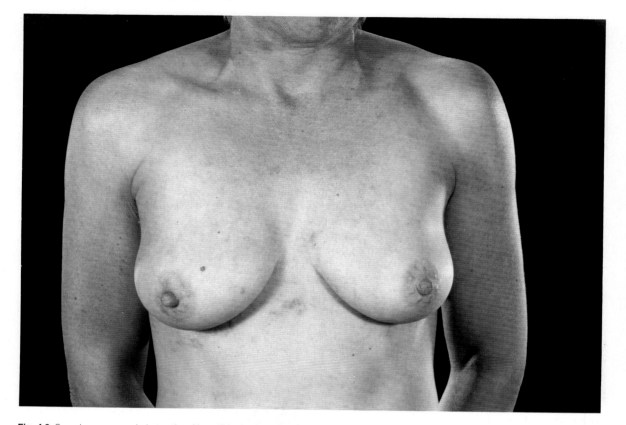

Fig. 4.3 Superior vena caval obstruction. Note dilated veins on chest and upper abdomen with dilated external jugular veins.

the chest: mild forms of pectus carinatus (pigeon chest) (Fig. 4.4) and pectus excavatus (funnel chest) (Fig. 4.5) are quite common. Pectus carinatus, with its prominent sternum and costal cartilages, may be congenital or secondary to severe childhood asthma, rickets or congenital heart disease. When the cause is asthma, Harrison's sulci may also be present — these are horizontal grooves at the bottom of the rib-cage in children caused by persistent indrawing of the ribs. Pectus excavatus (Table 4.13) is a congenital deformity and not secondary to lung disease. It is usually seen as a depressed lower end of the sternum, though in severe forms the whole sternum and costal cartilages are sunken.

Scoliosis (Table 4.14) is a lateral curvature of the spine. At the apex of the curve, the vertebral bodies are rotated so that they face the convex side of the curve. The ribs therefore protrude backwards on the convex side (Fig. 4.6). Kyphosis, on the other hand, is an increase in the anteroposterior curvature of the spine (Fig. 4.7) probably most frequently seen in elderly people with osteoporosis or much less commonly in younger men with ankylosing spondylitis. Both deformities, but scoliosis especially, can lead to serious respiratory disability and sometimes respiratory failure.

Note any scars indicating previous chest operations or signs of trauma. You may still see patients who

Table 4.13. Points about pectus excavatus
May cause
Displaced apex beat
Cardiac murmur
Apparent enlarged heart on chest x-ray
Only affects lung function if very severe

Table 4.14. Causes of scoliosis (see also Table 17.2)
Idiopathic — commonest
Congenital
Neuropathic, e.g. poliomyelitis
Myopathic, e.g. muscular dystrophy
Traumatic

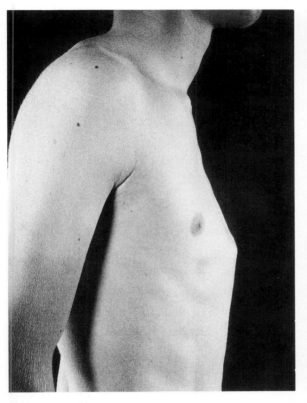

Fig. 4.4 Pectus carinatus.

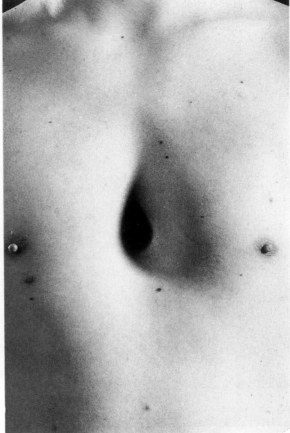

Fig. 4.5 Pectus excavatus.

have had a thoracoplasty (Fig. 4.8). This operation was done for tuberculosis in the days before chemotherapy was available and consisted in pushing in part of the ribcage to collapse part of the underlying lung. A thoracoplasty can lead to respiratory difficulties later in life.

Other chest wall lesions Look carefully at the skin. Assess any lumps in the usual way but remember also that occasionally chest wall lumps (such as lipomata) may cause a shadow on the chest x-ray which can trap the unwary into presuming that the patient has an intrapulmonary lesion. Feel for the crackling sensation of subcutaneous emphysema if you suspect pneumothorax or chest trauma. Is there any local tenderness? Dilated veins on the chest wall should prompt you to look for the other signs of SVCO (see above).

Observation of respiration

Rate The normal respiratory rate is about 10–15 breaths/min, anything above 20/min being abnormal (tachypnoea). Don't make it obvious to your patient that you are watching his breathing since anxious patients readily increase their respiratory rate while being observed. Tachypnoea is otherwise an important sign and can sometimes be the only clue to the presence of respiratory disease. Almost any respiratory disease can cause an increased respiratory rate but an increase is sometimes found with fever due to non-respiratory causes.

Pattern of breathing Observe the pattern of breathing carefully as it may give important diagnostic clues. Shallow breathing is seen when breathing is restricted either by certain types of pulmonary disease (e.g. fibrosis) or chest wall disease, or by pain. A large increase in the depth of respiration (Kussmaul breathing) is often due to metabolic acidosis such as in renal failure or diabetic ketoacidosis. Cheyne–Stokes or periodic breathing is a cyclical variation in depth and rate of breathing. Each cycle can last up to two minutes and involves a period of apnoea followed by a gradual return of respiration before this declines again to another period of apnoea. Cheyne–Stokes

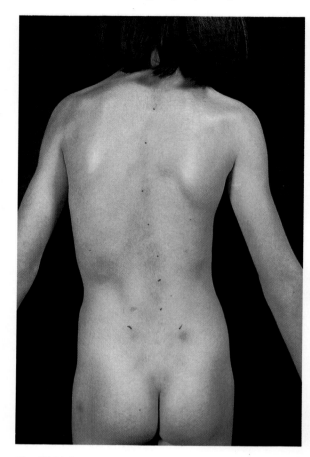

Fig. 4.6 Scoliosis.

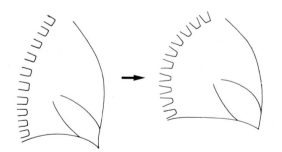

Fig. 4.7 Schematic lateral view of chest to show development of kyphosis due to wedging of thoracic vertebrae.

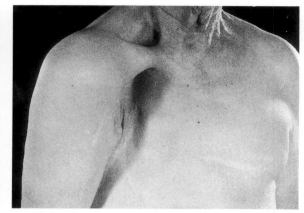

Fig. 4.8 Right thoracoplasty (and mastectomies).

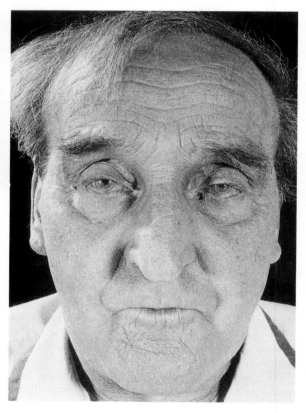

Fig. 4.9 Pursed-lip breathing.

breathing usually indicates serious brainstem dysfunction. It is quite normal to sigh from time to time but when your patient sighs frequently while you are examining him, there is likely to be a psychogenic component to his symptoms. Pursed-lip breathing (Fig. 4.9) is a sign of severe airflow obstruction. If on lying flat your patient becomes breathless or pre-existing breathlessness worsens (orthopnoea) then you should particularly think of pulmonary oedema or bilateral diaphragmatic paralysis, though any breathless patient will usually prefer the upright position.

Chest wall movements

Chest expansion may be assessed by placing the hands on the lateral chest wall, picking up a fold of skin medially with the thumbs and watching the thumbs move apart in inspiration (Fig. 4.10). Normal chest expansion, measured with a tape-measure at the level of the nipples, is usually not less than 5 cm. Frankly, however, in routine clinical practice it is sufficient merely to note on inspection whether expansion appears normal or is obviously reduced; exact measurement of expansion is unnecessary being crude and of little diagnostic help since any cause of diffuse lung or chest wall disease can reduce expansion. Much more importantly you should look for unilaterally reduced expansion which will point to local pathology whether this be consolidation, fibrosis, effusion or pneumothorax. Paradoxical inward movement of part of the rib-cage during inspiration indicates a flail segment (Fig. 4.11). This arises when a group of ribs are fractured along two lines creating a segment of ribs without support which is then sucked inwards by the negative intrathoracic pressure during inspiration. The high negative pressure created in the face of airflow obstruction can similarly lead to intercostal recession on inspi-

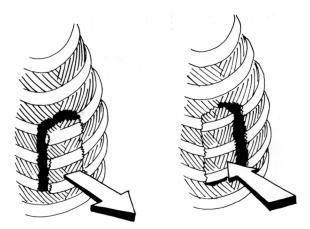

Fig. 4.11 Paradoxical movement of flail segment, moving *out* on an expiration (left) and *in* on inspiration (right).

ration. Normally during inspiration the lower ribs move outwards but when the lungs are hyperinflated due to airflow obstruction the diaphragm now becomes flat and may cause indrawing of the ribs (Fig. 4.12). Watch the abdominal movement during respiration. Normally the abdomen moves out due to diaphragmatic descent as the rib-cage expands; inward or asynchronous abdominal movement can indicate diaphragmatic paralysis or fatigue which may herald respiratory failure. Finally, in severe airflow obstruction, you may see the accessory muscles, scalenus anterior and sternomastoid, in action to help in the work of breathing. Such patients may also use their arms to fix the shoulder girdle further to increase the effectiveness of the accessory muscles.

Palpation of the trachea

You should next assess whether the trachea is central. There are several different ways to do this, each with its own adherents. The easiest way is to put your index finger centrally in the suprasternal notch and gently move it backwards until the tip of your finger meets the trachea (Fig. 4.13), feeling then whether it is central or deviated to one side. This is a crude test and you are unlikely to be able to detect minor degrees of tracheal shift. Don't, therefore, spend a long time on the trachea — decide briskly whether you think it is central or not and move on. Further information about the position of the mediastinum is also gained from the position of the apex beat of the heart. Thus a large right pleural effusion may cause the heart and apex beat to be displaced to the left (Fig. 4.14). Displacement of the apex beat, however, is far more commonly due to cardiac than respiratory disease.

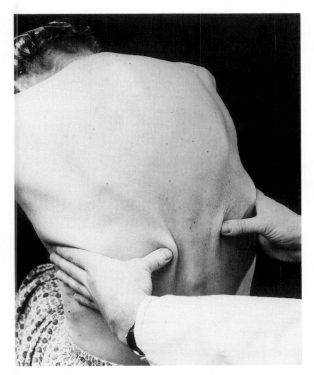

Fig. 4.10 Assessing chest expansion (see text).

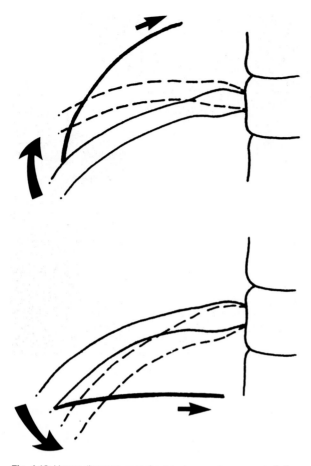

Fig. 4.12 Upper diagram: normal out and upward movement of ribs on inspiration with normal diaphragm (small arrow). Lower diagram: paradoxical inward movement of ribs when diaphragm flat as in hyperinflation.

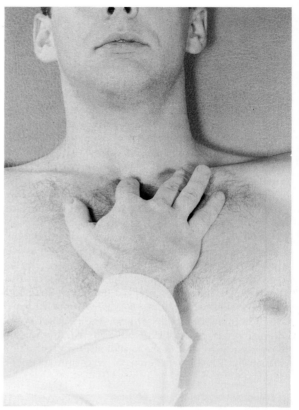

Fig. 4.13 Palpation of trachea.

opposite sides of the chest. If your attention is drawn to a particular area of the chest by an altered percussion note or by other signs or local symptoms then you will need to examine that area in greater

Percussion of the chest

The technique of percussion requires practice but should become second nature. If you are right-handed put the middle finger of your left hand flat on the chest wall and strike its middle phalanx smartly with the tip of the terminal phalanx of your right middle finger (Figs 4.15 and 4.16). All the movement in your right hand should come from the wrist and you should assess the percussion note by a combination of the pitch of the noise produced and the vibrations detected under your left middle finger. You should percuss the clavicle directly with your right middle finger. Percuss over the sites shown in Fig. 4.17, the key point being that you must constantly compare the percussion note in the corresponding sites on

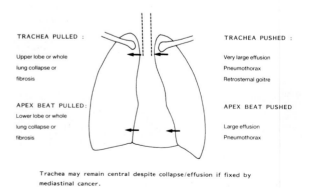

TRACHEA PULLED :

Upper lobe or whole
lung collapse or
fibrosis

TRACHEA PUSHED :

Very large effusion
Pneumothorax
Retrosternal goitre

APEX BEAT PULLED:

Lower lobe or whole
lung collapse or
fibrosis

APEX BEAT PUSHED

Large effusion
Pneumothorax

Trachea may remain central despite collapse/effusion if fixed by mediastinal cancer.

Fig. 4.14 Movement of mediastinum (trachea and apex beat) due to various pathologies.

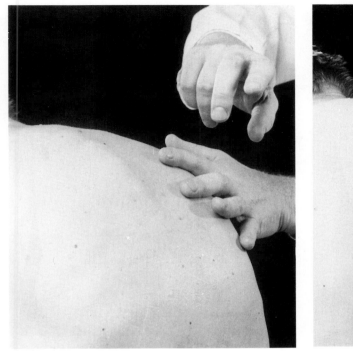

Fig. 4.15 Technique of percussion (see text).

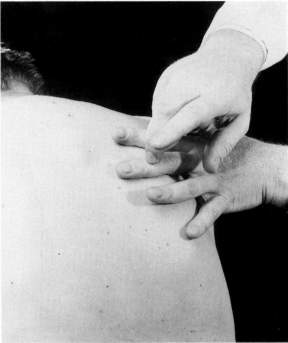

Fig. 4.16 Technique of percussion (see text).

detail. You should assess each percussion note as being normal, hyper-resonant, dull or stony dull (Table 4.15). The distinction between dull and stony dull will seem difficult at first but will come with practice.

Remember that if the percussion note on one side is different to the other side, there is likely to be an abnormality, either hyper-resonance on one side or dullness on the other side. If, however, you find the same apparent abnormality on both sides, then it is much less likely that you are dealing with a significant problem. Thus while bilateral basal dullness

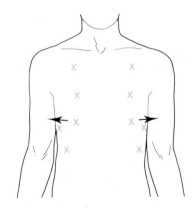

Fig. 4.17 Approximate sites for routine percussion (posterior similar).

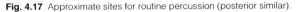

may be due to bilateral pleural effusions, it may simply be due to obesity. Diaphragmatic movement is usually difficult to detect by percussion but basal dullness on the right sometimes reflects a raised right hemidiaphragm and basal hyper-resonance on the left a raised left hemidiaphragm.

Table 4.15. Percussion note	
Hyper-resonant	Hyperinflation as in emphysema, asthma
	Pneumothorax
	Very thin people
Dull	Consolidation, collapse, fibrosis
	Obesity
Stony dull	Pleural effusion

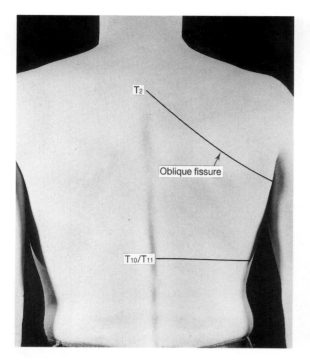

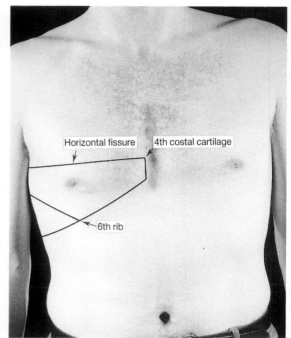

Figs 4.18−4.20 Surface anatomy of right lung. Oblique fissure follows a line from T2 posteriorly to the sixth rib in the mammary line. Horizontal fissure follows lower border of fourth rib to meet the oblique fissure in the mid-axillary line. Surface anatomy on the left is the same but there is no horizontal fissure.

Fig. 4.19 See caption to Fig. 4.18.

Surface anatomy

While percussing or listening to the chest, you should bear in mind what part of the lung it is that you are examining (Figs 4.18−4.20 and Table 4.16). You will normally find that liver dullness to percussion can be detected below the level of the sixth rib in the mid-clavicular line although the upper border of the liver extends to just above the level of the fifth rib. With hyperinflated lungs this upper border of liver dullness will be pushed lower.

The breath sounds

Sounds heard at the mouth

With a healthy person breathing at rest, you should not be able to hear the breath sounds at the mouth. By contrast, in airways obstruction (e.g. chronic bronchitis, asthma) the breath sounds will often be easily heard; in general the worse the airway narrowing the more noisy is the breathing. These

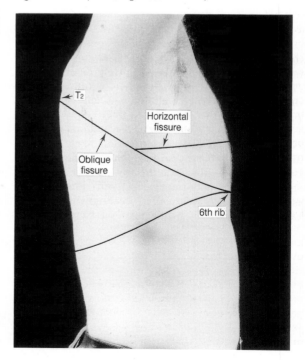

Fig. 4.20 See caption to Fig. 4.18.

Table 4.16. Simple guide to surface anatomy of the lung

Right	Anterior	Upper chest	Upper lobe
		Below horizontal level of fourth costal cartilage	Middle lobe
	Posterior	All apart from apex	Lower lobe
Left	Anterior	Almost all apart from lateral base	Upper lobe
	Posterior	All apart from apex	Lower lobe

sounds arise from increased turbulence of the gas flow in the main airways and noisy breathing should be considered separately from wheeze though the two may coexist. Stridor is a harsh, often musical note heard at the mouth, most marked on inspiration and denoting major airway obstruction — we will consider it further below.

Auscultation

How to listen The diaphragm of the stethoscope is better suited to listening to high-frequency sounds and the bell to lower-frequency sounds. Many prefer to use the diaphragm to listen to the breath sounds but the bell can be useful in patients with hairy chests (to reduce the crackling sounds produced by movement of hair) and in very thin patients in whom it may be difficult to get the diaphragm flat on the chest wall. Ask your patient to 'take some deep breaths in and out with your mouth open'. Make sure the pattern of breathing is otherwise normal but be gentle with your patients with pleuritic pain who may be unable to take the deep breaths that you ask for.

Where to listen Once again it is vitally important to compare the two sides. At each position at which you listen, you should then compare this with the corresponding position on the opposite side. Listen more than 2–3 cm away from the mid-line, to listen over lung rather than central airways. The number of sites in which you listen and the number of breaths to which you should listen at each site will depend on your experience and whether you think your patient could have a respiratory problem. For example, for a preoperative assessment for an inguinal herniorrhaphy in a fit young male it would be quite sufficient to listen in three or four positions on both sides from just below the clavicle anteriorly and the apex posteriorly down to the lung base, and

laterally. Similar sites to percussion can be chosen (Fig. 4.17). By contrast a woman on the contraceptive pill who has chest pain and breathlessness may require much more careful auscultation including a search for a pleural rub.

What to listen for (Table 4.17) You must train yourself to concentrate on both parts of the respiratory cycle separately and to ask yourself at each site:

- are the breath sounds of normal intensity?
- are the breath sounds normal in character, or bronchial?
- are there any added sounds?
- if added sounds are present, in which part of inspiration or expiration are they?

With practice these questions are automatically answered by the ear and brain, but it is all too easy to lose concentration and thereby to lose information.

Table 4.17. Auscultation

Breath sounds
    Normal or reduced/absent
    Bronchial
Added sounds
    Wheeze
    Crackles
    Rub

Normal and bronchial breath sounds

Normal breath sounds These are the sounds you hear over normal lung. Sometimes they are termed 'vesicular' but 'normal' is far preferable. The sounds probably arise from turbulent airflow in major airways rather than from movement of air in the alveoli. These sounds are then transmitted across intervening lung to the chest wall, with resulting loss of the higher frequencies. The sounds increase in inspiration but fade away soon after expiration (Fig. 4.21).

The normal sounds may be reduced or absent if there is a barrier to their transmission as in pleural effusion or pneumothorax, or when airflow is reduced locally to a part of the lung, as in collapse. The breath sounds will be quiet bilaterally in obesity, hyperinflation and when respiration is depressed as in an unconscious patient. It may sometimes be difficult to be sure if the breath sounds are quite normal but if they are the same on both sides then there is a good chance that they are indeed normal.

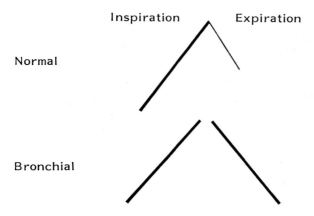

Fig. 4.21 Normal and bronchial breath sounds.

Bronchial breath sounds   When the lung between the large airways and the chest wall is relatively solid the breath sounds are transmitted with much less loss than normal and are called 'bronchial'. You will hear bronchial breathing, therefore, over consolidation, collapse and sometimes fibrosis (but see Table 4.18 and Fig. 4.22). The sound resembles that heard by listening directly over the larynx or trachea.

Table 4.18. Points about bronchial breathing (BB)

1. Absence of BB does not rule out presence of consolidation
2. BB will *not* be heard over consolidation or collapse in lower lobes if the main bronchus is obstructed (Fig. 4.22)
3. BB may be heard over consolidation or collapse in upper lobes even if the main bronchus is obstructed (tracheal sounds being transmitted directly across adjoining lung) (Fig. 4.22)

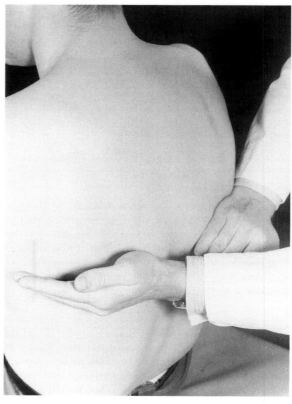

Fig. 4.23 Eliciting tactile vocal fremitus (see text).

The breath sounds in bronchial breathing are distinguished from normal sounds (Fig. 4.21) since they:

- are harsher with their higher frequencies preserved
- have a definite pause between inspiration and expiration
- can be heard throughout expiration

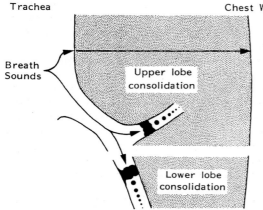

Upper lobe bronchus obstructed : BB still heard (sounds transmitted from trachea).

Lower lobe bronchus obstructed : BB not heard

Fig. 4.22 Transmission of breath sounds when central airways obstructed.

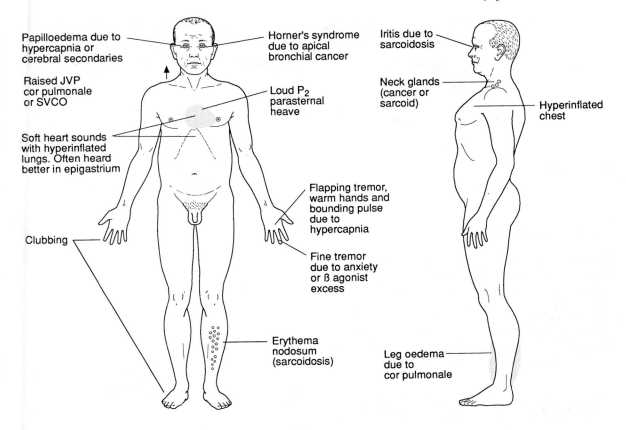

Fig. 4.24 Extrathoracic signs associated with respiratory disease.

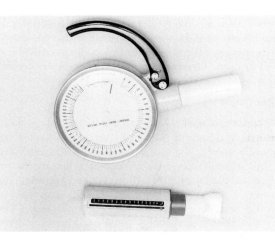

Fig. 4.25 Two common types of peak flow meter.

Added sounds

In recent years, the classification of added sounds has become much simpler. You can forget rhonchi, rales and crepitations (both wet and dry!) and concentrate on three sounds: wheezes, crackles and rubs.

Wheezes Wheezes are musical sounds produced by airway walls oscillating between the open and nearly closed positions. Wheeze indicates narrowing of an airway and usually occurs mainly on expiration but also on inspiration in severe airway narrowing. When there is generalized airway narrowing (Table 4.19) you will hear wheeze composed of sounds of many different pitches (polyphonic) during respiration. Remember, however, that in very severe airflow obstruction, wheeze may be absent. If you hear a localized wheeze of single pitch unaltered by coughing (monophonic, fixed) you should strongly suspect a local airway obstruction, most commonly due to tumour.

Wheeze or stridor? Stridor is a loud, mainly inspira-

Table 4.19. Causes of wheeze on auscultation		
Generalized	Asthma ⎫ Chronic bronchitis ⎬ and emphysema ⎭	Common
	Left ventricular failure	Occasional
	Bronchiolitis	In children
Localized	Tumour Foreign body	

tory noise, usually heard at the mouth. It is produced by the potentially serious situation of laryngeal, tracheal or major airway obstruction and must therefore be recognized. Like wheeze, stridor can often be a musical noise and may be difficult to recognize in patients with coexisting generalized airway narrowing. Always suspect stridor if the inspiratory noise of wheeze is louder than the expiratory sound.

Crackles Crackles are most often due to the sudden opening of lightly occluded airways when gas passes through, though may sometimes be produced by secretions in main airways. When listening to crackles, note their position in the respiratory cycle and whether they are localized to a certain area in the lung (Table 4.20). Be careful the crackles are not being produced by hair moving under your stethoscope! With experience you will be able to describe crackles as being fine or coarse but this distinction often adds little. Nevertheless, certain crackles are characteristic — those of fibrosing alveolitis for example, are like unfastening Velcro.

Pleural rub This is a coarse, creaking sound said to be produced by the irregular movement of the visceral and parietal pleura on each other when the surfaces are inflamed. You may hear it both in inspiration and expiration but rarely when a substantial pleural effusion is present. Any cause of pleural inflammation can cause a rub (commonly infection,

pulmonary infarction or pleural trauma, including biopsies).

Other added sounds Rarely a bruit will be heard and this is likely to be due to an arteriovenous communication such as an aneurysm. Certainly you should listen carefully for a bruit if the patient has a rounded opacity on the chest x-ray of uncertain aetiology, particularly before biopsy! Occasionally clicks may be heard over a left-sided pneumothorax — these are of little significance.

Voice sounds and tactile vocal fremitus

Since normal lung transmits the higher frequencies very poorly, speech is unintelligible and whispering inaudible when you listen with a stethoscope at the chest wall. The presence of solid lung (e.g. consolidation) allows these higher frequencies to be transmitted and so speech becomes intelligible (bronchophony) and whispering clearly audible (whispering pectoriloquy). These two signs, however, are only present when bronchial breathing is present (since they share the same mechanism) and since they therefore add no further information, they are nowadays redundant.

The transmission of voice sounds to the chest wall is palpable as low-frequency vibration. This is tactile vocal fremitus (TVF) and as always the key to this sign is comparison of the two sides, preferably simultaneously. Put the sensitive part of the palms of both hands on the chest wall and ask your patient to say '99' (Fig. 4.23). TVF is palpable over normal lung and remains palpable or increased over consolidated lung but is always reduced over an effusion.

The present-day value of the voice sounds and TVF is doubtful. However when you find a reduced percussion note for which the reason is unclear, either because there is no bronchial breathing or the breath sounds are only slightly reduced, then a reduction in voice sounds or especially a reduction in TVF strongly favours a pleural effusion or thickening.

Other signs

Since lung disease, such as cancer, may have widespread systemic effects and systemic diseases frequently involve the lungs, you will need to complete a full examination with particular reference to the signs in Fig. 4.24. You should also examine your patient's sputum if available. Finally, just as you would test your patient's urine for glucose if you were suspecting diabetes mellitus, so you should measure your patient's peak expiratory flow rate (PEFR) if you suspect airflow obstruction. Using a

Table 4.20. Causes of crackles	
Late inspiratory crackles	
Pulmonary oedema (e.g. LVF) ⎫ Fibrosing alveolitis ⎬ Asbestosis ⎭	Typically bilateral and basal
Early inspiratory and expiratory	
Bronchiectasis Chronic bronchitis	Localized coarse scanty
Inspiratory	
Pneumonia	Localized

peak flow meter (Fig. 4.25) ask your patient to take the biggest breath in that he can manage and to blow out as hard as he can into the meter with lips tightly round the mouthpiece. The meter will record the maximum airflow in the first 10 ms, so a short sharp blow is essential. Take the best of three readings and express the mean as a percentage of your patient's predicted value (calculated for height, sex and age). This provides a measure of the degree of airflow obstruction at that time. Graphs and charts of predicted values of PEFR are widely available. Note, however, that a single reading may often be normal in asthma — the hallmark of this disease being its variability.

Synthesis of physical signs in common respiratory conditions

The next few pages bring together the physical signs we have discussed above. The principal signs of the following respiratory conditions are shown:

- airflow obstruction (Fig. 4.26)
- consolidation right middle lobe (Fig. 4.27)
- collapse left upper lobe (Fig. 4.28)
- collapse right lower lobe (Fig. 4.29)
- massive right pleural effusion (Fig. 4.30)
- moderate left pleural effusion (Fig. 4.31)
- Large right pneumothorax (Fig. 4.32)
- Fibrosing alveolitis (Fig. 4.33)

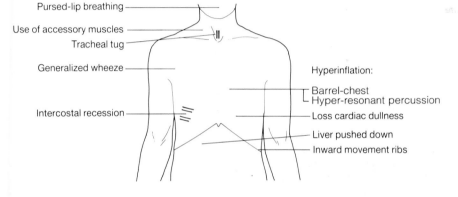

Fig. 4.26 Signs seen in airflow obstruction.

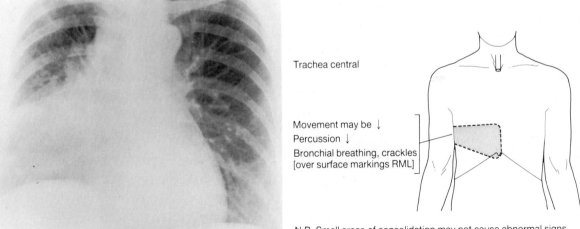

(a)

(b)

Fig. 4.27 Consolidation right middle lobe (a) chest x-ray; (b) signs.

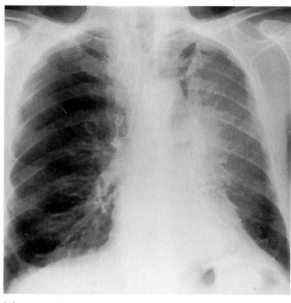

(a)

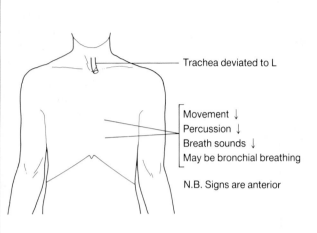

Trachea deviated to L

Movement ↓
Percussion ↓
Breath sounds ↓
May be bronchial breathing

N.B. Signs are anterior

(b)

Fig. 4.28 Collapse left upper lobe (a) chest x-ray; (b) signs.

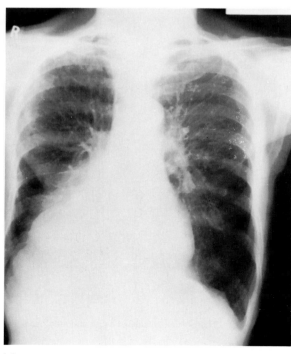

(a)

N.B. Respiratory signs
are posterior

Movement ↓
Percussion ↓
Breath sounds ↓
Bronchial breathing only
if patent bronchus

Apex beat may be
deviated to R

(b)

Fig. 4.29 Collapse right lower lobe (a) chest x-ray; (b) signs.

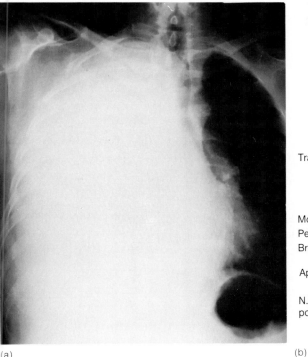

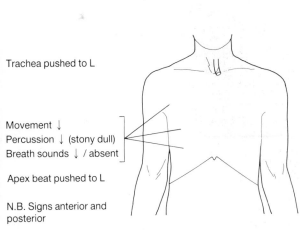

Trachea pushed to L

Movement ↓
Percussion ↓ (stony dull)
Breath sounds ↓ / absent

Apex beat pushed to L

N.B. Signs anterior and
posterior

(a)   (b)

Fig. 4.30 Massive right pleural effusion (a) chest x-ray; (b) signs.

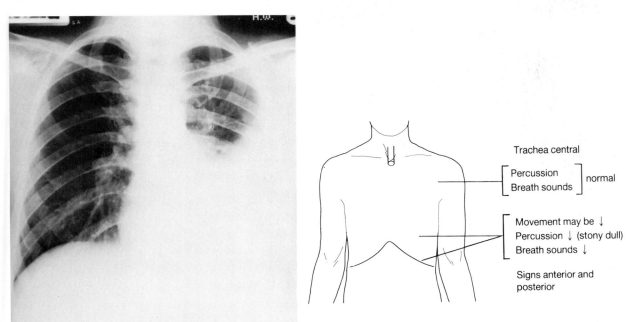

Trachea central

Percussion
Breath sounds   normal

Movement may be ↓
Percussion ↓ (stony dull)
Breath sounds ↓

Signs anterior and
posterior

(a)   (b)

Fig. 4.31 Moderate left pleural effusion (a) chest x-ray; (b) signs.

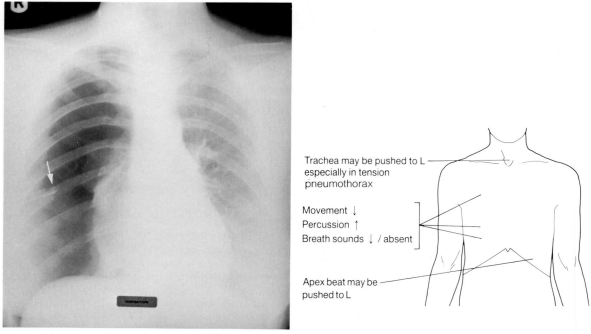

(a)   (b)

Fig. 4.32 Large right pneumothorax (note blocked drainage tube) (a) chest x-ray; (b) signs.

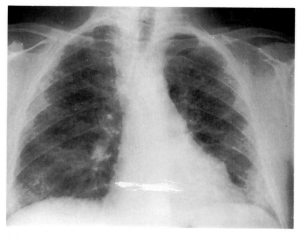

(a)   (b)

Fig. 4.33 Fibrosing alveolitis (a) chest x-ray; (b) signs.

References and further reading

Brewis RAL, Gibson GJ, Geddes DM. *Respiratory Medicine*.
   London. Bailliere Tindall, 1990.
Forgacs P. *Lung sounds*. London: Bailliere Tindall, 1979.

5

The mouth

P. J. Toghill

Symptoms
Physical signs
References and further reading

Patients open their mouths and stick out their tongues for inspection as an expected and essential part of physical examination. Obviously much useful information can be gleaned from this manoeuvre but the state of the tongue cannot be used as an index of health in the way that many patients naïvely believe.

Examination of the mouth allows the doctor to:

- assess the degree of hydration from the state of the tongue and mucous membranes
- look at specific lesions that are drawn to attention such as ulcers, sore patches and lumps
- search for local and additional clues that may help in the diagnosis of systemic diseases. The finding of Koplik's spots in a child in the prodromal stage of measles is a good example of this

Symptoms

Certain symptoms are related to the mouth but must not be taken in isolation; frequently they are features of generalized disease.

Thirst and dryness of the mouth

These apparently simple symptoms may need clarification. Many patients describe themselves as being thirsty when they really mean that their mouths are dry. This may be because they have defective salivary secretion because they have been taking certain drugs or because they have had local radiotherapy. Some of the commoner causes of dryness of the mouth (xerostomia) are shown in Table 5.1.

Table 5.1. Causes of dryness of the mouth

Emotion
Drugs (e.g. atropine, tricyclics, inhalers, antidepressives)
Mouth breathing
Local radiotherapy
Diseases of the salivary glands (e.g. Sjögren's disease)
Old age
Dehydration

When thirst is the primary symptom patients need to be questioned about other symptoms such as polyuria — which would occur with hypercalcaemia and diabetes mellitus and insipidus — and nocturia which might be the first evidence of chronic renal failure. Whereas thirst is a prominent symptom of dehydration in the young and middle-aged it may be less evident in the elderly or the confused. Do not forget to enquire about diuretics as a possible cause. Excessive thirst may also be a symptom of psychiatric disease as in compulsive water drinking.

Soreness of the tongue and mucous membranes

A wide variety of haematological and systemic diseases including severe iron-deficiency anaemia, pernicious anaemia and mucositis due to chemotherapy may cause soreness of the tongue and mouth. The physical changes are discussed later. Soreness of the tongue is not infrequently a symptom for which no organic cause can be found. However, in recent years attention has been drawn to a condition in which there is generalized soreness of the mouth which has been termed the 'burning mouth syndrome'. This was thought to be related to psychological factors but it is known that many aetiological components including monilia, allergies, poor salivary secretion and diabetes mellitus may all play a part.

Bad taste and foul breath

A disagreeable odour to the breath is often a feature of infections of the mouth, such as gingivitis, or of the respiratory tract, such as bronchiectasis. These may, but not necessarily, be complained of by the patient but are usually more evident to his or her companions. Many normal people have bad breath for which no cause is found and conversely many others complain of their own bad breath that cannot be smelt by those nearby. A bad taste in the mouth may be caused by diseases such as uraemia, and drugs, such as metronidazole. Many patients complain of a bad taste for which no cause can be found. With advancing years the ability to appreciate saltiness and bitterness declines though the ability to detect sweetness and sourness persists. Dental prostheses also impair the sensation of taste. Loss of taste may complicate serious illnesses and may be a toxic effect of drugs such as penicillamine.

Physical signs

When you examine the mouth remember you need:

- a good light
- a spatula to depress the tongue and retract the cheeks
- a pair of gloves to palpate lesions bimanually

The lips

Painful fissuring with scaling and crust formation (cheilitis) is a common feature of physical damage to the lips by sunlight, cold or wind and those enjoying unusual exposure to the elements, such as skiers, may suffer nasty temporary attacks. Cracks at the corners of the lips (angular stomatitis or cheilosis) are common. They may be due to anaemia and malabsorption states but they are more usually caused by overlapping of the lips in edentulous patients or those with ill-fitting dentures. The infolded skin becomes sodden and macerated and sometimes harbours secondary monilial infection (Fig. 5.1).

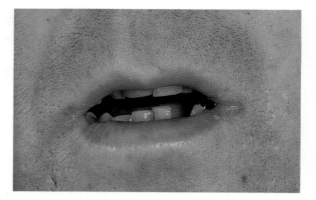

Fig. 5.1 Angular stomatitis or cheilosis. The cracks at the angles of the mouth may become infected with monilia.

The commonest infection to affect the lips is herpes simplex which results in clusters of vesicles on the lips and surrounding skin. Crops of herpes simplex may erupt in healthy but vulnerable individuals but they are often precipitated by exposure to the sun or coincidental febrile states such as the common cold or pneumonia (Fig. 5.2).

Localized chronic ulceration of the lips may be due to a carcinoma which may appear as a thickened plaque or warty growth. The lower lip is a common site for carcinoma particularly in men (Fig. 5.3). Pipe-smoking and exposure to sunlight are common associated factors. Do not forget to examine the patient for possibly enlarged submental nodes. Primary syphilitic chancres may be seen on the lip where they appear as button-like nodules which crust and ulcerate. If you have any suspicions about the nature of any lip lesion make sure that you put on

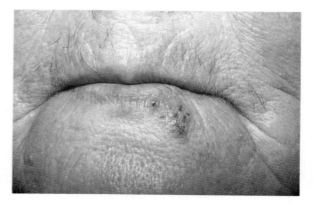

Fig. 5.2 Herpes labialis. The lesions are preceded by a tingling and burning sensation. They then blister and later become crusted; the whole cycle lasts a few days.

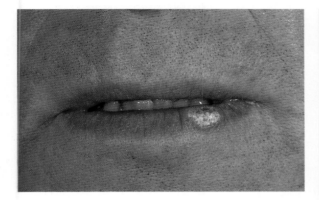

Fig. 5.3 Carcinoma of lip.

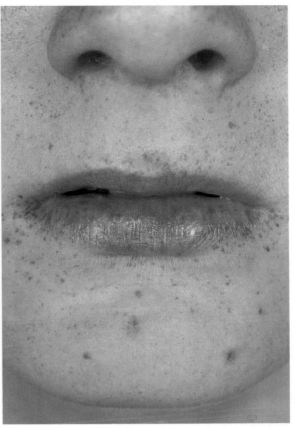

Fig. 5.5 Peutz−Jeghers syndrome.

gloves before examining the patient. Chancres are highly contagious.

Of particular interest to the gastroenterologist are the lesions of hereditary haemorrhagic telangiectasia. These appear as bluish spots on the lips, tongue, buccal and nasal mucosa (Fig. 5.4). Similar lesions are found in the upper gastrointestinal tract as far as the stomach while bluish lesions are seen in the anterior nares and on the finger ends. The great importance of these lesions is that they bleed intermittently and produce a chronic iron-deficiency anaemia. The lesions may not be immediately obvious and need to be sought for carefully in any patient with an unexplained and intractable iron-deficiency anaemia.

Also of interest to the gastroenterologist, but much rarer, are the lesions of the Peutz−Jeghers syndrome. These often appear as brownish flecks of pigmentation at the mucocutaneous junction of the lips or around the mouth (Fig. 5.5). Their importance is the association with small intestinal polyps that may cause intestinal obstruction or intussusception.

The gums and teeth

Although the teeth and gums (gingivae) are the province of the dental surgeon there are many signs that are relevant to the general health of the patient.

The earliest features of gingivitis, often the result of irritative calculus formation, are swelling and redness of the margins of the gums which bleed easily. Gingivitis may progress to periodontitis which is inflammation of the deeper tissues round the teeth and is a very common cause of teeth loss in adults.

Swelling of the gums (Table 5.2) occurs physiologically in puberty and pregnancy but also develops with long-term anticonvulsant therapy with phenytoin. Gross hypertrophy, infection, bleeding and necrosis of the gums is a feature of acute leukaemia, particularly of the acute monoblastic variety (Fig.

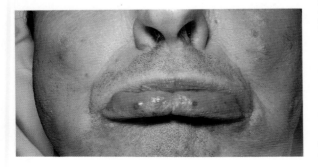

Fig. 5.4 Hereditary haemorrhagic telangiectasia (Osler−Weber−Rendu syndrome). The mucosal lesions on the everted lower lip are characteristic.

Table 5.2. Swelling of gums
Puberty
Pregnancy
Drugs
Phenytoin
Nifedipine
Cyclosporin
Gingivitis*
Acute leukaemia*
Scurvy*

* Associated with bleeding and infection

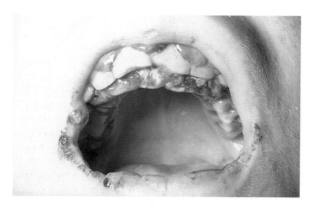

Fig. 5.6 The gums in acute monoblastic leukaemia.

5.6). Bleeding gums due to vitamin C deficiency (scurvy) are rarely seen now in the Western world except in those living on bizarre diets limited in fresh fruits and vegetables.

Acute necrotizing ulcerative gingivitis is a painful infection characterized by sloughly ulceration at the gum margins and halitosis.

A brownish pigmentation due to melanin is frequently seen on the gums of negroes and other dark-skinned individuals. It is unusual but may occur in healthy light-skinned people; it may also be seen in Addison's disease in which the more characteristic buccal pigmentation is located opposite the upper molar teeth. Melanotic gum pigmentation must be distinguished from the extremely rare line 1 mm from the gum margin that is seen in lead or bismuth poisoning.

For the physician the state of the teeth often gives a good indication of his patient's general state of oral hygiene. Nevertheless with advancing years irreversible changes take place which are beyond the control of the patient. Recession of the gum margins

exposes the necks of the teeth hence the expression 'long in the tooth'. In elderly people the teeth are worn down by chewing and the consequent flattening of the biting surfaces is referred to as attrition. These changes are accompanied by exposure of the underlying dentine by the wearing away of the enamel.

Certain changes in the teeth are of interest to the physician. The domed, notched and widely spaced teeth of congenital syphilis (Hutchinson's teeth) are now rarely seen in the Western world. Enlargement of the mandible with underbite and increasing spacing of the lower teeth may be seen in acromegaly (Fig. 5.7). Tetracyclines are deposited in growing bone and may stain the teeth and cause dental hypoplasia when given to young children or pregnant women. Chronic ingestion of fluorides in moderate amounts causes mottling of dental enamel (fluorosis).

The tongue

As mentioned earlier, the appearance of the tongue does not necessarily reflect the well-being of the patient. A dirty, coated tongue may be compatible with good health and conversely a clean, moist tongue may be retained in spite of advancing disease. There are wide variations in the appearance of the normal tongue.

Irregular painless clefts may develop, sometimes with advancing age giving rise to what has been termed a 'scrotal tongue'. Such changes have no significance. Other normal tongues have scattered irregular red areas, denuded of papillae, producing a map-like appearance on the dorsum. These areas may change from time to time but the cause of this so-called geographical tongue is not known (Fig. 5.8)

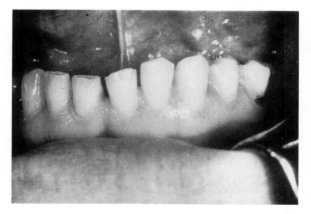

Fig. 5.7 Widening of the teeth in the lower jaw in a patient with acromegaly.

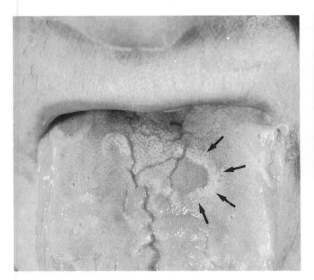

Fig. 5.8 The geographical tongue. The arrows surround an area of epithelium denuded of papillae.

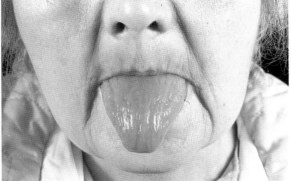

Fig. 5.9 The raw, red tongue. This patient had a chronic iron-deficiency anaemia of 7.0 g/dl.

and it should be regarded as a normal variant. Another normal variant is the black, hairy tongue caused by elongation of the filiform papillae on the dorsum. It may, but not necessarily, follow antibiotic therapy. Many elderly patients have varicosities on the undersurface of the tongue; these have given rise to the picturesque concept of the 'caviar tongue'. Some people have an ovoid bare area in the mid-line of the posterior third of the tongue; this should be regarded as a congenital abnormality and it has been termed median rhomboid glossitis.

The condition of the tongue and the turgor of the skin reflect the degree of hydration of an ill patient. In severe diabetic ketoacidosis, for example, the tongue may feel as dry as a bone. But not all dry tongues indicate dehydration, and mouth breathing, absence of salivary secretions and drugs may convey false impressions (Table 5.1). A dirty, dry tongue is a common feature of acute febrile illnesses particularly of gastrointestinal origin.

Whilst a coated tongue may be normal, a smooth, red, depapillated tongue is certainly not. Such a raw, red tongue (Fig. 5.9) should suggest possible deficiency syndromes like iron-deficiency anaemia, pernicious anaemia, malabsorption and pellagra. Similar changes of the tongue and mouth follow the mucositis of radiotherapy or chemotherapy. Tongue changes of this type, though conspicuous and striking, have no other specific or diagnostic features.

White patches on the tongue are important.

Leukoplakia is a premalignant condition characterized by white streaks and patches with sharply defined edges, like streaks of white paint (Fig. 5.10). The creamy white, curdy patches of moniliasis (thrush) are usually easily recognized and are frequently seen in sick babies, immunosuppressed individuals, debilitated elderly patients and people on antibiotic therapy (Fig. 5.11). The appearance of thrush in an apparently well young man should raise suspicions of the AIDS-related complex (see Chapter 21). Moniliasis may even flourish on dentures which may have to be cleaned as part of the patient's therapy. Chronic irritation of the tongue as with a broken tooth may produce white hyperkeratotic patches that are termed pachyderma oralis. They quickly heal when the irritant is removed.

Ulceration of the tongue (Table 5.3) may be a feature of most of the ulcerative conditions affecting the mouth (see later). Of the chronic ulcers, carcinoma of the tongue is the most important. It is commonly sited along the edges or base of the tongue where it is less readily detected. Most carcinomas of the tongue

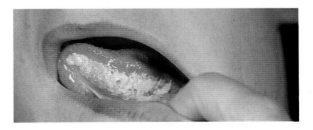

Fig. 5.10 Leukoplakia of the under surface of the tongue.

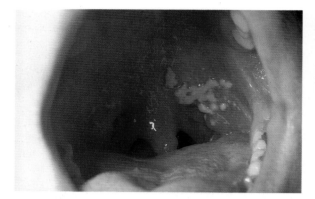

Fig. 5.11 Moniliasis of the mouth. The lesions are mainly on the soft palate but extend to the dorsum of the tongue. This patient had been receiving chemotherapy for non-Hodgkin's lymphoma.

Table 5.4. Causes of macroglossia

Children	Congenital hypothyroidism (cretinism)
	Haemangiomata
	Lymphangiomata
Adults	Myxoedema
	Acromegaly
	Amyloidosis
	Massive infiltration with tumours

Table 5.3. Ulcers of tongue

Acute	Aphthous
	Herpetic
	As a feature of stomatitis (see Table 5.5)
Subacute and chronic	Irritative (usually from teeth)
	Tuberculosis
	Chancre
	Carcinoma
	Non-Hodgkin's lymphoma

present the characteristic features of a malignant ulcer with indurated everted edges and a sloughy ulcerated base. Carcinoma of the tongue initially metastases to the submental nodes and then to the cervical nodes. It is important to look for leukoplakia which may be associated with the cancer. Lymphomatous ulcers of the tongue are rare, being usually high-grade non-Hodgkin's lymphomas that develop as bulky tumour masses which quickly ulcerate.

Tuberculous ulcers of the tongue are rarely seen in the Western world but small lesions may be associated with gross submental and cervical lymphadenopathy.

Patients rarely complain themselves of an unduly large tongue but macroglossia may be noted as part of the routine examination of the patient and may suggest or confirm a diagnosis of systemic disease. Some of the causes of macroglossia are listed in Table 5.4.

Stomatitis

This very generalized term covers a wide variety of conditions in which there may be ulceration, infection, necrosis and desquamation of the mucous membranes. It may range from the trivial, though uncomfortable, idiopathic aphthous ulceration to the potentially fatal cancrum oris. As with the wide range of severity there is a similarly wide range of causes including infections, drugs and haematological malignancies. A list of some of the more important causes of stomatitis is shown in Table 5.5. Some of these deserve special mention.

In children and young adults infective causes of stomatitis predominate. Glandular fever (infectious

Table 5.5. Stomatitis

Infective	Acute herpetic gingivostomatitis
	Glandular fever
	Vincent's infection
	Herpangina
	Hand, foot and mouth disease
	Monilia
Uncertain aetiology	Stevens–Johnson syndrome
	Behçet's syndrome
	Aphthous ulceration
Toxic agents	Radiotherapy
	Chemotherapy
Haematological conditions	Acute leukaemia
	Agranulocytosis
	Aplastic anaemia
	Scurvy
Drugs	Gold
	Methotrexate
	Etoposide
Generalized debility	Carcinoma
	Lymphoma
Immunosuppression	AIDS
Skin diseases (see Chapter 13)	Pemphigus/pemphigoid
	Lichen planus

mononucleosis) may produce a nasty ulcerated throat with a sloughy grey tonsillar exudate, tonsillar enlargement and palatal petechiae. Although palatal petechiae are frequent at the end of the first week of the illness they are by no means pathognomonic of the disease as has been suggested in the past. The oral features of the disease are usually associated with generalized lymphadenopathy.

Herpes simplex may also be responsible for stomatitis in both healthy and immunosuppressed patients.

Diphtheria due to *Corynebacterium diphtheriae* is now uncommon in the Western world but is common in undeveloped countries. Recently there has been a resurgence of the disease in Russia. The symptoms depend on the site of primary infection but often the

disease affects the pharynx, larynx, nose and tonsils. When established there is a thick, grey membrane which may be firmly attached to underlying tissues so that removal results in bleeding. With severe disease there is much oedema and lymphadenopathy giving a 'bull-neck' appearance.

Aphthous ulceration is one of the commonest, if relatively minor, causes of oral ulceration. These ulcers mainly affect women and often appear in crops in relation to menstruation. Each ulcer starts as a tender whitish-grey nodule, a few mm in diameter, which quickly ulcerates and then heals in a few days. The ulcers may appear anywhere on the buccal mucosa on tongue and may be so extensive as to interfere with eating and drinking. In a few patients

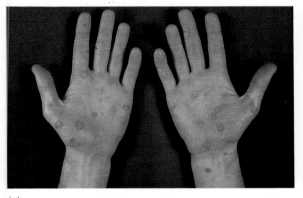

(a)

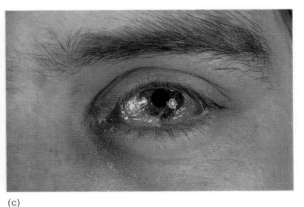

(c)

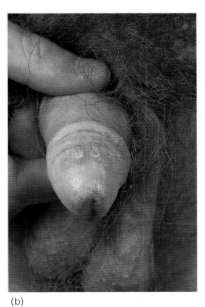

(b)

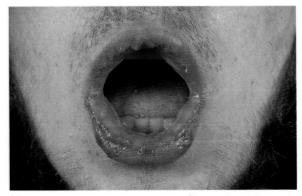

(d)

Fig. 5.12 A patient with Stevens–Johnson syndrome: (a) target lesions of the hands; (b) genital lesions; (c) severe conjunctivitis; (d) stomatitis.

they may be associated with coeliac disease in which case the institution of a gluten-free diet sometimes results in a gratifying reduction in the ulceration.

A rarer but serious form of stomatitis is seen in the Stevens–Johnson syndrome. This is a disorder of uncertain aetiology, sometimes related to drugs, in which stomatitis is associated with skin, genital and ocular lesions. The skin lesions are those of erythema multiforme and are mainly on the extremities of the upper limbs. As the term erythema multiforme suggests, these lesions may be macular, papular, blistering or purpuric but most typically of 'target' form. Sometimes the eye lesions may result in iritis, uveitis and panophthalmitis (Fig. 5.12) (a–d)). Recurrent eye and oral ulceration characterizes another rare disease, Behçet's syndrome, a curious disorder seen mainly in the Middle East and Japan. In this disorder other manifestations include arthritis, skin lesions, neurological and vascular lesions.

In hospitals in the Western world one of the commonest causes of stomatitis is chemotherapy for haematological and other malignancies. Multiple factors may be responsible including dryness of the mouth following radiotherapy, leucopenia, opportunistic infections and the direct effects of some chemotherapeutic agents. Of these methotrexate and etoposide seem to have a particular predilection towards oral toxicity and mucositis.

The most extreme form of oral ulceration is in cancrum oris where there is complete necrosis around the mouth. This may be seen in debilitated children with systemic diseases such as measles in undeveloped countries.

Oral fetor

Much can be learned from the breath of the ill patient. Nasal, oral, dental and respiratory infections may be identified by the foul breath (Table 5.6). Let us remember Sir William Osler's comments 'Learn to see, learn to hear, learn to feel, learn to smell and to

Table 5.6. Causes of foul breath

Local	Infections of mouth, gums, teeth and sinuses
	Tonsillitis (particularly tonsillolithiasis)
Respiratory tract	Bronchiectasis
	Lung abscess
Systemic	Hepatic fetor
	Uraemic fetor
	Altered blood in stomach
	Appendicitis

know that by practice alone you can become expert'; the sense of smell is rarely used in clinical diagnosis but it has good discriminatory powers. The stench of an anaerobic infection of a lung abscess is characteristic as is that of a Vincent's infection. The breath in hepatic coma often has a sweet, sickly aroma and some claim that the breath in uraemia has a fishy, uriniferous smell. It is important for the physician to recognize the smell of ketosis and this may be a skill which some students and doctors find difficult to acquire. Certainly the recognition of the sweet, sickly smell of ketones in the breath of a patient with diabetic coma may give early warning of the severity of the metabolic crisis.

References and further reading

Beaven DW, Brooks SE. *A colour atlas of the tongue in clinical diagnosis.* London: Wolfe, 1988.
Buxton PK. *ABC of dermatology.* London: British Medical Association, 1988.
Lamey PJ, Lamb AB. Prospective study of the aetiological factors in the burning mouth syndrome. *British Medical Journal.* 1988; **296**: 1243–6.
Tyldesly WR. *Oral medicine.* London: Wolfe, 1988.

6

The abdomen

P. J. Toghill

Symptoms
Examination
Further reading

In this section we are going to deal with those problems primarily referable to the gastrointestinal tract.

Symptoms

Many of the terms that patients use to describe digestive disorders are vague and imprecise. The patients know what these terms mean and assume we, as doctors, do too! Let us take as an example the symptom of heart-burn. Some patients use this term to describe the reflux of acid fluid into the mouth; others use it to describe retrosternal burning after food. Similar confusion may exist with indigestion. Does this mean abdominal pain, fullness after meals or nausea? We have to ask to find out.

Other patients may attribute their symptoms to 'stomach upsets' but yet have serious disease elsewhere. The retired clergyman with nausea and vomiting may have uraemia due to his enlarged prostate whereas the lady at the supermarket check-out desk may have similar problems because of hypercalcaemia due to myelomatosis. Gastrointestinal symptoms are not necessarily due to disease of the alimentary tract.

Let us consider some of these gastrointestinal symptoms in more detail.

Pain

Here a few minutes of careful history-taking may yield more dividends than hours of expensive investigation. Of course, sudden catastrophic pain, usually the province of the surgeon, demands immediate attention. Intense, constant, generalized abdominal pain of quick onset often implies perforation of a peptic ulcer, acute pancreatitis, or a ruptured aortic aneurysm. Do not forget that the pain of myocardial infarction may be felt in the epigastrium. Waxing and waning pain felt diffusely over the abdomen suggests gut colic, as with intestinal obstruction. If acute colicky pain is associated with diarrhoea and vomiting it is likely to be due to an enteric infection such as *Salmonella*. When the colicky pains start in one or other flanks and radiate to the lower abdomen or genitalia, ureteric colic must be considered. Severe, upper abdominal, colicky pain radiating to the right upper quadrant and through to the back at the angle of the right scapula suggests biliary colic and gall-bladder disease. Acute, central abdominal pains shifting after a few hours to the right iliac fossa are likely to be due to appendicitis. Sometimes metabolic diseases such as porphyria and diabetic ketoacidosis may present with severe abdominal pain.

Some chronic pains have helpful diagnostic features. Patients with peptic ulcer disease, particularly duodenal ulceration, may have bouts of pain lasting for a few days at a time with complete remissions for weeks or months. This relapsing/remitting pattern may extend over many years and may be accepted by the patient as a normal feature of life. The pain in peptic ulceration is usually epigastric but may radiate through to the back; not infrequently the patient is unable to define its site of origin. Worsening of pain before meals, nocturnal waking and relief with food may characterize duodenal ulceration. Colicky abdominal pains associated with disturbances of bowel habit and abdominal distension point to obstructive lesions of the gut such as colonic cancer of Crohn's disease. Concurrent weight loss, anaemia and anorexia with abdominal pain should always alert to you to the possibility of underlying malignancy.

Remember that residents and visitors returning from tropical areas may have other causes of abdominal pain that do not necessarily spring to mind when those patients are seen in a Western setting. Sickle-cell crises, splenic infarcts and amoebic liver abscess must be considered (see Chapter 19).

Nausea and vomiting

These common symptoms may be difficult to evaluate. Nausea as an isolated symptom, without vomiting, is much more likely to be due to depression or neurosis than primary gastrointestinal disease. Just 'feeling sick' is often an expression of non-specific ill-health. When the nausea is associated with vomiting, careful enquiry must be made about associated symptoms such as weight loss and abdominal pain which may lead on to the diagnosis of peptic ulceration or carcinoma. The vomiting of gastric outlet obstruction is profuse and the vomit may contain undigested food taken many hours previously. Substernal burning or 'heart-burn' after meals characterizes gastro-oesophageal reflux; this may be aggravated on lying down or bending over doing tasks such as gardening or brick-laying. The hot burning fluid may regurgitate into the mouth but is rarely actually vomited. Fresh or altered blood in vomit (haematemesis) is usually a serious symptom indicative of ulcerative lesions of the upper gastrointestinal tract as far as the second part of the duodenum. However, severe retching, as with an alcoholic binge, may tear the mucosa at the gastro-oesophageal junction to cause fresh bleeding; this is known as the Mallory–Weiss syndrome.

Do not forget that recurrent, periodic, and sometimes profuse, vomiting is a feature of migraine in children and young adults; so it is essential to enquire about associated headaches with the bouts of vomiting. The effortless and unexpected vomiting of raised intracranial pressure is relatively uncommon and is usually accompanied by other more prominent features of the primary disease. Other non-gastrointestinal causes of nausea and vomiting include uraemia, hypercalcaemia and digoxin toxicity. Remember the possibility of pregnancy as a cause of vomiting in women in the reproductive years.

Problems with swallowing

Common problems are those of 'food sticking' and pain on swallowing. The term dysphagia is often used by doctors to cover both symptoms but it is better to restrict it to the former. The complaint of food sticking in the throat or gullet must always be taken seriously, particularly when it is of recent onset and of increasing severity. In the second half of life it is often caused by a carcinoma of the pharynx, oesophagus or gastro-oesophageal junction; sometimes an adjacent invading tumour such as a bronchial carcinoma may also announce its presence by dysphagia. Chronic and/or intermittent dysphagia may be due to benign oesophageal stricture or achalasia of the cardia. Most patients with swallowing problems have more difficulty with solids than liquids but sometimes with achalasia the reverse is true. Often patients point to the site of apparent obstruction but this does not always relate accurately to the subsequently demonstrated anatomical site.

Discomfort or pain on swallowing is usually due to oesophagitis and it is always important to ask about associated gastro-oesophageal reflex or heart-burn (see later). A not uncommon problem, encountered often in young women of nervous disposition, is an apparent need to swallow frequently to overcome what seems to be an obstruction in the upper gullet. When, as is usually the case, nothing is found to account for this, it is termed globus hystericus.

Choking on swallowing is another serious symptom implying a neurological lesion affecting the larynx or pharynx or a fistula between the upper gastrointestinal tract and the bronchi or lungs.

Bowels

The extent to which people inspect their motions or complain about their bowels varies greatly amongst both individuals and cultures. Nevertheless, any changes in bowel habit must be critically assessed bearing in mind patients' limitations in language, vocabulary and background (see Chapter 1). For some patients to defecate 2–3 times each day may be normal whereas in others just two or three bowel actions per week is compatible with normal health. Remember to ask about medication which may cause altered bowel habit.

The passage of blood and mucus must always be taken seriously except in the context of what is obviously an acute, infective diarrhoea. Fresh red blood passed with the stools which spatters the lavatory pan and is present on the toilet paper is likely to be due to bleeding piles. However, this diagnosis must only be made after careful examination including sigmoidoscopy. Blood and mucus usually points to chronic inflammatory bowel disease, diverticulitis, polyps or cancers of the colon or rectum. Blood and mucus with diarrhoea and a sensation of incomplete emptying of the rectum is almost pathognomonic of a rectal tumour. Ask your patient about the consistency of the diarrhoea. Is it watery and very frequent as in colitis? Are the motions porridgy, bulky, pale and offensive as with steatorrhoea? Is nocturnal diarrhoea a problem? Diarrhoea that wakes a patient from sleep is nearly always of an organic basis whereas a flurry of two or three bowel actions on rising in the morning is often of nervous origin. Many textbooks write of alternating constipation and diarrhoea as being a symptom of colonic cancer; this is rarely so in practice. Long, thin stools are also rarely of significance. Some patients may not necessarily equate the black, tarry motion of melaena with blood loss and you need to ask about this carefully. Diabetics often have disturbances of bowel function but, of course, they are not immune to other gut disorders such as bowel cancer.

Find out about recent travel in patients from abroad but bear in mind that parasites or infections in the gut may not necessarily be the cause of your patient's symptoms (see Chapter 19). Tropical gut infections such as amoebiasis and strongyloidiasis together with other sexually transmitted diseases such as gonorrhoea and syphilis may form part of the 'gay-bowel' syndrome in male homosexuals (see Chapter 20). If in doubt you must ask (tactfully) about sexual activity and proclivities.

Wind

This is a common dyspeptic symptom not often of great significance. You need to know what your patient really means by it. Mostly flatulence means bringing wind up (belching) and flatus means passing wind down below (farting) but many patients and their doctors are not always clear what they mean by these terms. Excessive belching usually means that the patient is an air-swallower. Excessive flatus may be due to alactasia but it is rarely a symptom of complaint from those working alone in the open who can with ease and without embarrassment relieve themselves! Borborygmi is a lovely onomatopoeic word that doctors often use to describe the gurgling and rumbling abdominal noises that arise from peristalting bowel and which may be heard to excess in patients with obstructive gut lesions.

Heart-burn

Mention has already been made of this term which is widely used. Many people correctly recognize the sensation of acid secretions regurgitating into the gullet. Some describe it as waterbrash. Nevertheless, it is dangerous to assume that the discomfort that the patient describes is, in fact, due to gastro-oesophageal reflux. Question your patient carefully and make sure you do not fail to diagnose angina.

Examination

Abdomens, like their owners, come in all shapes and sizes. In the slim, thin or wasted the anterior wall is often scaphoid whereas in the grossly obese an apron of fat may hang down over the pubic region. With such gross variation from one patient to another it is difficult, and indeed nonsensical, to divide the abdomen into nine separate regions as has been medical tradition. For descriptive purposes most clinicians refer to quadrants of the abdomen (Fig. 6.1) or describe pains or masses as being in the epigastric or suprapubic regions or in right or left iliac fossae.

Short, squat patients tend to have wide subcostal arches whereas tall, thin patients have narrow subcostal margins. With advancing age, shortening of the spine and progressive dorsal kyphosis contracts the area of the abdominal wall available for examination. With this trunk shortening the ribs ride on the iliac crest or funnel into the false pelvis, whilst the skin of the abdominal wall creases into a transverse fold (Fig. 6.2 (a)(b)).

Position of patient

Attention to simple points is essential. Physical signs are easily missed with the patient in a bad position, often hunched up with too many pillows. This reduces the size of the area available to palpation (the abdominal window) and may tuck enlarged livers and spleens out of reach under the costal margin. The patient must be:

- warm, comfortable and relaxed
- supine, with one pillow only and arms by the side
- lying in good light with abdomen exposed from xiphoid to pubis

The examiner must:

- put the patient at ease
- have warm hands
- enquire about sites of pain or tenderness

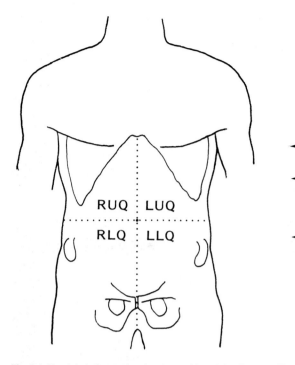

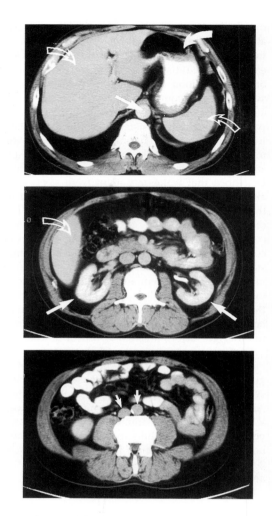

Fig. 6.1 Normal abdomen showing the position of the viscera at T11, L2 and L5 on CT scan. CT scans are viewed as though one is looking up from the feet of the patient.
The upper cut at T11 shows the position of liver and spleen (open curved arrows), the aorta (solid white arrow) embraced by the crura of the diaphragm and the stomach filled with contrast (solid curved arrow).
At L2 the straight arrows indicate the kidneys and the open curved arrow indicates the lower limit of the right lobe of the liver.
At L5 arrows indicate the aorta (circular) and the inferior vena cava (oval) in front of the lumbar vertebra.

- monitor the progress of the examination by the patient's facial responses. This means and ensures that you don't hurt him!

Inspection of the abdomen

An initial glance takes in the general contours, scars and abnormal masses. Tangential views from a sitting position may show up visible peristalsis and abnormal pulsations.

A fine leash of blue venules is commonly seen over both costal margins in thin elderly patients. Distended veins over the lower abdomen with leg oedema may indicate inferior vena caval obstruction. These dilated veins run upwards from the femoral region (Fig. 6.3). Very rarely veins may be seen radiating out from the umbilicus to form the so-called caput Medusae. This unusual physical sign

occurs with portal hypertension when anastomoses develop between the portal and systemic circulations along the round ligament of the umbilicus.

Silver striae or stretch marks over the lower abdomen are often seen in women who have borne children. However, any rapid weight gain, as in pubescent girls, may produce red or purple striae which subsequently fade to a silver-grey colour. They are also seen in patients on high-dosage steroid therapy and in Cushing's syndrome (Fig. 6.4).

Scars and associated incisional herniae must be noted. Keloid change in a scar is extension of the fibrous tissue beyond the extent of the original incision. Some patients, particularly Negroes, are particularly prone to develop keloid scars.

A careful search must be made in each groin for herniae or enlarged lymph nodes. Sweaty, obese patients with poor hygiene may have intertrigo

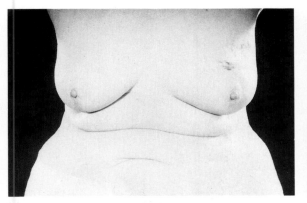

(a)

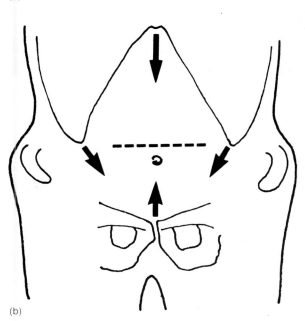

(b)

Fig. 6.2 (a) Reduction of the 'abdominal window' with shortening of the trunk due to osteoporotic collapse. Note the transverse skin fold. (b) Shortening of the trunk and funnelling of ribs into pelvis.

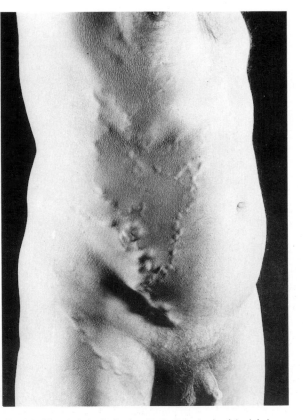

Fig. 6.3 Dilated abdominal veins due to thrombosis of the inferior vena cava in polycythaemia rubra vera.

affecting the groins. The skin in the groins and often the natal cleft, becomes red, macerated and weepy and may become secondarily infected with monilia.

Careful inspection of the umbilicus yields dividends. It is frequently the site of a hernia, this being a true umbilical hernia in babies and a paraumbilical hernia in obese adults. A horny, sebaceous plug is often seen in the elderly, particularly those unable (or reluctant) to immerse themselves in soap and water. Gross abdominal distension may result in transverse stretching, 'the grinning umbilicus', or herniation.

Pigmentation around the umbilicus due to altered blood may be seen with intraperitoneal haemorrhage or, more rarely, with carcinoma of the pancreas or acute pancreatitis (Cullen's sign) (Fig. 6.5). Another unusual sign in acute haemorrhagic pancreatitis is bruising in the flanks (Grey–Turner's sign).

The interpretation of visible peristalsis often gives rise to difficulties. In thin elderly subjects peristalsis is often normally visible. Visible peristalsis in the upper abdomen from left to right is seen with gastric outlet obstruction as with a stenosing duodenal ulcer or a pyloric carcinoma. Here the stomach is distended with fluid and may give rise to a succussion splash when the patient is rocked from side to side. Whereas the visible peristalsis of pyloric stenosis is not difficult to identify, the ladder pattern of small intestinal peristalsis may be perplexing. Large gut peristalsis is described as extending from right to left but this is only so when the peristalsis is seen extending along the transverse colon.

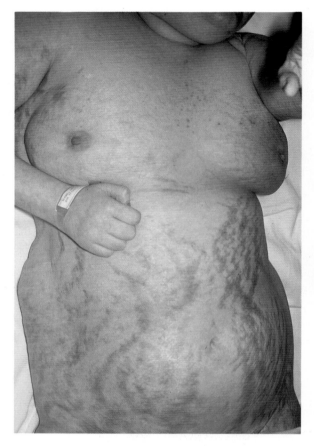

Fig. 6.4 Gross abdominal striae in a patient with Cushing's syndrome.

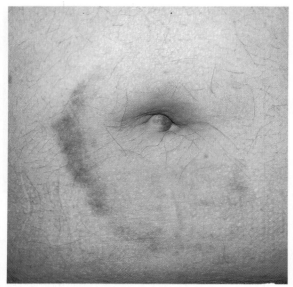

Fig. 6.5 Periumbilical bruising in acute pancreatitis (Cullen's sign).

Palpation

For the examination of the abdomen palpation usually follows inspection with, later, percussion and auscultation to clarify, bolster or confirm those signs detected earlier.

Palpation of the abdomen is performed predominantly using the right hand with the examiner on the right side of the patient. Avoid digging into the patient's abdomen with the fingertips and palpate with the pads of the fingertips with the forearm and hand horizontal. This may mean raising the bed if it is low; alternatively do not hesitate to kneel down alongside the patient's bed to palpate. Ask the patient about painful areas and then begin palpation well away from the sites of tenderness or pain. Start by feeling all over the abdomen, preferably talking to the patient to gain his or her confidence.

Several structures may be normally palpable in the slim abdomen (Fig. 6.6). In particular a descending colon full of hard faeces may be palpable in the constipated patient and a tender, gurgly caecum may be felt in the right iliac fossa, particularly in women. Curiously, the caecum is usually larger in women than in men. The pulsation of the abdominal aorta is often much in evidence and should be regarded as normal unless there is associated lateral, expansile pulsation. The sacral promontory can be felt in women with a marked lumbar lordosis. Care should be taken not to misinterpret a lumbar lordosis and scoliosis as a sinister retroperitoneal tumour.

Auscultation

Auscultation of the abdomen is particularly useful in acute surgical emergencies where the silent belly indicates ileus due to perforation, and/or peritonitis. Bowel sounds are heard normally every few seconds with prolonged gurgles or borborygmi less frequently. These may be excessively loud in intestinal obstruction.

Most arteriopathic patients will have bruits in the abdomen but it is impossible to localize them accurately clinically. This does not mean that the clinician should ignore vascular bruits, rather that he

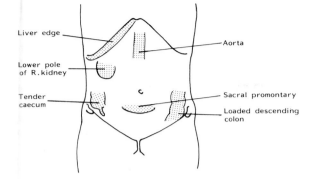

Fig. 6.6 Structures often palpable in the normal abdomen.

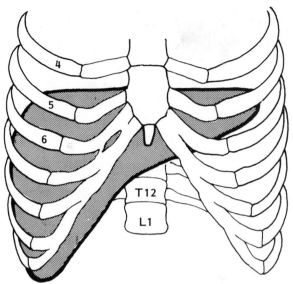

Fig. 6.7 Surface markings of the liver.

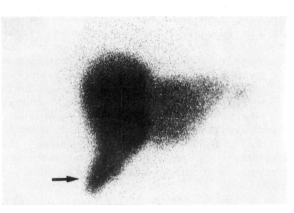

Fig. 6.8 ^{99m}Tc scan of liver showing Riedel's lobe.

should be cautious in ascribing them to a particular vessel.

Rarely venous hums may be audible over patent, dilated umbilical veins in patients with cirrhosis and portal hypertension. The names of Cruveilhier and Baumgarten have been attached to this syndrome. Their names are well remembered by students but the syndrome is extremely rare!

The liver

Before starting to examine the liver it is important to visualize its position in the body (Fig. 6.7). Its upper border usually extends to 1 cm above the upper border of the right fifth rib in the mid-clavicular line but this surface marking is greatly dependent on body shape and on underlying lung conditions. For instance, with hyperinflated lungs as in emphysema, the upper border of the liver may be two rib spaces lower. The left lobe of the liver extends to just outside the left mid-clavicular line and the oblique lower border tends to follow the right costal margin, though it may be palpable on inspiration below the costal margin in normal subjects.

Liver scanning has shown that liver shape is extremely variable even in health. One of the commonest variations is a tongue of liver tissue, termed a Riedel's lobe, extending downwards towards the right iliac fossa (Fig. 6.8).

Hepatic enlargement

When the liver is enlarged its lower border is best defined with the fingertips with the fingers parallel to the rectus muscle (Fig. 6.9). Even in health, on inspiration the liver edge may nudge the fingers and may sometimes produce a distinct flip of which the patient may be conscious. Once the liver edge has been defined many examiners find it easier then to palpate the liver edge with the radial border of the hand parallel to the costal margin. Liver enlargement should be recorded accurately in centimetres below the costal margin in the right mid-clavicular line and below the xiphoid in the mid-line. Assessments in finger-breadths are to be discouraged.

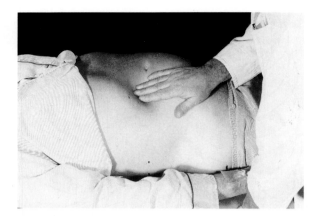

Fig. 6.9 Palpation of the liver.

with tricuspic incompetence systolic pulsation of the liver may be elicited. Gross enlargement of the liver with metastases often causes elevation of the right diaphragm simulating a right pleural effusion on clinical examination. Where the liver is diffusely enlarged by infiltrative disease such as lymphoma, amyloid or sarcoidosis a careful search for associated splenomegaly or lymphadenopathy should be made.

The physical signs of several conditions causing changes in liver size and shape are shown in Figs 6.10–6.16.

The fact that the liver edge is palpable well below the right costal margin does not necessarily mean that the liver itself is enlarged. As mentioned above, hyperinflation of the lungs as in asthma or emphysema may depress the liver. In end-stage cirrhosis the liver is usually shrunken but the left lobe may be palpable as a firm, and often irregular, edge in the epigastrium just below the xiphoid. Percussion of the liver may help to define the position of a shrunken cirrhotic liver and may have practical implications in liver biopsy which is normally performed through the eighth or ninth interspaces in the mid-axillary line. In cirrhosis the biopsy site may have to be adjusted to the appropriate level of dullness in the mid-axillary line percussed out during expiration. Some causes of reduced liver dullness are shown in Table 6.1

In right heart failure the liver is enlarged and often tender. Pressure over the liver may distend the jugular veins, the hepatojugular reflux. In heart failure

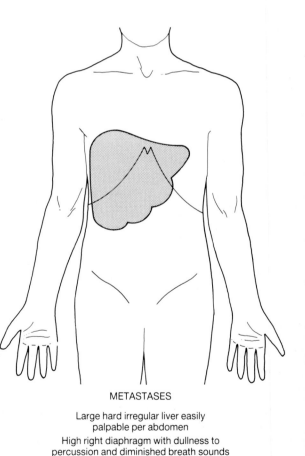

METASTASES

Large hard irregular liver easily
palpable per abdomen

High right diaphragm with dullness to
percussion and diminished breath sounds
over lower chest

Clinical signs may simulate pleural effusion
at right base posteriorly

Fig. 6.10 Diagrammatic representation of the physical signs of metastases in the liver.

Table 6.1. Causes of reduced liver dullness

Small liver	Cirrhosis
	Hepatic necrosis
Overinflated lungs	Asthma
	Emphysema
	Paralysed right diaphragm
Gas over liver	Perforated viscus
	Loop of colon

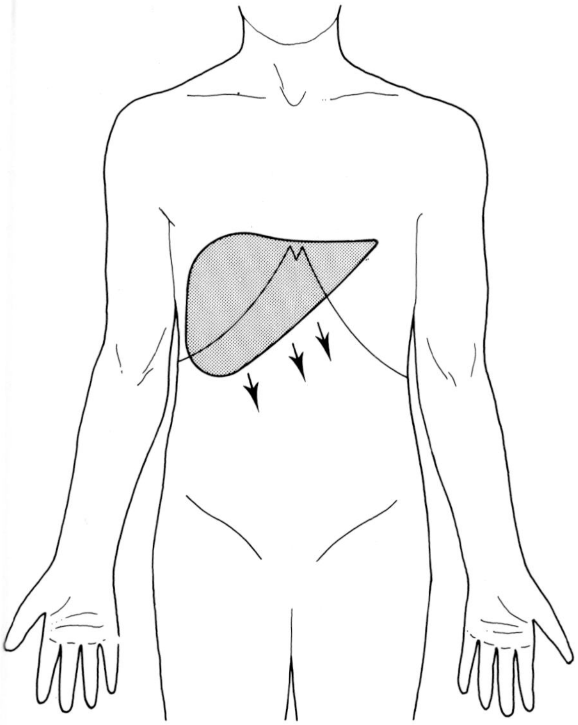

RIGHT HEART FAILURE

Tender enlarged liver
Right diaphragm not necessarily elevated
Hepatojugular reflux positive
Other signs of right heart failure
Systolic pulsation of liver if tricuspid
incompetence present

Fig. 6.11 Physical signs in right heart failure.

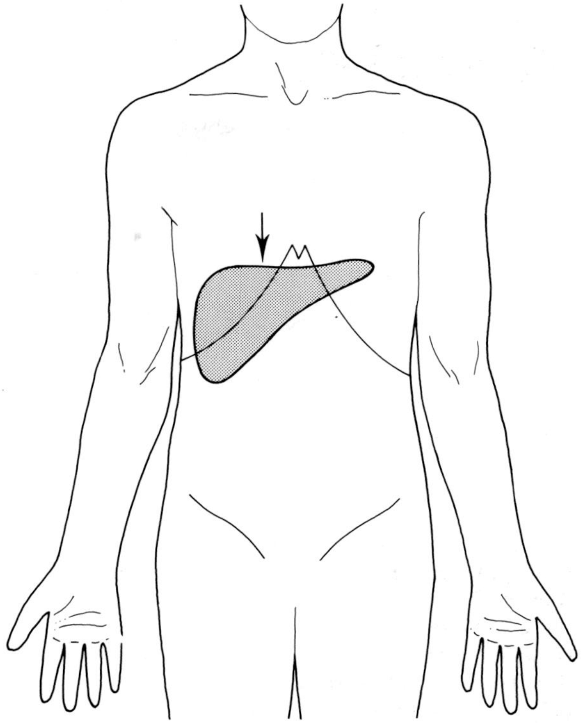

OVERINFLATED LUNGS

Liver edge soft and palpable per abdomen
Chest hyper-resonant with levels of liver
dullness depressed

Fig. 6.12 Physical signs with overinflated lungs.

Stigmata of chronic liver disease (CLD)

No examination of the liver is complete without a search for stigmata of chronic liver disease, including jaundice (Table 6.2). In the alcoholic cirrhotic the signs of liver disease may blur into those due to chronic alcoholism such as facial telangiectasia, rhinophyma and blepharitis.

Some of the signs of chronic liver disease are disease-specific. Kayser—Fleischer rings, for example, are light brown rings of copper chelates at the periphery of the cornea which are seen in Wilson's disease. These may be only visible on slit-lamp examination.

Other physical signs of liver disease are not disease specific and are common to a wide range of chronic liver diseases. Spider naevi may be markers of liver

disease and consist of a central dilated arteriole with radiating smaller vessels like spiders' legs (Fig. 6.17). A few vascular spiders may be seen in healthy men and women and they are common in pregnancy. They are usually spread over the upper half of the body, particularly over face, shoulders and hands. There is no evidence that spider naevi are distributed exclusively over the drainage area of the superior vena cava. Spider naevi are particularly prominent with immune active chronic hepatitis and crops come out with deteriorating liver function or with the development of hepatoma. Along with spider naevi there may be multiple small vessels in the skin of the arms and neck resembling silk threads (the paper money sign).

Men with chronic liver disease of varied aetiology become feminized whereas women tend to become masculinized. In the male, gynaecomastia is the

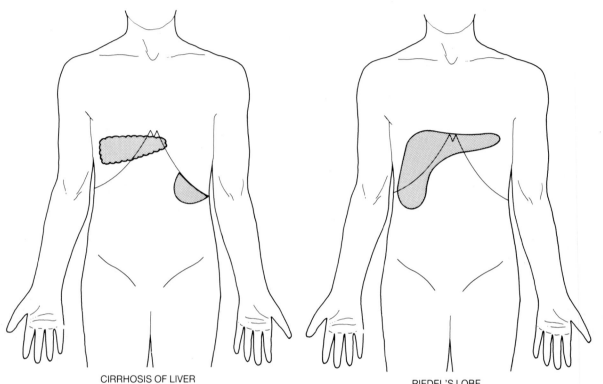

CIRRHOSIS OF LIVER

Small liver to percussion but a hard edge may be
palpable under the xiphoid
Spleen palpable
Other stigmata of chronic liver disease

RIEDEL'S LOBE

A tongue of liver extends downwards from
the right lobe

Fig. 6.14 Riedel's lobe.

Fig. 6.13 Cirrhosis of the liver. In many patients with cirrhosis the liver
may be enlarged or of normal size.

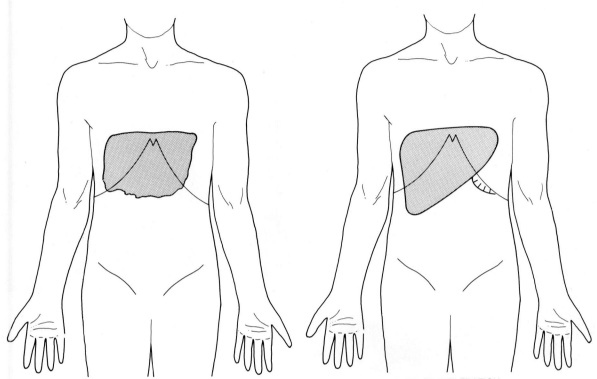

PRIMARY HEPATO-CELLULAR CARCINOMA

African patient   .
Tenderness in epigastrium
Wasting +

Fig. 6.15 Primary hepatocellular carcinoma.

DIFFUSE INFILTRATION

e.g. Amyloid or sarcoidosis
Generalized firm regular enlarged liver
Spleen may also be palpable

Fig. 6.16 Diffuse infiltration of the liver.

Table 6.2. Stigmata of chronic liver disease	
	Specific associations
Face	
Scleral icterus	
Telangiectasia	
Xanthelasma	Prolonged cholestasis
Paper-money sign	
Kayser–Fleisher rings	Wilson's disease
Cushingoid facies	Alcoholic liver disease
Hands	
Clubbing	
White nails (leuconychia)	
Liver palms	
Dupuytren's contracture	Possibly with alcoholic liver disease
Skin	
Spider naevi	
Scanty body hair	
Slaty-grey pigmentation	Haemochromatosis
Scratch marks	Cholestasis
Endocrine	
Gynaecomastia	
Atrophic testes	

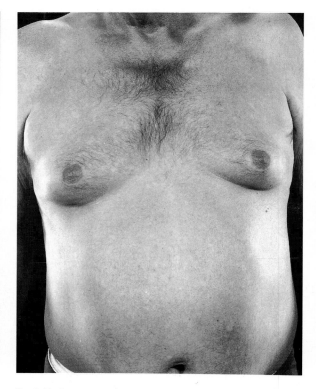

Fig. 6.18 Gynaecomastia.

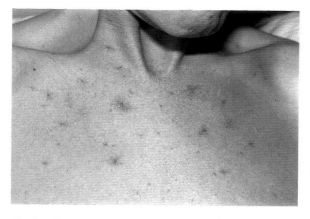

Fig. 6.17 Spider naevi on the chest of a young man with alcoholic liver disease.

most obvious manifestation. This sign is, of course, seen temporarily in the majority of normal pubertal males when it consists of a firm disc of ductal tissue behind the areola. In the gynaecomastia of the male cirrhotic the breasts are diffusely and bilaterally enlarged (Fig. 6.18). About 40 per cent of cirrhotic men have some degree of gynaecomastia. The state-ment that gynaecomastia occurs more commonly in alcoholic liver disease than in other forms of cirrhosis has been disputed. Spironolactone, a diuretic fre-quently used in cirrhosis, must be considered as an additional cause of gynaecomastia, as must other drugs including digoxin, steroids and pheno-thiazines. Other changes in the male cirrhotic include loss of body and facial hair, testicular atrophy and a lower incidence of benign prostatic hypertrophy.

The hand may yield supportive evidence of liver disease. Erythema of the thenar and hypothenar eminences, liver palms (Fig. 6.19), occurs in cirrhosis but is frequent in plethoric and otherwise normal persons. Clubbing, rarely gross, is common in all types of chronic liver disease. The nails may be white (leuconychia) and there may be a brownish crescent at the distal part of the nail (Fig. 6.20). Many patients with alcoholic cirrhosis commonly have Dupuytren's contracture. In chronic cholestasis, as in primary biliary cirrhosis, xanthelasmata may be seen (Fig. 6.21) and xanthomas may develop over extensor sur-faces such as wrist, elbow, knee and buttocks.

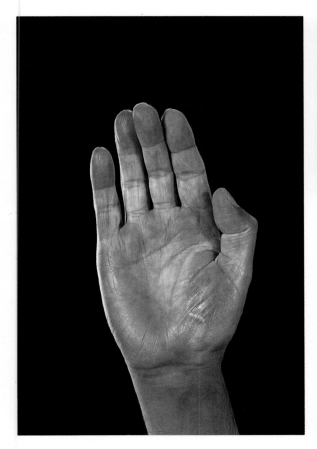

Fig. 6.19 Liver palms. Usually the erythema is limited to the thenar and hypothenar eminences. In this patient, who had alcoholic liver disease and a hepatoma, the changes were unusually striking.

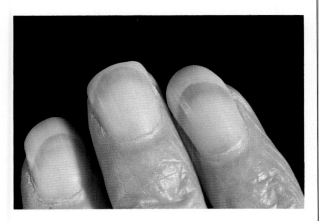

Fig. 6.20 Liver nails showing the typical pigmented crescent limiting the white nail (leuconychia). A similar crescent may be seen in the nails of patients with chronic renal failure.

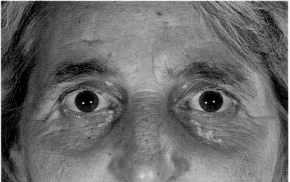

Fig. 6.21 Xanthelasmata in a lady with primary biliary cirrhosis.

Jaundice (Table 6.3)

Jaundice is obvious clinically when the total serum bilirubin rises above three times the normal level (50 µmol/l; 3.0 mg/100 ml). It is best detected in the sclerae where the bilirubin stains the elastic tissue but may also be seen at an early stage on the abdominal wall of white patients. Yellow fat in the sclerae of Negro patients may simulate jaundice. As jaundice deepens, the skin colour may change from a lemon

Table 6.3. Physical signs with main types of jaundice	
Cause	Physical signs
Haemolysis	Pallor
	Lemon-yellow tinge
	Often splenomegaly
	Often features of haemolytic anaemia, e.g. leg ulcers in haemoglobinopathies
Acute hepatocellular damage, e.g. infective hepatitis	Usually jaundice only
	Liver may be mildly enlarged
	Spleen may be palpable
Chronic hepatocellular damage, e.g. cirrhosis	Usually stigmata of CLD
	Hepatosplenomegaly
	Leg oedema + ascites
Cholestasis due to extrahepatic biliary obstruction	May progress to olive-green jaundice
	Scratch marks
	Palpable GB if obstruction due to carcinoma of pancreas
	Tender distended liver

tinge to deep yellow and eventually to a greenish-brown colour. In haemolysis, in which the jaundice is due to unconjugated hyperbilirubinaemia, the degree of jaundice is usually mild but the accompanying anaemia gives the patient a characteristic pale lemon-yellow tinge.

Where cholestatic jaundice is due to an obstruction at the lower end of the common bile-duct, as with carcinoma of pancreas or cholangiocarcinoma, the gall-bladder may be palpably distended. Corvoisier's law states that when the gall-bladder is palpable the jaundice is unlikely to be due to stones as the gall-bladder wall, in the presence of gallstones, would be fibrotic and non-distensible. The converse of the law, i.e. obstructive jaundice without a palpable gall-bladder does not necessarily imply that the jaundice is due to stones. A stone in the neck of the gall-bladder may cause a distended mucocele of the gall-bladder.

The gall-bladder when distended is palpable as a smooth, oval swelling emerging from below the right costal margin. The hemispherical fundus may sometimes be 'bobbed' by the examining fingers through the anterior abdominal wall like an apple floating in water.

With extrahepatic biliary obstruction the liver, distended with bile, is often smoothly enlarged with its lower edge a few cm below the right costal margin (Fig. 6.22).

Occasionally, in a thin patient, a gall-bladder packed with stones may be palpable. The remaining cause for a palpable gall-bladder mass is carcinoma. This occurs mainly in elderly patients.

The spleen

In the young healthy adult the spleen is approximately the size of a fist, 10 cm in its largest axis, which is parallel to the left tenth rib, 7 cm broad and 3−4 cm in thickness. What is not generally recognized is that the spleen atrophies from a maximum of 200 g in the twenties to 60−70 g in extreme old age. It is rarely palpable in health and palpability usually implies enlargement (Table 6.4). Nevertheless, some young adults have palpable spleens for which no cause can be detected. The statement that the spleen has to enlarge two to three times its normal size to become palpable is inaccurate and dependent on the age of the patient.

Table 6.4. Causes of splenomegaly	
Infective	Glandular fever
	Infective hepatitis
	Subacute bacterial endocarditis
	Malaria
	Kala-azar
	Tropical splenomegaly*
	Enteric fevers
Congestive	Cirrhosis
	Bilharzia
	Portal + splenic vein thrombosis
Haematological	Acute leukaemia
	Chronic granulocytic + lymphatic leukaemia*
	Myelosclerosis*
	Hereditary spherocytosis
	Thalassaemia
	Lymphoma
Infiltrations	Sarcoidosis
	Amyloidosis
	Gaucher's disease
Others	Cysts + tumours
	Felty's syndrome

* In these conditions the spleen may be hugely enlarged.

The first sign of splenic enlargement is an increase in the normal splenic dullness anterior to the mid-axillary line over the tenth rib, but this sign may be obscured by the tympany of the gastric air bubble (Fig. 6.23). With progressive enlargement, the spleen spreads downwards and medially and may, if enormously enlarged, reach the right lower quadrant of the abdomen. Palpation should, therefore, commence in this region to avoid missing monstrous splenomegaly.

To detect mild to moderate degress of splenomegaly the examiner's left hand should be placed in the patient's left loin to lift the spleen anteriorly. The right hand then palpates the spleen as it emerges

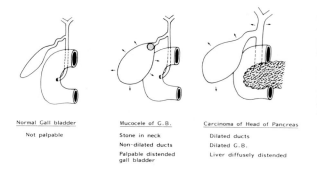

Normal Gall bladder — Not palpable

Mucocele of G.B. — Stone in neck / Non-dilated ducts / Palpable distended gall bladder

Carcinoma of Head of Pancreas — Dilated ducts / Dilated G.B. / Liver diffusely distended

Fig. 6.22 Mechanisms of distension of the gall-bladder.

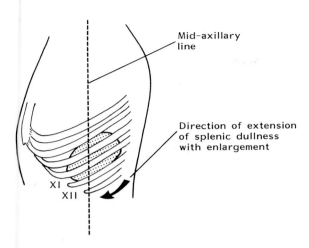

Fig. 6.23 The first sign of splenic enlargement. Extension of splenic dullness.

from below the left costal margin (Fig. 6.24). The anterior border of the spleen is always notched and this may prove useful for identification but may not be detected unless the spleen is appreciably enlarged. With inspiration the spleen moves downwards and medially. Dullness on percussion over an enlarged spleen distinguishes it from a renal mass which carries forward with it, as it enlarges, the resonant splenic flexure (Fig. 6.25; see also Fig. 7.7).

Occasionally a friction rub may be heard over the site of a splenic infarct.

Distension of the abdomen

A feeling of distension of the abdomen is common

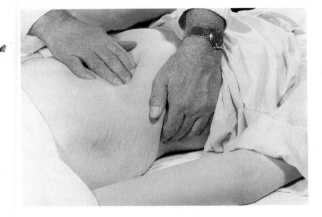

Fig. 6.24 Palpation of the spleen when it is only minimally enlarged.

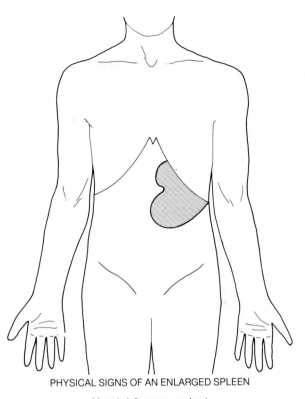

PHYSICAL SIGNS OF AN ENLARGED SPLEEN

Mass in left upper quadrant
Impossible to get above that mass
Dull to percussion
Notch
Can be lifted from loin laterally
Moves downwards on inspiration

Fig. 6.25 Diagrammatic representation of the physical signs of the enlarged spleen.

but not necessarily due to serious organic disease. Many patients complain bitterly of abdominal distension that is neither immediately apparent to the examining doctor nor adequately explained by subsequent investigations. In spite of this the five Fs — fat, fluid, faeces, flatus and fetus — taught to generations of students provides a useful check list. It is worth adding a sixth F 'fibroids' as a reminder that massive solid or semisolid tumours sometimes present with abdominal distension.

Fat

Obesity is usually not difficult to diagnose but is sometimes surprisingly localized to the abdomen in a patient who is not excessively fat elsewhere. Usually abdominal obesity is due to a combination of fat in the mesentery and in the abdominal wall which results in a firm protuberence which tends to flatten when the patient lies down. This may produce some flank dullness simulating ascites but unlike ascites, the flank dullness does not shift. Some patients, particularly women, accumulate enormous deposits of fat subcutaneously in the abdominal wall producing an apron which hangs over the pubis, groins and upper thighs. Truncal obesity with wasted limbs is a feature of Cushing's syndrome or of long-term, high-dosage steroid therapy.

Flatus

Excess gas in the alimentary tract produces a tympanitic distension of the abdomen. It may be due to air-swallowing, high-fibre diets, or alactasia. Gaseous distension due to more serious disorders, such as large-bowel obstruction, is usually generalized but may be localized as with a sigmoid volvulus. When mechanical obstruction of the gut is present loud borborygmi are audible and peristalsis is visible.

Faeces

Loading of the gut with impacted faeces rarely causes significant abdominal distension but when it does one may be able to indent the faeces in the descending colon by firm pressure. In children faecal distension is usually due to Hirschsprung's disease whereas in adults an acquired megacolon is most often seen in demented or psychiatrically disturbed patients with hard faeces in the rectum. When impaction of faeces in the rectum occurs the patient may complain of diarrhoea which is in fact spurious caused by seepage of mucus and soft faeces round the main rectal mass.

Ascites (fluid) (Table 6.5)

The correct detection of ascites, particularly when minimal, is a good deal harder than many of the textbooks suggest and several objective studies have shown a high rate of false-positives. The contour of the abdomen with fullness in the flanks and a curious floppy, splashy feel to the experienced examining hand often indicates ascites before the traditional physical signs of shifting dullness, which requires at least 500 ml fluid, to be present. Turning the patient allows the fluid to gravitate to the dependent half of the abdomen increasing the fullness there and rendering the upper flank resonant to percussion

Table 6.5. Causes of ascites

Associated with chronic diseases
  Cirrhosis of liver
  Heart failure   } Common causes
  Abdominal malignancy
  Liver disease without cirrhosis
  Hepatic vein occlusion
  Constrictive pericarditis
  Polyserositis (for example, systemic lupus erythematosus)
  Nephrotic syndrome
  Infections (for example, tuberculosis)
  Pancreatitis
Associated with acute abdomen
  Trauma (haemoperitoneum)
  Bacterial peritonitis
  Acute pancreatitis

(Fig. 6.26). With the patient in the knee-elbow position a puddle of ascitic fluid accumulates in the most dependent part of the belly and may be percussed out (Fig. 6.27). With moderate ascites a U-shaped area of dullness can be percussed out (Fig. 6.28).

With increasing distension with ascites the resonant central area (with the patient supine) shrinks and at this stage a fluid thrill can be elicited (Fig. 6.29). When this situation has been reached the diagnosis of ascites is usually obvious, not only from the bedside but from the end of the ward! The changes in abdominal signs with increasing ascites are shown in Fig. 6.30.

Central and mid-line abdominal masses

The physical signs of the more important central and mid-line abdominal swellings are summarized in Figs 6.31–6.34.

The fixed, hard, irregular epigastric mass in a

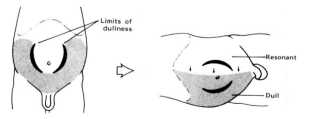

Fig. 6.26 Shifting dullness due to ascites.

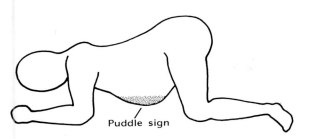

Fig. 6.27 The ascitic puddle.

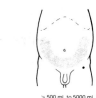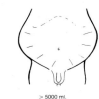

< 500 ml. ascites
Splashy. floppy abdomen
Fullness in flanks

> 500 ml. to 5000 ml. :
U-shaped dullness
Shifting dullness

> 5000 ml.
Tense abdomen
Fluid thrill

Fig. 6.30 The three stages of ascites.

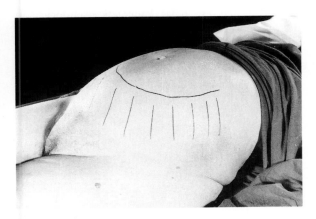

Fig. 6.28 U-shaped dullness to percussion in a lady with gross ascites.

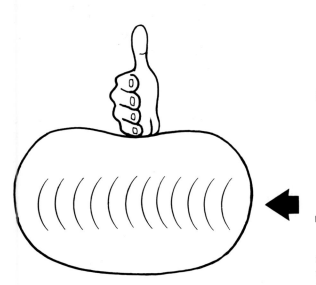

Fig. 6.29 With gross ascites a thrill may be obtained by tapping or flicking one flank and feeling the transmitted percussion wave, through the ascites, in the other flank. To avoid transmission of the wave across the abdominal wall a hand is placed as in the diagram.

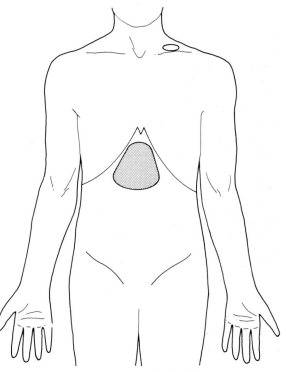

CARCINOMA OF STOMACH

Troisier's node
Hard irregular epigastric mass
Wasted patient

Fig. 6.31 Carcinoma of the stomach.

middle-aged or older patient in the Western world is most likely to be due to an advanced and almost certainly inoperable carcinoma of stomach (Fig. 6.31). This condition most commonly affects middle-aged or elderly men who, as the disease advances, will become wasted and anaemic. Where the tumour obstructs the outflow of the stomach the patient may have the features of pyloric stenosis with recurrent vomiting of large volumes of stale, undigested food and distension of the proximal stomach with visible peristalsis from left to right. Metastases may spread to the liver to cause associated hepatomegaly and jaundice. Frequently, nodes in the supraclavicular fossae are involved; a palpable left supraclavicular node constitutes Troisier's sign. Occasionally a carcinoma of pancreas may be palpable in the epigastrium. Primary or secondary tumours in the left lobe of the liver may cause confusion in this area though they usually move with respiration.

The diagnosis of aortic aneurysm depends on the finding of a mid-line pulsating swelling, usually, though not necessarily in an arteriopathic patient (Fig. 6.32). The lateral expansion on pulsation in addition to the forward pulsation is the critical diagnostic factor. Tumours or masses anterior to the aorta show transmitted pulsation only. Vascular bruits may be audible over an aortic aneurysm or over adjacent diseased vessels.

Masses of enlarged para-aortic or mesenteric glands may give rise to a lumpy central abdominal swelling (Fig. 6.33). These are usually due to lymphoma or chronic lymphatic leukaemia but may be secondary to a primary tumour elsewhere such as a seminoma. Iliac or inguinal nodes with an enlarged spleen may also be detected.

Cystic swellings in the abdomen are characterized by a tense, fluctuant feel. If large enough a fluid thrill may be elicited (Fig. 6.34). Pancreatic pseudocysts in the lesser sac are usually fixed and situated in the epigastrium. Mesenteric cysts usually move at right-angles to the axis of the mesentery and may be confused with hydatid cysts when they arise in this region. Cysts arising from the pelvis are most likely

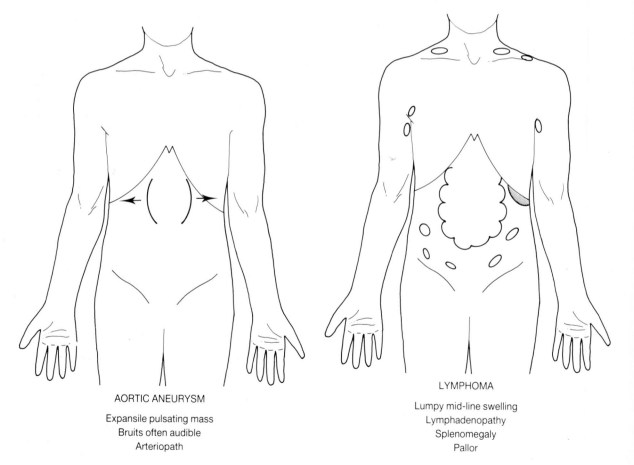

AORTIC ANEURYSM

Expansile pulsating mass
Bruits often audible
Arteriopath

Fig. 6.32 Aortic aneurysm.

LYMPHOMA

Lumpy mid-line swelling
Lymphadenopathy
Splenomegaly
Pallor

Fig. 6.33 Lymphoma.

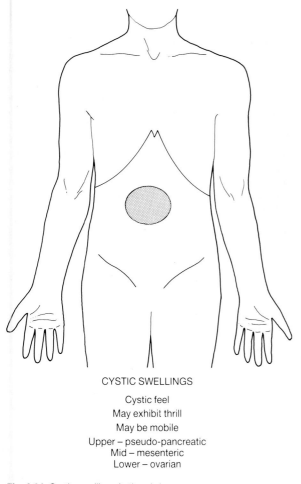

CYSTIC SWELLINGS

Cystic feel
May exhibit thrill
May be mobile
Upper – pseudo-pancreatic
Mid – mesenteric
Lower – ovarian

Fig. 6.34 Cystic swellings in the abdomen.

to be ovarian and, if malignant, are often associated with ascites.

Masses in the right iliac fossa

The diagnosis of a mass in the right iliac fossa is dependent upon the age, circumstances and racial background of the patient. Some of the conditions are listed in Table 6.6.

A child or a young adult in the Western world with a recent history of central abdominal pain followed by pain in the right iliac fossa is likely to have an inflammatory appendix mass. Additional features such as high fever, sweats and inflammation of the overlying skin indicate progression to an appendix abscess.

Table 6.6. Causes of a mass in the right iliac fossa

Appendix mass	
Appendix abscess	Common in Western
Crohn's disease	world
Carcinoma of caecum	
Tuberculosis	Seen mainly in
Amoeboma	undeveloped countries
Lymphoma	
Psoas abscess	
Mobile ovarian cyst	Less common
Retroperitoneal tumour	
Bony tumours	
Malignant undescended testis	Rare
Iliac artery aneurysm	

Subacute or chronic pain in the right iliac fossa, often of colicky type, with diarrhoea, anaemia and weight loss in a young or middle-aged patient may indicate Crohn's disease of the terminal ileum. Often the mass is composed of the diseased ileum with surrounding inflammation. A similar pattern of illness in an Indian or African patient is much more likely to be due to tuberculosis of the ileum or caecum with enlarged and inflamed lymph nodes. With a more acute illness, fever and diarrhoea in a patient in the tropics a mass might be due to an amoeboma.

Carcinoma of the caecum in middle-aged or old patients is often without local symptoms presenting with diarrhoea and iron-deficiency anaemia. A few patients may notice the mass themselves, whereas others may get intestinal obstruction.

The first sign of lymphoma may be a mass of nodes in the right iliac fossa. Here the lump may be relatively painless and may be associated with enlarged para-aortic or inguinal glands and an enlarged spleen. Such a mass of nodes is more likely to be a non-Hodgkin's lymphoma than Hodgkin's disease.

Masses in the left iliac fossa

As with right iliac fossa masses the diagnosis of the left-sided mass depends on factors such as race and age (Table 6.7). In the Western world a common cause is a diverticular mass or abscess. Such a mass may be associated with pain, fever and a disturbance of bowel habit. Progression to a vesicocolic fistula may give rise to frequency, dysuria, dirty smelly urine with the unusual symptom of gas in the urine, pneumaturia.

Table 6.7. Causes of a mass in the left iliac fossa

Diverticular mass or abscess	
Faeces in loaded colon	Common
Carcinoma of colon	
Crohn's disease	
Lymphoma	
Psoas abscess	Less common
Mobile ovarian cyst	
Retroperitoneal tumour*	
Bony tumours	Rare (as with
Malignant undescended testis	masses in
Iliac artery aneurysm	the RIF)

* See Fig. 6.35.

In constipated patients, hard faeces may accumulate in the descending colon to produce a mass in the left iliac fossa. Such changes occur with an organic obstruction as with a lower colonic or rectal carcinoma. Of course a large carcinoma of the descending colon may be felt in the left iliac fossa. Occasionally large retroperitoneal tumours may extend into the left iliac fossa (Fig. 6.35).

Anus and rectum

Inspection of the perineum and anus and digital examination of the rectum completes the clinical examination of the abdomen and gastrointestinal tract. Whilst routine rectal examination is unnecessary in children without relevant complaints it is essential in middle-aged and elderly adults. Without it the asymptomatic rectal carcinoma or polyp will be missed. The old adage 'If you don't put your finger in you'll put your foot in it' taught by generations of surgeons still holds good!

For the patient, rectal examination presents the most embarrassing and disagreeable part of the whole of a medical examination. It requires sympathetic explanation and gentleness in performance. The patient is placed in the left lateral position with hips and knees flexed and buttocks on the edge of the bed. Gloves are worn and the anus and perineum inspected in good light by lifting the right buttock. At this stage look for:

- soiling of the perineum or underwear with faeces, blood or mucus
- prolapsed piles
- papillomata, condylomata or anal warts (see Fig. 20.4)
- ulcers or fissures
- scarring and/or fistula formation (Fig. 6.36)
- skin rashes (Fig. 6.37)

The right index finger is lubricated with jelly and the pulp of the finger placed flat on the anus. Gentle pressure is exerted and the patient asked to push down as though having his bowels opened; the finger tip then slips into the anal canal and is inserted as far as possible into the rectum.

The examining finger then sweeps round the rectum to palpate surrounding structures, to assess the state of the mucosa and to search for specific lesions. Pelvic structures may be palpated bimanually

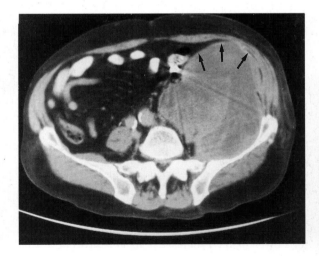

Fig. 6.35 CT scan of the lower abdomen showing a left retroperitoneal tumour presenting as a mass in the left iliac fossa (arrows point to the part of the mass that was palpable).

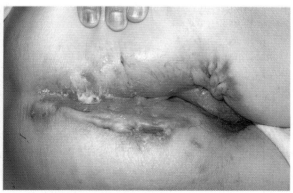

Fig. 6.36 Perianal fistulae and scarring in a patient with severe Crohn's disease.

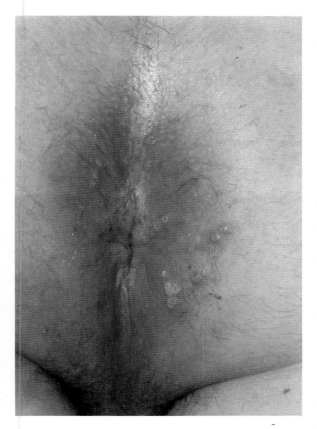

Fig. 6.37 Herpes simplex of the anus.

tumour produces 'winging' of the prostate as it extends beyond the confines of the gland. An acutely tender prostate suggests acute prostatitis.

Lateral to the rectum on both sides are the ischiorectal fossae which may be the site of ischiorectal abscesses. Posteriorly it is usually possible to palpate the concavity of the coccyx.

In the female the corresponding landmark to the prostate is the cervix which, depending on its size and maturity, feels like a firm nodule, like the end of a nose, anteriorly. The uterus, depending on its size, may be palpated bimanually. Pelvic tumours such as ovarian masses may be palpated on either side of the rectum.

In both sexes the character of the rectal wall must be assessed. When inflamed as with ulcerative proctitis it may have a 'velvety' feel. Careful search must be made for polyps or rectal carcinomas. In fact about 90 per cent of rectal carcinomas can be felt digitally. Small lesions may be papilliferous or nodular but often only the edge of large, ulcerating rectal carcinomas can be felt. As the tip of the examining finger crosses the edge of the tumour there may be a sensation as though it is then entering a cavity; in fact this is the necrotic floor of the ulcer.

On withdrawing the finger, examine the glove for mucus and blood and note the characteristics of the faeces. Bloody mucus suggests either an ulcerating tumour of the colon or rectum or chronic inflammatory bowel disease such as ulcerative colitis. Copious mucoid watery discharge may suggest a colonic villous adenoma. In the debilitated or senile patient spurious diarrhoea may be the result of impacted faeces; a mass of hard faeces filling and distending the rectum yet not capable of being evacuated by the patient. Softer faeces seep round the impacted mass producing incontinence. Smelly, pale, sticky faeces may indicate malabsorption as in coeliac disease whereas putty-coloured stools are a feature of obstructive jaundice.

Further reading

Pounder RE, Allison MC, Dhillon AP. *A colour atlas of the digestive system*. London: Wolfe.

Allison MC. Gastroenterology. London: Wolfe, 1991.

by placing the left hand on the anterior abdominal wall suprapubically and in both iliac fossae.

In the male the primary landmark is the prostate gland which is normally the size of a chestnut and of firm consistency but with a shallow central groove. The nodular seminal vesicles may be palpable at the full extent of the finger on each side. With advancing age the prostate hypertrophies with enlargement and progressive protrusion into the rectum. The enlargement may be asymmetrical. Carcinoma of the prostate starts as a hard nodule in the gland which may be impossible to differentiate clinically from an area of calcification. As the carcinoma enlarges it produces a hard, bumpy, irregular tumour with obliteration of the median groove. With extension laterally the

7

The kidneys and bladder

P. J. Toghill

Symptoms
Physical signs
The urine
Further reading

Although this chapter deals primarily with symptoms and signs relating to the kidneys and bladder it must be remembered it overlaps with other sections such as those dealing with the abdomen and genitourinary disease.

Symptoms

Effects of renal failure

Uraemia is the term which is applied to the clinical syndrome found in patients suffering from severe loss of renal function. Symptoms appear when the glomerular filtration rate (GFR) falls below 20–25 per cent of normal. These symptoms are often ill-defined and may persuade the patient that other systems are involved. For example, the anorexia and vomiting that are often prominent features of uraemia may suggest to the patient, and his doctor, a disturbance of the gastrointestinal tract such as peptic ulcer or gastric cancer. Other patients may have symptoms such as breathlessness on exertion, paroxysmal nocturnal dyspnoea and leg swelling that may point to a cardiac basis for the problems. With long-standing, but not necessarily severely impaired renal function, metabolic bone disease may supervene and give rise to musculoskeletal aches and pains. Ultimately in renal failure there is lack of concentration, drowsiness and confusion progressing to coma.

Oedema

In some patients the gross, generalized oedema of the nephrotic syndrome is the first symptom to draw attention to a renal problem. Here the massive loss of protein into the urine leads to hypoproteinaemia and a consequent increase in the transudation of fluid into the tissues. In practice the syndrome is defined as a loss of more than 3.5 g protein in 24 h though it may be up to 10 or even 20 g/24 h as compared with a normal of less than 250 mg/24 h. The nephrotic syndrome may be due to primary renal disease or may be the renal complication of another systemic disease such as diabetes (Table 7.1). Although it is often taught that the oedema of the nephrotic syndrome tends to be less influenced by gravity than cardiac oedema this is not necessarily true. Most patients

Table 7.1. The causes of the nephrotic syndrome

Primary renal disease
  (glomerulonephritis)
Secondary to systemic diseases
  SLE
  Amyloidosis
  Diabetes
  Myelomatosis
  Infections (e.g. streptococcal, hepatitis B, malaria
    (see Fig. 19.14)
Secondary to drugs
  Gold
  Penicillamine
  Captopril

with the nephrotic syndrome present with leg swelling. Milder degrees of oedema characterize acute nephritis or chronic renal failure.

Pain

Gross structural disease of the kidney causes pain. This is usually felt in the renal angle which is the region in the loin between the twelfth rib above and the edge of the erector spinales muscles medially (Fig. 7.1). Sometimes the pain from massive renal swellings or malignant tumours may be felt anteriorly. Try not to use the term 'renal colic' which is often applied to the excruciating pain of a stone or blood-clot passing down the ureter. Colic is pain due to contraction of smooth muscle in an obstructed hollow tube — so the correct term is 'ureteric colic'. This is intensely severe pain starting in the renal angle, which may be tender, and radiating round the flank into the groin and thence into the penis, scrotum or labia majora (Fig. 7.2). Ureteric colic is true colic with each bout reaching a crescendo and then fading away, only to recur again in a minute or so. During the paroxysms of pain the patient may roll on the floor prostrated by the severity of the pain which may be associated with sweating and vomiting. With the passage of the stone or clot into the bladder the pain stops abruptly to the profound relief of the patient.

During an attack of ureteric colic the patient may experience strangury which is an intense desire to

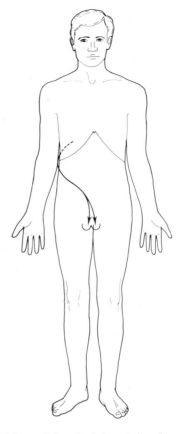

Fig. 7.2 The radiation of pain in ureteric colic.

pass urine, a few drops at a time, even though the bladder may be almost empty.

Hypertension

Although not strictly a symptom, the presence of renal disease is often brought to light by the finding of hypertension on routine examination. Here the associated presence of protein in the urine may be an essential clue.

Problems with micturition

The final group of symptoms which most commonly draw attention to disease of the renal tract are those related to disturbances of micturition. We have invented hybrid terms for our own medical shorthand to describe these symptoms. Most end in 'uria' — i.e. they relate to the urine — but their use is not entirely precise. So as well as knowing what our patients mean by their symptoms we need to know what we

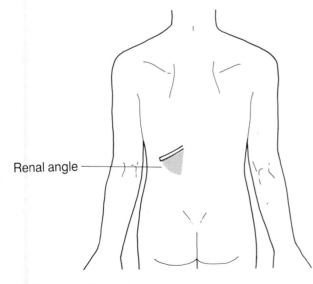

Renal angle

Fig. 7.1 The renal angle.

mean! Question your patients meticulously. Use plain words! Circumlocutions are confusing and unnecessary.

Polyuria means the passage of excessively large volumes of urine both day and night. Some of the conditions causing polyuria and thirst will be dealt with in Chapter 12 and are listed in Table 12.5. Of these probably the commonest is diabetes mellitus. Strictly speaking chronic renal failure does not cause polyuria; because of the loss of concentrating power of the kidney the normal circadian rhythm is lost and the patient develops nocturia. Compulsive water-drinking is a not uncommon cause of polyuria.

Of course, patients with polyuria will have frequency of micturition but the term frequency implies more than it actually says. It is used to mean the frequent passage of small amounts of urine as would occur with a urinary tract infection. Sometimes it is useful to record in the notes the degree of frequency. Thus D/N = 6/3 means that the patient is passing urine six times in the day and three times in the night (nocturia).

Dysuria is another term which is often inappropriately used. Strictly speaking it should mean difficulty in micturition but in fact it usually is held to mean stinging, scalding or pain on micturition.

Oliguria is the passage of small volumes of urine in

24 h (and is usually defined as less than 400 ml/day). When no urine is produced the patient is described as being anuric, or having anuria. Really this term is best applied to patients who have acute renal failure and it is of critical importance to distinguish this from retention of urine in which there is lower urinary tract obstruction. With retention the urine is produced by the kidneys but cannot be passed because of mechanical or neurogenic difficulties.

For the patient haematuria or blood in the urine is an alarming symptom. To some extent a description of the urine helps to define the site of blood loss. Blood uniformly mixed with urine suggests bleeding from the kidneys whereas fresh blood or clots, not uniformly mixed with the urine suggests bleeding from the bladder. In the tropics frank blood at the end of micturition may be due to *Schistosoma haematobium* infection. Urethral blood, as from a perineal injury is washed out before the main urine stream. Some of the causes of haematuria are listed in Table 7.2.

Remember that what the patient thinks is blood may not necessarily be so. Certain foods like beetroot stain the urine red and drugs such as L-dopa and rifampicin may confer a pinkish tinge. Gross intravascular haemolysis will produce haemoglobinuria; this is seen in its most extreme form in blackwater fever (see Chapter 19) but may be seen in the Western world when it occurs with paroxysmal nocturnal haemoglobinuria or exertional haemoglobinuria. In some forms of porphyria the urine turns dark on standing.

Urinary incontinence is another symptom requiring careful interrogation. Constant dribbling incontinence is unusual and nearly always means that there is a fistula present, usually between bladder and vagina. Intermittent incontinence is common and its causes are multiple ranging from dementia, cerebrovascular disease, paraplegia, multiple sclerosis, prolapse and perineal weakness. Some of these problems causing incontinence in the elderly will be discussed in Chapter 13. When urine leaks away on coughing, sneezing or straining this is described as stress incontinence: it is usually due to prolapse.

Urgency of micturition means that the patient has very little warning of the need to empty his or her bladder. Unless this is done quickly urine is voided without control. This symptom has numerous causes but is common in multiple sclerosis and in benign prostatic hypertrophy.

'Key in the door' incontinence is a common condition in which patients, often elderly, who may have urgency or incomplete control of micturition,

Table 7.2. Some conditions causing haematuria

Site	Cause
Anywhere in urinary tract	Haemorrhagic disorders such as thrombocytopenia, overdose of anticoagulants, haemophilia
Kidney	Polycystic kidneys Trauma Tuberculosis Tumours (carcinoma of kidney and of renal pelvis) Renal infarction (e.g. sub-acute bacterial endocarditis) Stones
Ureter	Stones Neoplasms
Bladder	Stones Trauma Acute infections (e.g. *E. coli*) Chronic infections (in tropics bilharzia) Tumours
Prostate	Benign and malignant disease

become incontinent when they anticipate emptying their bladders but are foiled by a last-minute delay.

Physical signs

General appearance

In chronic renal failure the physical signs are largely non-specific. A combination of anaemia and pigmentation gives the patient a muddy, sallow complexion. In advanced renal failure loss of weight and dehydration may be combined with rapid respiration (Kussmaul's breathing), a pericardial friction rub, generalized twitching of muscles and drowsiness. More often the features of uraemia may be swamped by the physical signs of the basic disease such as diabetes, malignant hypertension and myelomatosis. The generalized oedema of the nephrotic syndrome has been alluded to earlier but other features such as muscle wasting related to hypoproteinaemia may be a striking feature (Fig. 7.3). Some of the diseases commonly leading to chronic renal failure are listed in Table 7.3.

The kidneys

Being posterior wall structures the kidneys are palpated bimanually. Thus for examination of the left kidney (Fig. 7.4) the left hand is placed in the left loin with the fingers in the angle formed by the twelfth rib and the erector spinales muscles. The right hand palpates anteriorly in an attempt to catch the left kidney between the two hands. The right kidney is palpated in a similar way with the left hand in the right loin (Fig. 7.5). In thin patients the lower pole of the normal right kidney may be felt but the left rarely so. Renal swellings are palpable from the loin and move with respiration. They are thus palpable bimanually but are not strictly 'ballottable' in that

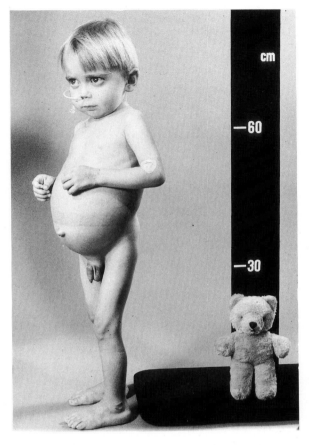

Fig. 7.3 A child with the nephrotic syndrome. Note the gross ascites with relatively little leg oedema. The gross muscle wasting and feeding nasogastric tube emphasize the need for good nutrition in such cases.

they cannot be bounced from one hand to another (Fig. 7.6).

The colon lies anterior to the left kidney and the splenic flexure is pushed forwards when that kidney enlarges. Because of the presence of gas in the colon in front of the kidney, left renal swellings are usually resonant on percussion (Fig. 7.7).

The finding of bilateral renal swellings indicates either polycystic disease or bilateral hydronephroses. About 30 per cent of patients with adult polycystic disease have hepatic cysts which may cause enlargement of the liver (Fig. 7.8). Bilateral hydronephrosis usually indicates obstruction of the lower urinary tract and in men this is likely to be due to benign prostatic hypertrophy or carcinoma of the prostate or bladder. In women the lower ureters may be invaded by pelvic tumours such as carcinoma of the uterus, ovaries or bladder. With the syndrome of idiopathic

Table 7.3. Causes of chronic renal failure	
Chronic glomerulonephritis	(40%)
Chronic pyelonephritis	(15%)
Hypertension and other vascular diseases	(10%)
Diabetes	(10%)
Polycystic disease	(10%)
Analgesic nephropathy	
Obstructive uropathy, e.g. prostatic enlargement	(15%)
Miscellaneous other causes	

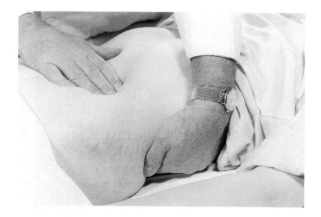

Fig. 7.4 Palpation of the left kidney with the examiner's left hand in the loin and right hand anteriorly.

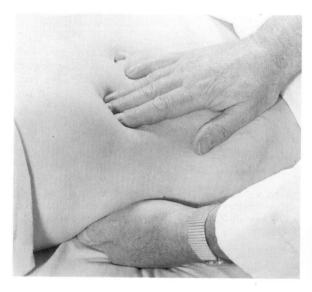

Fig. 7.5 Palpation of the right kidney.

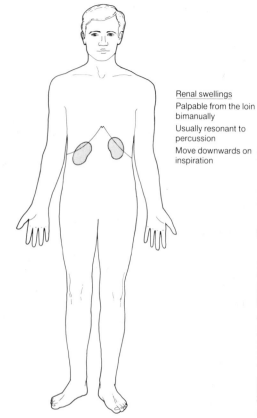

Renal swellings

Palpable from the loin bimanually

Usually resonant to percussion

Move downwards on inspiration

Fig. 7.6 The physical signs of renal swellings.

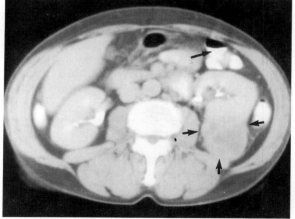

Fig. 7.7 CT scan with short arrows showing a left renal tumour (hypernephroma). The anterior longer arrow shows gas visible in the gut demonstrating why left renal masses are usually resonant to percussion.

retroperitoneal fibrosis the inferior vena cava may also be obstructed to give leg oedema, collateral veins on the lower abdominal wall and varicoceles in the male. Some causes of renal swellings are shown in Table 7.4.

Bladder

Palpation of the bladder is critical in any assessment of a patient's renal function. Acute retention of urine produces an exquisitely painful, tender bladder and pressure on the bladder increases the overwhelming

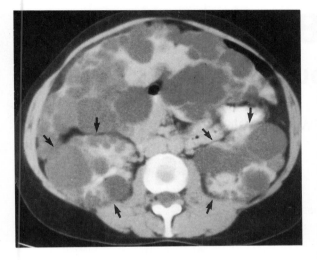

Fig. 7.8 CT scan showing polycystic disease of the kidneys (arrowed) and the liver.

Table 7.4. Renal swellings

Unilateral	Bilateral
Hydronephrosis	Polycystic diseases
Pyonephrosis	Hydronephroses
Cysts	
Abscess	
Tumour	

sensation to micturate. By contrast chronic retention of urine is painless and produces a large floppy leaky bladder. This is the syndrome of retention of urine with overflow. Your patient may be able to pass normal amounts of urine but is left with an overfilled bladder. In the male the diagnosis of chronic retention of urine is usually straightforward but it must be remembered that it is virtually impossible to define the size of the prostate gland when the bladder is full. In women a pregnant uterus and an ovarian cyst may feel like a distended bladder. If in doubt ask your patient to try to empty her bladder before re-examining her.

With the advent of haemo- and peritoneal dialysis few patients are being seen in the developed countries with the physical signs of advanced renal failure.

The patient on haemodialysis can be identified by an arteriovenous fistula or shunt. A thrill can be palpated and a loud bruit heard at the site of anastomosis. After transplantation the new kidney can be palpated under the scar in one or other iliac fossae.

The urine

Although the text deals primarily with symptoms and signs, examination of the urine is such an integral part of the physical examination that it is included at this point.

Appearance

Comment has already been made on the effects of blood in the urine and also on unusually coloured urines. Freshly passed urine is usually clear but deposits of urates and phosphates appear on standing and render the urine cloudy. Heavily infected urines are usually smelly and turbid on passing. Care must be taken to collect urine cleanly to avoid contamination with discharges.

Specific gravities

The specific gravity of urine varies from 1.015 to 1.025 (usually styled 1015 to 1025). Very dilute urines with specific gravities of 1010 occur with chronic renal failure, after diuretic therapy and after fluid loads. After fluid deprivation the urine specific gravity rises to above 1025.

Special testing

The chemical testing of urine has been simplified by the use of dip-strip testing. The tests are based on colour changes in a strip of absorbent cellulose which has been impregnated by an appropriate test solution. In this way the following tests can be performed on a single strip:

- pH
- protein
- glucose
- ketones
- bilirubin
- blood
- urobilinogen

Of particular importance is the recording of very low levels of protein in the urine. In diabetes, for example, this has important prognostic implications.

Further reading

Whitworth JA, Lawrence JR. *A textbook of renal disease.* Melbourne: Churchill Livingstone, 1987.

8

The nervous system

R. B. Godwin-Austen

Symptoms
The examination
General medical examination
The unconscious or poorly responsive patient
The diagnosis of brain death
References and further reading

Patients with neurological symptoms have earned the reputation with medical students of being 'difficult to diagnose'. This stems, at least partly, from the fact that there are a large number of physical signs that may be elicited on examination — far more than in the relatively simple task of examining the heart or abdomen. In a neurological case the diagnosis can usually be made on the basis of the history alone and the examination of the patient may confirm the anatomical diagnosis but only defines pathology in the minority. It is therefore very important to develop skills in history-taking as discussed in Chapter 1. Armed with a suspected diagnosis and a differential diagnosis you will then be able to focus your examination to confirm or refute your suspicions. Let us first consider some of the common neurological presenting symptoms.

Symptoms

Black-outs

This is a term that has only entered our vocabulary in the last 20 or 30 years. Strictly speaking it should mean loss of vision but almost everyone takes the term 'black-out' to mean loss of consciousness. Much information has to be taken from eye-witnesses. Did they observe colour change, convulsions and incontinence? Was the patient actually unconscious (that is not recording continuous memory), was he standing or lying down at the time, did he fall? What were the sequelae?

Circumstances are important (see also Chapter 15). The guardsman standing to attention on a hot day, who goes pale and sweaty before falling is most likely to have had a syncopal episode; the elderly clergyman bidding his parishioners farewell after matins who pales and falls to the ground unconscious, to recover in a minute or so, is more likely to have had a Stokes—Adams attack. The teenager at a pop concert who becomes dizzy and faint is likely to be hyperventilating; the obese, plethoric barrister who snores and has funny turns in the night is likely to be suffering from the sleep apnoea syndrome.

Epilepsy presents in many guises. Most witnesses will recognize immediately the generalized tonic—clonic seizure. What may be more difficult is the interpretation of complex partial epilepsy in which the patient loses conscious contact with his surroundings but may, at the same time, be able to undertake complex activities such as driving a car. Here questioning of the patient subsequently may reveal premonitory symptoms (the aura) which include unusual smells or curious sensations that may, to the patient, be familiar yet indescribable. A combination of both the patient's and the witnesses' accounts is essential. Terms such as grand mal and petit mal have now largely been abandoned and a scheme for the classification of epilepsy is shown in Table 8.1.

Sudden collapses in the elderly may commonly be associated with serious brady- or tachyarrhythmias but when collapses occur on getting up from a lying

Table 8.1. The classification of epilepsy

GENERALIZED

- Tonic–clonic (grand mal)
- Tonic
- Atonic
- Absence (petit mal)
- Atypical absence
- Myoclonic

PARTIAL (focal)

A Without impairment of consciousness (simple partial seizures)
B With impairment of consciousness (complex partial seizures)
  - With motor signs (e.g. Jacksonian, versive)
  - With sòmato- or special sensory symptoms (e.g., olfactory, visual)
  - With autonomic features) (e.g. epigastric sensations)
  - With psychic symptoms (e.g. fear, déjà vu)
  - With automatisms (complex partial, psychomotor)

PARTIAL SEIZURES SECONDARILY GENERALIZED
  i.e. clinical or electrical evidence of focal discharge before, during or after the generalized seizure

UNCLASSIFIED

From Laidlaw J, Richens A. *Textbook of epilepsy.* Edinburgh: Churchill Livingstone, 1982.

Table 8.2. Some important causes of recurrent or persistant headache

*Migraine *Tension headaches *Extracranial causes (i.e. cervical spondylosis) Hypertension Raised intracranial pressure Cranial arteritis	These can almost always be diagnosed from the history and physical signs

* Common causes.

or sitting position postural hypotension must be considered.

Do not forget that severe fluid depletion after severe gastroenteritis is a common cause of fainting in young and previously healthy young folk.

Headaches

The patient complaining of headaches seldom shows any abnormality on physical examination and the diagnosis is normally reached on the history. The differential diagnosis of headache is very large but tension headaches, migraine and extracranial causes account for the majority (Table 8.2). Patients with brain tumours presenting with headaches usually have associated symptoms or signs on examination to indicate the cause. In the elderly, cranial arteritis is a fairly common cause of headache and the patients do not necessarily localize tenderness over the temporal arteries. Hypertension is frequently blamed, but is not often the cause for headaches. The typical hypertensive headache is worse on waking, occipital in site and pounding in character; mild hypertension never causes headaches and severe hypertension is not necessarily associated with them!

Problems with vision

These are dealt with in more detail in Chapter 22. Acute and catastrophic loss of vision quickly brings the patient to his or her doctor for advice and demands urgent attention and diagnosis the same day. Primary ocular events such as vitreous haemorrhage or retinal detachment may be associated with floaters, zig-zag lines and flashing lights as well as field loss. Attacks of migraine often start with visual loss or with zig-zag lines (fortification spectra) that persist for $\frac{1}{4}-\frac{1}{2}$ hour and are followed by headache, often hemicranial in site.

The symptom of double vision (diplopia) rarely presents difficulties in interpretation but older folk often misinterpret a homonymous hemianopia as blurred vision, complaining that they just cannot see properly. Apparent movement of the visual image (oscillopsia) or central visual acuity impairment may also be described as blurring.

Dizziness

The complaint of dizziness taxes the most sympathetic and patient doctor. Is the patient describing true vertigo (hallucination of movement) or something else (impairment of consciousness or a feeling of depersonalization)? True rotational vertigo can usually be identified by careful interrogation in many patients but symptoms such as giddiness, floating on air, 'mazy heads' and faint-headedness may not infrequently deny their origins to the most astute diagnostician. Nevertheless, disagreeable feelings of dizziness may be due to a multiplicity of causes as disparate as anaemia, postural hypotension and phenytoin toxicity, so a careful history is essential.

Weakness and difficulty in walking

Here it is, of course, essential to establish the time-course of the symptoms. Slowly progressive weakness of the limbs over a period of many years in a young person may point to a muscular dystrophy whereas recent weakness of the legs may indicate cord compression or a demyelinating disorder. Where a cord lesion is suspected, further questions must be directed towards associated sensory disturbances and bladder function. Patients with Parkinsonism, by contrast, complain of weakness when, in fact, their limbs are strong. In the very old the leg weakness may be just part of the feebleness of senile cachexia.

In patients with multiple sclerosis a meticulous history has to be extracted from the patient. Because of the variable and flunctuating course of the disease, questions have to be posed about apparently unrelated symptoms, almost forgotten in the distant past. The 40-year-old teacher with weakness of his legs may not regard a transient bout of tingling in the left arm ten years earlier as being particularly relevant; blurred vision in his right eye 10 years before that might seem to him to be an even more tenuous association. We must remember that patients, unlike their doctors, do not package, symptoms neatly under a CNS enquiry.

Confusion

The history becomes unreliable or impossible when the patient is demented, or has impairment of consciousness or speech or memory defect. In these cases an independent history is obviously essential. But in many other cases where the patient is capable of providing the history, the account of a close member of the family or a friend may also be very valuable.

Changes in personality and mood, and the observed effects of the symptoms, may be put in clearer perspective by an independent history. In hospital practice, when a patient is to be admitted, it is particularly important to ask relatives to wait until they have been seen and a history taken.

The examination

The examination must be 'directed' so that at completion a working diagnosis and assessment can be made. It begins as the patient enters the consulting room. Observe the patient's gait, posture, facies and mood. Abnormal involuntary movements may be obvious and an attempt should be made to classify them (Table 8.3).

Paroxysmal symptoms (such as pain in the face from trigeminal neuralgia) may become evident during the history-taking.

When you begin the formal examination of the patient note whether he can undo his buttons or remove his shoes and assess his general mobility (especially where pain in the back or neck is the chief complaint). Any tendency to favour the use of one side more than the other, should be observed.

The examination of the patient must concentrate on those physical signs relevant to the history that has been elicited. There is no 'routine neurological examination'; in each cases the examination has to

Table 8.3. Abnormal involuntary movements

Abnormal movements	Definition
Tremor	Regular rhythmical repetitive oscillations at a joint
Chorea	Jerky, random, non-repetitive movements (Ballism = chorea affecting predominantly proximal limb joints)
Athetoid dystonia	Slow, writhing, non-repetitive movements associated with disturbance of posture
(Tic or habit spasm)	Repetitive (but often complex) jerking movements which can be voluntarily suppressed (at least temporarily), and associated with a conscious urge to move and a sense of relief when the movement has been carried out
Myclonus	Jerky repetitive movements (irregular or rhythmic), outside voluntary control and arising in the central nervous system (to exclude myokymia)
Fasciculation	Irregular and diffuse muscular twitching where the contractions involve the motor unit
Myokymia	Repetitive irregular muscle twitches localized to one part of muscle and usually involving several motor units
Asterixis	Brief lapses of sustained posture

be adjusted to that particular patient's problem and adjusted according to his personality and behaviour. Some assessment of general intelligence, memory and mood will have already been made while taking the history. These observations should be recorded at the start of the examination and, where relevant, with the patient still seated, tests of higher mental function, memory, reading and writing should be performed. Where the history has suggested dementia or a confusional state tests of minor hemisphere function are indicated (see Chapters 13 and 14).

Patients, and their relatives, often confuse memory defects (amnesia or dysmnesia) with disturbance of language (dysphasia). Thus a patient with dysphasia may be thought to be losing his memory because he is unable to say the name of a person or place. But amnesic syndromes generally develop in isolation from language defects so first test for speech deficits and then investigate the patient's memory.

Dysphasia

Dysphasia is usually a combination of a receptive defect, i.e. difficulty in understanding the spoken word, and an expressive defect, i.e. difficulty in putting thoughts into words.

Dysphasia indicates damage to, or disturbance of, function in the dominant temporal lobe (angular or supramarginal gyrus) or the dominant premotor cortex (third frontal convolution) (Fig. 8.1a). The dominant hemisphere is almost always the left in right-handed individuals and is also the left in about 60 per cent of left-handers.

Dysphasia may be obvious when severe but minor degrees of dysphasia have to be sought. In spontaneous speech the patients may use an inappropriately restricted vocabulary paraphrasing when they cannot remember words. Occasional mispronunciations or neologisms (words that do not exist) may be noted and some patients with dysphasia develop a slight stammer. The receptive component of dysphasia can be tested by asking the patient to do something, e.g. 'hold out your hand' or more complicated 'touch your left ear with your little finger'. Problems with expressive speech can be tested by asking the patient to name objects. Again begin with simple objects: finger, glasses, orange. Then graduate to more difficult ones: rim, lens, petals.

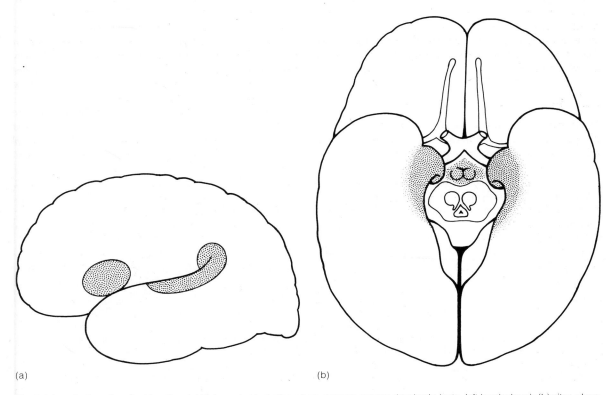

(a)   (b)

Fig. 8.1 Localization of cortical function. (a) Main anatomical sites where damage causes dysphasia (note, left hemisphere); (b) sites where damage causes memory loss.

Memory impairment

When a patient complains of memory impairment, or when a memory defect is suspected, it is usually easy, but none the less important, to exclude disturbance of consciousness as the cause. Thus a short loss of memory may be due to concussion or epilepsy. A continuing memory defect may be isolated or part of a diffuse cerebral disorder. In the latter case dysphasia, perceptual defects and general cognitive defects will contaminate the memory disturbance making testing more difficult and indeed unnecessary when the deficit is severe and causing dementia.

When testing memory distinguish between: immediate recall, recent memory and remote memory.

Immediate recall is tested by asking the patient to repeat back a series of numbers in the order given; and then another series in reverse order. Patients can normally recall at least six digits forwards and four backwards. Alternatively the patient can be asked to repeat the 'Babcock sentence' — 'One thing a nation needs to be rich and great is a large, secure supply of wood'. Four repetitions should achieve a correct response. Failure of immediate recall usually indicates either some impairment of consciousness (and is therefore very useful in assessing patients with recent concussion for degree of recovery) or it may indicate a failure of attention, either through emotional preoccupation with other symptoms or for other reasons.

Recent memory is tested first by orientation in time, place and person. Then give the patient a name and an address and a flower asking him to recall these after five minutes. An alternative is to tell a short story and to question the patient after five minutes. Patients with the specific amnesic syndromes with damage to the hypothalamus, mamillary bodies and temporal lobes (hippocampus) (Fig. 8.1(b)) will characteristically show a severe defect of recent memory.

Remote memory forms part of a permanent store of information in the brain. Defects of remote memory imply a failure of retrieval. It is difficult to test remote memory although a difficulty recalling general information such as the names of the Queen's children, president of the USA, seven common flowers, etc. may indicate a general decline in memory. Failure in these tests with relative preservation of recent memory implies the early stages of a diffuse cerebral disturbance such as a dementia.

Personality changes

These may characterize frontal lesions. The patient may become apathetic and disinhibited. He may give his history with an inappropriate lack of concern or anxiety; he may be dirty or untidily dressed and occasionally childish; silly behaviour or boorishness may be noted.

Parietal lobe lesions

Complex disorders of higher mental function may characterize parietal lobe lesions especially in the non-dominant hemisphere. Thus while the left hemisphere is mainly concerned with symbolic thought such as speech, writing, reading, calculation, musical notation, etc., the right hemisphere is concerned with spatial, topographical and constructional skills. Damage to the right parietal lobe by stroke or tumour may lead to difficulties in dressing, finding the way about the house or laying the table. Traditionally we ask the patient to copy a star diagram or draw a bicycle.

Articulation and voice production

It is customary to record abnormalities of speech before the cranial nerve examination.

Dysarthria is a disorder of the articulation of speech and there are three main varieties. First the patient with bilateral pyramidal deficit above the tenth nerve nucleus (as in motor neurone disease or after bilateral strokes) may exhibit a spastic dysarthria, where speech seems to require more effort and is 'squeezed out' with little modulation of speed or pitch and lacking the gaps between words. The voice is 'flat' and slow. Secondly cerebellar dysarthria is 'drunken speech' with slurring of the words and uncontrolled changes in pitch, speed and volume. Thirdly in extra-pyramidal disorders, such as Parkinson's disease, speech becomes soft and monotonous often with a slight stammer.

Of course a facial weakness, or weakness of the muscles of the palate, from myasthenia gravis may cause dysarthria but these conditions seldom present with the isolated symptoms and signs of a dysarthria. *Dysphonia* is a disturbance of sound production, which leads to a hoarse or soft voice. This is mainly due to local abnormalities of the larynx but sometimes due to problems with the recurrent laryngeal nerve (see below).

Cranial nerves

The detail with which the cranial nerves are examined depends as elsewhere on the symptoms. Don't waste time on tests of hearing when the patient complains of paraesthesia in the feet! Unnecessary examination exhausts patient and doctor alike, scores no points with the consultant and may confuse you. But when the symptoms indicate the possibility of dysfunction in a cranial nerve, detailed examination is necessary.

Before examining the cranial nerves you must know their anatomical relationships (both within and outside the brain) and their function. Of particular importance is the anatomy of the visual pathways (see Chapter 22) the functions of the IIIrd, IVth and VIth nerves, the cutaneous and buccal distribution of the main divisions of the Vth nerve, and the muscles supplied by the Vth, VIIth, Xth, XIth and XIIth nerves.

I. The olfactory nerve

Patients with loss of sense of smell (anosmia) will frequently report an associated loss of taste. This is because the appreciation of flavour of food depends on olfaction. Testing of primary taste with sweet/sour/salt/bitter test substances will be normal where the apparent loss of taste is due to first cranial nerve damage. The olfactory nerve is sometimes damaged in head injury (especially frontal or occipital injuries) or in frontal tumours where the nerve on one or both sides may be directly compressed.

Olfaction is most reliably tested with familiar smells such as orange, perfume or coffee powder. Where feigned anosmia is suspected, asafoetida powder or solution has a sufficiently pungent odour for most patients to recoil involuntarily. Ammonia vapour is detected by its effect on the nasal mucosa (Vth nerve) and will therefore be perceived by the patient with a genuine anosmia.

II. The optic nerve

This is examined under three headings: the fundus, visual acuity and visual fields.

The fundus The use of the ophthalmoscope and the recognition of abnormalities in the fundus depends on practice and experience. Do not miss an opportunity to examine the fundus.

This then is the exception to the rule stated above; always examine the fundi even when there are no relevant symptoms. Only in this way can you learn to recognize the range of the normal and minor deviations from it.

The right eye should be examined holding the ophthalmoscope to your right eye; and the left eye using your left eye, to avoid rubbing noses with the patient. Lighting in the examination room should be reduced so that the pupil is large. Short-acting, weak mydriatics, such as tropicamide, can be safely used in the vast majority of patients to allow better views of the fundus. However, they are best avoided in those predisposed to narrow-angle glaucoma.

Approach the pupil of the eye on the equator and about 15° lateral to the axis of fixation (Fig. 8.2). This allows you to see the region of the optic disc immediately. Follow any blood vessel towards the disc as it gets larger and then structure your examination as follows:

Is papilloedema present?

- is the disc margin distinct or blurred?
- are small vessels at the margin obscured?
- are veins on the disc distended and not pulsating?
- is the disc abnormally pink?
- is the physiological cup filled?

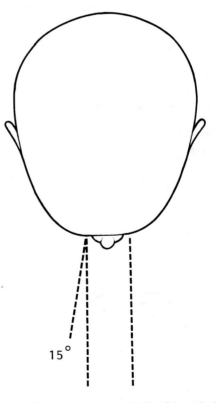

Fig. 8.2 Ophthalmoscopic examination of the optic disc. An approach 15° to the axis of fixation will allow sight of the optic disc immediately.

Is the disc atrophic?

- is the disc abnormally pale?
- are the arteries abnormally attenuated?
- is the disc margin sharp or blurred?
  (primary or secondary optic atrophy respectively)
- are there retinal abnormalities present which are associated with optic atrophy, i.e. retinitis pigmentosa.

Are there other abnormal features of the disc? Abnormalities noted at this stage might be medullated nerve fibres or drusen. The former present as irregular white patches with feathered margins which obscure the disc and vessels but are of no significance. The latter (colloid bodies) are seen as small, yellowish-white spots which are a concomitant of normal ageing.

After the optic disc, examine the retina and finally the fovea. The retina is best searched by following out from the disc each of the four main retinal vessels to about three or four disc diameters. The fovea can be examined reducing the size or intensity of the light source on the ophthalmoscope and asking the patient to look just to one side of the light. A 'blind spot' noticed by the patient close to central vision may be due to a retinal lesion near the macula. And the same lesion may give symptoms of unilateral impairment of central visual acuity.

Visual acuity Distance vision is measured using the Snellen chart. Near vision is measured using the Jaeger or Rayner Test Types. In either case the patient should be tested using his appropriate spectacles or contact lens (i.e. reading glasses for near vision). If, as is often the case, the patient has forgotten to bring his distance glasses the Snellen visual acuity can be tested asking the patient to view the chart through a pinhole in a card (see Chapter 22).

Any patient with visual symptoms should have his visual acuity recorded in the notes so that a comparative record over time can be kept. The same applies to records of the visual fields.

Visual fields The normal testing of visual fields depends on confrontation although this may need to be supplemented with more detailed charting using the Bjerrum screen, grey screen, Goldmann apparatus or perimeter (see Chapter 22).

Confrontation depends on comparing the extent of the patient's visual field with that of the examiner. Its great advantage is that the patient's attention and visual fixation can be assessed throughout the procedure.

The patient is first asked to fixate the bridge of the examiner's nose. While the examiner fixates the patient's eye he moves a finger in each of the four peripheral quadrants of the visual field, asking the patient if he can detect the movement (Fig. 8.3). In this way a homonymous field defect can be recognized.

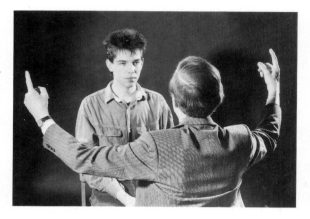

Fig. 8.3 The initial stage in testing visual fields.

Simultaneous movement of the finger in the periphery of right and left field will exclude a 'visual attention defect'. Then use the same method on each eye separately with the other closed to exclude a monocular peripheral visual field defect.

The central visual field and the blind spot has to be tested using a coloured pin-head 4 mm in diameter. With one eye covered and the patient fixating the examiner's eye, the pin-head is moved in such a way that the patient can report the area affected by the blind spot. The examiner can compare the size or shape of his own blind spot with that of the patient and in the normal the two should precisely coincide.

Using the red pin-head abnormal defects in the central visual field of each eye separately can be similarly plotted and should be recorded with a diagram in the notes (Fig. 8.4). Remember that the patient's field of vision is a lateral inversion of the field of vision of the examiner. It is easy to draw a defect in the notes 'back to front'!

III, IV and VI. The oculomotor, trochlear and abducent nerves

These nerves individually or collectively are responsible for (a) the pupillary responses; (b) eye movement and (c) elevation of the upper eyelid. Under (a) and (c) we are not only testing for a lesion of these cranial nerves but may also be testing for a defect of

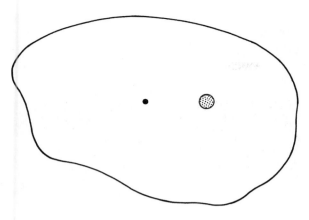

Fig. 8.4 The normal visual field of the right eye plotted with the examiner's left eye.

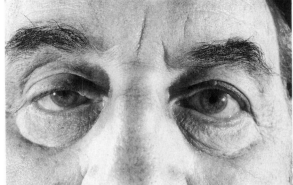

Fig. 8.5 Right Horner's syndrome. Note the ptosis and small right pupil. Other features which may be difficult to elicit include enophthalmos and absent sweating on the affected side.

the sympathetic or parasympathetic nervous system. Under (b) likewise we may elicit nystagmus or a disorder of conjugate eye movement (failure of the eyes to deviate together) indicative of disturbance of the cerebellum, brainstem or the 'supranuclear' pathways in the cerebral hemispheres.

Pupils The pupils should be equal (E) and react (R) directly and consensually to light (L) and convergence (C). This may be abbreviated in notes to 'PERLC'.

The consensual light response is the pupillary constriction that occurs when a light is shone in the opposite eye. Observations on each of these characteristics should be carried out in order ending with direct stimulation of each pupil with a bright torch shone obliquely at the eye.

If the pupils are unequal and irregular this may indicate damage or disease of the iris (e.g. due to surgery or iritis). Neurosyphilis may cause small irregular unequal pupils (Argyll—Robertson pupil). A unilateral small pupil may indicate Horner's syndrome (Fig. 8.5) which is the combination of a small pupil, drooping of the eyelid, loss of sweating in the face and slight retraction of the eye. This syndrome results from dysfunction of the sympathetic nervous system on that side. The sympathetic supply to the head leaves the spinal cord at T1 and ascends to the bifurcation of the carotid artery where the fibres to the pupil and upper eyelid separate from those concerned with sweating. A lesion below this point will therefore give the full syndrome, whereas a lesion above this point will only affect the pupil and the eyelid.

A unilateral large pupil may indicate a lesion of parasympathetic nerve supply (Holmes—Adie syn-

drome) or a lesion of the oculomotor (IIIrd) nerve which carries the pupilloconstrictor fibres to the eye from the brainstem. In the Holmes—Adie syndrome the large pupil reacts sluggishly to direct and indirect stimulation whereas in the latter situation the dilated pupil will be associated with the disorder of eye movement due to weakness of the muscles supplied by the third nerve.

Eye movements are tested by asking the patient to look at your finger and follow it first up and down and then laterally to the limits of binocular gaze. Any defect of eye movement should then be re-tested with one eye closed. The control of eye movements by the IIIrd, IVth and VIth nerves is summarized in Fig. 8.6. Finally where visual symptoms have been mentioned your patient should be asked whether double vision develops at any point of lateral or vertical deviation of the eyes.

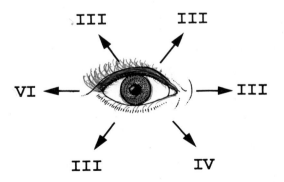

Fig. 8.6 The action of the IIIrd, IVth and VIth nerves on eye movements of the right eye.

In this way it should be possible to identify the following abnormalities of eye movement:

(i) Weakness in one eye of elevation and adduction indicating a IIIrd nerve lesion. This is usually associated with drooping of the eyelid (ptosis) and a large unreactive pupil and results in the eye looking downwards and outwards (Fig. 8.7).

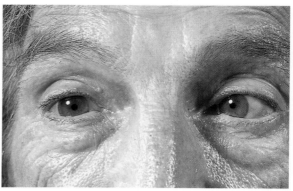

Fig. 8.8 Left VIth nerve lesion showing weakness of abduction of the eye (left lateral rectus muscle weakness).

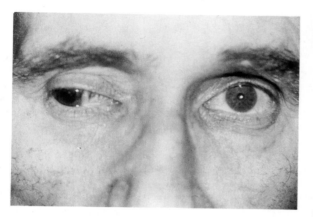

Fig. 8.7 Right IIIrd nerve lesion showing ptosis, large pupil and deviation of the eye downwards and outwards.

(ii) Weakness of abduction of one eye indicating a VIth nerve palsy (Fig. 8.8).
(iii) Double vision and torsion of the globe of the eye on downward gaze indicating a IVth nerve lesion.
(iv) Loss or impairment of conjugate vertical or horizontal gaze indicating a lesion above the level of the brainstem oculomotor nuclei.
(v) Weakness of adduction in one eye with nystagmus (jerky, unsustained eye movement) in the abducting eye on lateral gaze indicating a lesion of the median longitudinal bundle in the brainstem between the IIIrd and the VIth nerve nuclei (Fig. 8.9). This is usually due to multiple sclerosis but may occur with vascular or structural lesions.
(vi) Vertical nystagmus indicating an intrinsic lesion either high in the brainstem (vertical nystagmus on upward gaze) or low in the brainstem (vertical nystagmus on downward gaze).

(i), (ii) and (iii) usually indicate lesions of these nerves outside the brainstem due to compression or

stretching of the nerve or disturbance of its blood supply.

(iv)–(vi) indicate disturbance of brainstem function either through a lesion of the brainstem or mechanical distortion of its structure.

Elevation of the eyelid may be weak resulting in ptosis (see Table 22.4). This occurs in IIIrd nerve palsy and Horner's syndrome on the same side. It may occur bilaterally although not always symmetrically in disorders of muscle such as myasthenia gravis or the ocular myopathies where it is generally associated with some weakness of the upper facial muscles (frontalis and orbicularis oculi) (Fig. 8.10).

Lid retraction and lid lag is characteristic of thyroid disease and is considered elsewhere (Chapter 12).

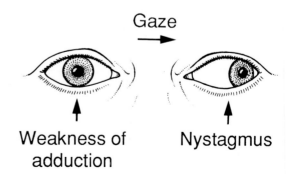

Fig. 8.9 Eye movements indicating a lesion of the median longitudinal bundle. With gaze to the left the right eye fails to adduct whereas the abducting left eye shows nystagmus.

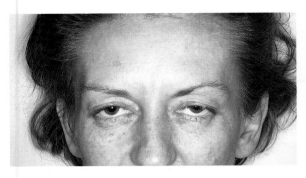

Fig. 8.10 Bilateral asymmetrical ptosis in myasthenia gravis.

V. The trigeminal nerve

The sensory loss of trigeminal nerve lesions conforms precisely to the territory of the trigeminal nerve and it is therefore important to know the exact distribution of the ophthalmic, maxillary and mandibular divisions (Fig. 8.11).

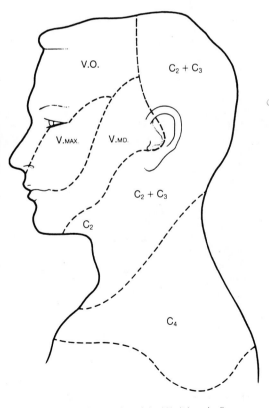

Fig. 8.11 The sensory innervation of the Vth (trigeminal) nerve.

As with testing other sensory nerves, pain is tested by pinprick using a disposable pin (not a hypodermic needle where the point is sharpened to a cutting edge). Helpful patients will often report parts of the face where the pin feels 'less sharp'. This is usually not significant. Loss of the perception of pain especially when associated with loss or impairment of cotton wool light touch in the same area is usually significant especially when it fills an anatomical territory recognizably that of a branch or branches of the trigeminal nerve.

The corneal reflex tests the sensation of the corneal conjunctiva supplied by the ophthalmic division. It is elicited by touching the cornea with a wisp of cotton wool having first warned the patient and asked him to look up. Loss of the reflex blink is abnormal. In this case the patient should be asked whether pain is felt (the corneal sensory receptors are only sensitive to pain).

The terminal parts of the mandibular division in its lingual branch carry taste sensation from the tongue but loss of taste due to damage to this branch will be associated with loss of pain and touch over that part of the front of the tongue.

Damage to the maxillary nerve in the sinuses or facial bones may affect the superior dental nerves giving anaesthesia in the upper teeth and hard palate on one side. Sensory loss in this area is tested with a pin and/or a stick.

Occasionally weakness of the muscles of mastication may occur when hollowing of the temporal fossa may be seen; the masseter muscle on the surface of the mandible may feel thinner than the other side. When the patient is asked to open his mouth against resistance unilateral pterygoid weakness will cause the jaw to deviate to the same side.

The jaw-jerk is obtained by tapping with the patella hammer on the point of the chin, with the patient asked to hold his mouth slightly open. In the normal reflex, closure of the mouth is just detectable. Where the jaw-jerk is increased it implies a bilateral pyramidal lesion above the Vth nerve nucleus in the brainstem. Conversely brisk jerks in the limbs with a normal jaw-jerk suggests a pyramidal lesion in the cervical region.

VII. The facial nerve

The facial nerve supplies the muscles of the face and runs a complicated anatomical course accompanied initially by the sensory fibres subserving taste.

Weakness of half the face may occur as the result of a lesion of the facial nerve but may also result from an upper motor neurone (pyramidal) lesion above the VIIth nerve nucleus.

To test facial movement the patient is asked to screw up his eyes 'as if soap might get into them', bare his teeth (or gums) 'in a big grin' and to puff out his cheeks. Observations of asymmetry and the absolute bilateral weakness should be made although the latter may be very difficult to detect. Strength of closure of the eyes can be tested by trying gently to prize the eyes open. Note if the eyelashes are buried symmetrically.

Upper motor neurone weakness (UMN) of the facial muscles is characteristically predominantly lower facial in distribution sparing frontalis. This is because there is bilateral innervation of the muscles of the upper part of the face. Emotional movements such as smiling may be spared with cortical lesions. By contrast a lower motor neurone lesion (LMN) will cause weakness of the upper and lower face on the affected side (Table 8.4).

The commonest cause of a lower motor neurone facial weakness is the idiopathic Bell's palsy (Fig. 8.12(a) and (b)) — a benign condition where pain in the region of the ear is followed by the development of a unilateral facial weakness often associated with unilateral impairment of taste on testing and the symptom of hyperacusis due to damage of the branch

Table 8.4. Causes of a lower motor neurone facial weakness
*Bell's palsy
*Middle ear disease
Ramsey–Hunt syndrome (geniculate herpes)
Acoustic neuroma
Non-Hodgkin's lymphoma
Sarcoidosis (uveoparotid fever)
Carcinoma of parotid
Damage following surgery to ear or parotid gland
Leprosy (in tropics)

* Common causes

of the facial nerve to the stapedius muscle. With attempted closure of the eyelids the eye on the paralysed side rolls upwards (Bell's phenomenon) (Fig. 8.12(c)).

VIII. The auditory and vestibular nerves

The severity of the hearing loss can most conveniently be assessed at the bedside by the following test. The

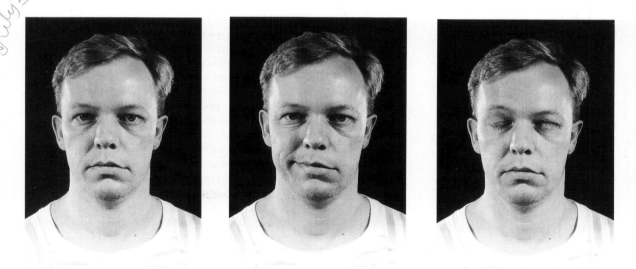

(a)   (b)   (c)

Fig. 8.12 Left Bell's palsy. (a) Minimal evidence of weakness at rest; (b) note the left absent nasolabial fold on smiling; (c) Bell's phenomenon: with attempted eye closure the globe rolls upwards.

opposite ear is occluded by shaking a finger in the external meatus; at the same time hearing is tested in the deaf ear by softly whispering a series of numbers in a progressively louder voice at a distance of about 1 m. It is important to cover your mouth with your other hand so that the patient cannot lip-read.

Conductive deafness, due to damage to the conducting mechanism in the external ear, eardrum, or middle ear must be distinguished from perceptive or nerve deafness where the lesion affects the cochlea or the auditory nerve itself. This distinction is made by doing Weber's test. A high-pitched tuning-fork (>512 Hz) when placed on the middle of the forehead is heard louder in the deaf ear when deafness is conductive, or mixed; and louder in the opposite ear when the deafness is perceptive.

Rinne's test of bone conduction is only necessary where a mixed bilateral deafness is suspected. In this case the patient is asked where the tuning-fork seems louder — in front of the ear (air conduction) or when placed on the mastoid process (bone conduction). The test should indicate perceptive or conductive deafness respectively but false results may occur; for example, a severe nerve deafness none the less allows the patient to perceive the tuning fork when it is ringing on the mastoid process by bone conduction to the other side (see also Chapter 23).

In any case of conductive deafness examine the external meatus and tympanic membrane with the auroscope. Any case of perceptive deafness, unless the cause can be readily identified on clinical grounds, should be referred for detailed testing of caloric responses and cochlea function.

The vestibular nerve and otolith apparatus of the inner ear may be tested at the bedside by examination for nystagmus and by positional tests. Thus horizontal nystagmus on lateral gaze with a rotary component usually indicates a recent disturbance of the vestibular nerve, its central nuclei or connections; or occasionally the semicircular canals. Long-standing peripheral lesions are not associated with nystagmus.

Positional tests may allow the symptom of positional vertigo (vertigo induced by sudden head movement) to be distinguished into central and benign peripheral types (see also Chapter 23).

The patient is moved quickly from the sitting position to lying with his head back and turned to one side. This change of posture may either (a) give rise to immediate vertigo and nystagmus indicative of a central cause, or (b) lead to vertigo and nystagmus after a latent interval of about 5 s and which stops after about 15 s. This latter response is indicative of a disturbance of the otolith apparatus in the inner

ear and is usually a benign, self-limiting condition attributable to a viral infection or a head injury.

It is noteworthy that structural lesions affecting the auditory nerve in the posterior fossa such as an acoustic neuroma give rise to a perceptive deafness usually associated with some degree of trigeminal sensory loss and facial weakness. Where a unilateral perceptive deafness is therefore found very careful testing of the corneal reflex and facial movement is mandatory.

IX and X. The glossopharyngeal nerve and the vagus nerve

Tests of sensation and movement in the pharynx are only relevant where there are symptoms of dysphagia, dysphonia or dysarthria; or where there are other signs of lower brainstem involvement.

Sensation in the pharynx (IXth nerve) is tested by getting the patient to open his mouth wide, depressing the tongue with a spatula and then touching each side of the posterior wall of the pharynx with an orange stick. The patient is then asked whether the sensation was similar on the two sides.

Reflex gagging to this stimulus is associated with elevation of the soft palate and lifting of the posterior wall of the pharynx; these movements should be central. Deviation of the uvula to one side indicates a Xth nerve lesion on the opposite side.

Bilateral Xth nerve weakness gives rise to nasal speech and (where the recurrent laryngeal nerve is involved) to dysphonia. Early degrees of weakness of the larynx are best tested by asking the patient to cough. The vocal cords must be examined in any patient suspected of unilateral or bilateral vocal cord paralysis (see Chapter 23).

XI. The accessory nerve

This is a motor nerve supplying the sternomastoid and trapezius muscles.

The sternomastoids are tested by asking the patient to turn his head to one side while the movement is opposed by pressing on the side of the chin. The opposite sternomastoid can be seen to contract and unilateral weakness can be confirmed by asking the patient to push his head forward against resistance placing the examiner's hand on the forehead and observing both muscles in the front of the neck.

The upper fibres of trapezius are tested by asking the patient to shrug his shoulders 'up to the ear'. The muscle can be seen and felt running between the upper part of the neck and the spine of the scapula.

A unilateral lesion of the accessory nerve implies compression or damage to the nerve in or near the jugular foramen or in the neck.

XII. The hypoglossal nerve

This nerve is a pure motor nerve to the tongue. It is tested first by observing the tongue when the patient is asked to open his mouth. Look for any sign of unilateral wasting or generalized fasciculation. Fasciculation is a continuous, random, irregular contraction of groups of muscle fibres (comprising a motor unit) and gives the appearance of tiny twitches and momentary dimpling of the tongue surface. The patient is then asked to protrude the tongue. Fasciculation and wasting is again looked for and if there is a weakness of one side of the tongue it will deviate to that side (Fig. 8.13).

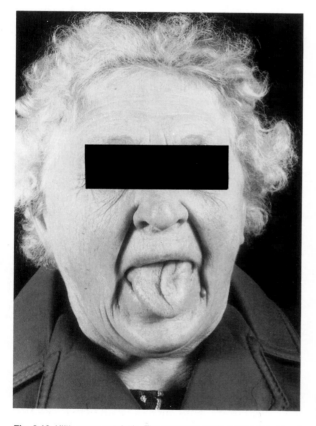

Fig. 8.13 XIIth nerve paralysis. The tongue is protruded to the side of the weakness.

The patient is then asked to flick the tongue rapidly from side to side and a slowness or paucity of movement suggests either an upper motor neurone lesion or an extrapyramidal deficit, as in Parkinson's disease.

Unilateral lower motor neurone weakness of the tongue is rare and suggests damage to the nerve in the base of the skull. Fasciculation and atrophy of the tongue indicate a lesion of the anterior horn cells, usually motor neurone disease.

Motor system

The examination of the motor system aims to establish whether there is weakness, whether there is an abnormality of cerebellar function or whether there is an extrapyramidal disturbance. If there is a weakness examination of the patient must establish whether the weakness is due to an upper motor neurone lesion, a lower motor neurone lesion or whether it is primarily due to disease of the muscle itself (myopathy).

The history will already have alerted you to the likely possibilities; watching the patient walk into the examination room may establish that one ankle appears to be weak and 'floppy', that the patient walks in an unsteady inco-ordinated manner as if drunk, or that he or she does not swing one arm.

Upper limb

Examine the arm first for signs of muscle wasting. Careful scrutiny of the small hand muscles is necessary if there is a possibility of median or ulnar nerve damage or a T1 root lesion (Fig. 8.14). Don't forget to look for wasting of other muscles of the limb girdle (Fig. 8.15). Look for fasciculation, especially if motor neurone disease is possible. This is seen as small irregular twitches in the muscle flitting from place to place in a random way. Irregular, coarse twitches recurring in the same place usually indicates myokimia which is a normal phenomenon.

Muscle tone may be increased (hypertonia) or decreased (hypotonia).

Hypertonia may be spastic (pyramidal) or rigid (extrapyramidal). In spasticity the resistance to passive movement increases initially and as the movement is continued the resistance falls away — the 'clasp-knife phenomenon' referring to the resistance experienced when the blade of a penknife is opened. Rigid hypertonia produces a resistance that feels uniform throughout the range of movement although it may be slightly jerky or 'cogwheel' in Parkinson's

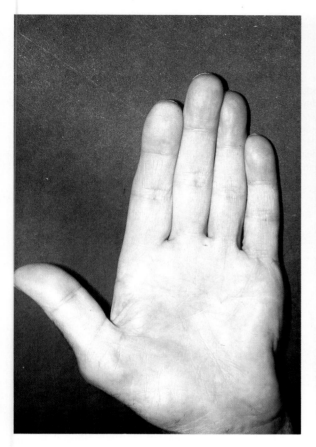

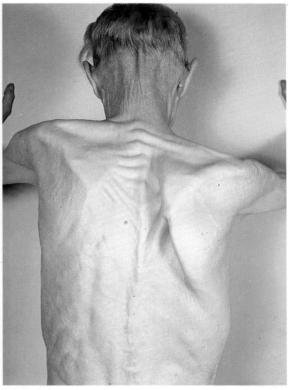

Fig. 8.15 Wasting of latissimus dorsi muscle (C6,7 and 8).

Fig. 8.14 Wasting of the thenar muscles in a median nerve lesion.

disease. Test tone by alternately flexing and extending the patient's elbow and wrist. A brisk movement is more likely to initiate the clasp-knife phenomenon and the patient must remain with the muscles relaxed throughout. Nervousness, cold, and actual or expected pain will cause the patient voluntarily to resist the movements imposed by the examiner and make testing for muscle tone impossible. If the patient is unable to relax the arm, distract his attention with conversation while continuing the examination.

Power should next be tested and this must be done in a methodical manner always concentrating your attention on the limb or group of muscles likely to be affected (Table 8.5). If an upper motor neurone lesion is suspected the deltoid, triceps and forearm extensors are the muscles more likely to be weak. Commit to memory the segmental root supply of the main muscles of the shoulder, elbow, wrist and hand. If a cord or root lesion is suspected work down through the segmental supply testing C6 muscles first and T1 muscles last. Before testing for a median, ulnar or radial neuropathy, bear in mind which muscles are likely to be affected and compare one side with the other. Thus where a median nerve lesion at the wrist is likely from the patient's history of painful nocturnal paraesthesiae test abduction of the thumb first on the normal side so that the patient understands what is required. And then compare the strength of the same movement on the side of the symptoms. When the strength exerted by the patient varies from moment to moment, it is the greatest power that he can exert, if only momentarily, that is significant. Scoring of muscle power is defined in Table 8.8.

Tenderness to palpation of a weak muscle may occur in some neuropathies (e.g. alcoholic) and in inflammatory diseases of muscle (myositis).

Co-ordination tests in the upper limb seek to identify

Table 8.5. Root supply of muscles in the upper limb

Joint supply	Muscle	Action	Root supply	Peripheral nerve
Shoulder	*Deltoid*	Abduction	C5,6	Circumflex nerve
	Infraspinatus	External rotation	C5,6	Suprascapular nerve
Elbow	Biceps	Flexion	C5,6	Musculocutaneous nerve
	Brachioradialis	Flexion	C5,6	Radial nerve
	Triceps	Extension	C7,8	Radial nerve
Wrist	*Ext. carp. radialis longus*	Extension	C6,7	Radial nerve
	Extensor and flexor carpi ulnaris	Ulnar deviation	C7,8	Radial and ulnar nerves
	Extensor digitorum		C7,8	Radial nerve
Fingers	Flexor digitorum profundus and sublimis		C8	Median nerve
	Thenar muscles		T1	Median nerve
	Other intrinsic hand muscles		T1	Ulnar nerve

Muscles selected for their usefulness in localizing a lower motor neurone weakness. Those muscles which tend to be weak in a mild pyramidal deficit are in italic.

either impairment of cerebellar function or extrapyramidal deficits as in Parkinson's disease. Tests of cerebellar function cannot be done when there is severe weakness. Occasionally severe joint-position sense loss will give inco-ordination indistinguishable from cerebellar ataxia.

First ask the patient to touch the tip of his nose with the forefinger and then to touch your finger held about 70 cm from his face and then to go backwards and forwards a few times. Normally the alternating movements should be smooth but in cerebellar ataxia the movement becomes jerky and the patient may 'overshoot' the target (past-pointing). 'Terminal intention tremor' describes a tremor of the hand as it approaches the target and is characteristic of cerebellar disease (for discussion of tremor see below). Alternating movements such as tapping one hand on the back of the other, or alternating pronation–supination movements of the forearm become jerky and irregular (dysdiadokokinesia).

Fine-controlled, manipulative movements of the upper limb are characteristically impaired in extrapyramidal disorders but pyramidal deficit may also lead to slowness and awkwardness in these movements. In the absence of signs of spastic weakness therefore, an inability to perform nimbly discrete finger movements is suggestive of Parkinson's disease. Ask the patient to touch each fingertip to the thumb in turn and then repeat the movement: or to tap rapidly with the forefinger with the hand resting on the desk. Writing is probably the best test of fine movement in the dominant hand.

Tendon reflexes are elicited with the patient again relaxed and at ease. Hold the limb at the wrist, which should be slightly extended. The supinator- (or brachioradialis-) jerk is obtained by tapping the region of the head of the radius at the wrist with the patella hammer. A contraction of brachioradialis can be seen but also look for simultaneous finger flexion which may imply an increased finger-jerk. The biceps-jerk is obtained by tapping your left index finger placed on the patient's biceps tendon at the elbow; and triceps-jerks by tapping the triceps tendon at the elbow. The finger-jerk may be difficult to obtain and needs practice. With the patient's arm pronated the hand is held with the fingers semiflexed and the wrist slightly extended. An upward tap on the fingertips will lead to a reflex jerk of the forearm finger flexors.

The segmental level for these jerks is shown in Table 8.5. A useful checklist for testing various aspects of motor function is shown in Table 8.6.

When it is difficult to obtain a reflex, or the reflex appears to be absent, an attempt should be made to 'reinforce' the tendon-jerk. This can be done by forcible contraction of muscles remote from those being tested. Thus to reinforce the knee- or ankle-jerks the patient can be asked to hook his hands together and then to try to pull them apart; for the upper limb reflexes he can be asked to clench his jaw.

Table 8.6. Assessment of motor function

Check list for assessing motor function	Wasting
	Tone
	Power
	Co-ordination
	Reflexes

The phenomenon of reinforcement only lasts for a second or two.

Trunk and neck

Occasionally in a patient with suspected Parkinsonism tone in the neck muscles may be increased and may be examined by rolling the head from side to side on the pillow. Power in the neck is tested by opposing voluntary flexion of the neck by pressing on the forehead; the trunk muscles are tested by asking the patient to sit up from lying flat with his arms folded. Deviation of the umbilicus during this movement implies weakness of the anterior abdominal muscles on one side.

The abdominal reflexes should be tested by stimulating the skin in each quadrant of the abdomen with a stick and observing for contraction of the underlying muscles. The abdominal reflexes are abolished in pyramidal deficits or in lower motor neurone weakness. They may also be difficult to elicit in patients who are obese or during pregnancy and shortly after childbirth.

Lower limbs

The same order of examination is adopted in the lower limbs as for the upper limbs — inspection, then muscle tone and power, co-ordination and finally reflexes.

Fasciculation in the leg muscles may be of no significance but asymmetry of muscle bulk may indicate a lower motor neurone lesion. Arthritis of the knee may also cause wasting of the quadriceps but the reflexes are normal and muscle power if testable is also well preserved.

Muscle tone is tested at the knee and ankle by holding the leg at the knee and the front of the foot and feeling for resistance to flexion at the knee and ankle. As in the arm, rigid (extrapyramidal) or spastic (pyramidal) hypertonia may be found. Quick dorsiflexion of the ankle may cause a few beats of 'clonus' or involuntary jerks of plantar flexion at the ankle usually indicating a pyramidal deficit but occasionally these may be seen in very tense individuals. Patellar clonus may be elicited with the knee fully extended and a sudden downward movement to the patella stretching quadriceps and provoking involuntary repetitive jerking contractions.

Power in the leg muscles should be tested methodically as in the arms. In Table 8.7 10 selected muscles are listed which usually allow an anatomical diagnosis of a lower motor neurone lesion. Assessment of

Table 8.7. Root supply of muscles in the lower limb

Joint	Muscle	Action	Root supply	Peripheral nerve supply
Hip	*Ilio-psoas*	Flexion	L1,2,3	Femoral nerve
	Adductors	Adduction	L2,3,4	Obturator nerve
	Rectus femoris	Flexion	L3,4	Femoral nerve
	Gluteus maximus	Extension	L5;S1	Inferior gluteal nerve
Knee	*Quadriceps*	Extension	L3,4	Femoral nerve
	Hamstrings	Flexion	L5;S1	Sciatic nerve
Ankle	Tibialis anterior	Dorsiflexion	L4,5	Anterior tibial nerves
	Peronei	Eversion	L5;S1	Common peroneal nerve
	Gastrocnemius/soleus	Plantar flexion	S1,2	Medial popliteal nerve
Foot	*Extensor digitorum brevis*	Hallux dorsiflexion	S1	Anterior tibial nerve

Muscles selected for their usefulness in localizing a lower motor neurone weakness. Those muscles which tend to be weak in a mild pyramidal deficit are in italic.

what is normal in terms of muscle strength is largely acquired by experience but comparison of the normal side with the abnormal is useful in detecting slight weakness.

Weakness should be graded and recorded so that serial observations allow assessment of the rate of progression or recovery (Table 8.8). It is often helpful also to assess upper neurone lesions (especially in the lower limb) in terms of disturbance of function. How far can the patient walk on the flat; can he manage stairs, or getting out of a bath; what appliance (stick, crutch, frame) is necessary for walking? In the arm the grading system is most applicable to weakness in the shoulder or elbow, for example, in cases of progressing polyneuritis or myasthenia gravis.

Table 8.8. Grading of muscle power

Grade 5 — Normal power
Grade 4 — Weak but power sufficient to overcome gravity and resistance
Grade 3 — Very weak but just able to overcome gravity
Grade 2 — Able only to move the limb if supported against gravity
Grade 1 — Flicker or trace of contraction
Grade 0 — Total paralysis

Co-ordination tests in the legs must include tests of balance, gait and stance off the examination couch and these may most conveniently be done at the start of the examination when it is clear from the history or preliminary observations that such tests are important. In Romberg's test the patient is asked to stand with feet together and eyes closed. Impaired position sense in the feet or severe vertigo or cerebellar ataxia will cause the patient to sway. 'Tandem walking' — that is heel-to-toe walking — will reveal minor degrees of ataxia of gait. On the couch the patient is asked to place the heel of one foot on the knee of the other leg and then slowly and neatly slide it down and up the front of the shin. In cerebellar disturbance the heel will wobble off the front of the shin. Repetitive tapping movements of the foot may be impaired in patients with Parkinson's disease when no other deficit is noticeable in the legs.

The patella and ankle reflexes are tested as follows. Support the semiflexed knees with your left forearm and tap the patella with the patella hammer. The ankle-jerks can be elicited either with the leg slightly

flexed at hip and knees and externally rotated at the hip, or alternatively with the legs together and straight on the bed. In the first case tap the Achilles tendon directly with the front of the foot supported with your left hand; in the second case tap your hand which is supporting the front of the foot. In all situations the force of the tap to elicit a jerk should begin quite gently and be reduced or increased according to whether a reflex is obtained or not.

Examination of the reflexes is completed with the plantar (Babinski) response. The normal reflex to stimulation of the sole of the foot is flexion of the big toe. In pyramidal lesions the big toe extends and this is a reliable indicator of corticospinal tract disturbance when the test is correctly performed. Holding the foot in a neutral position at the ankle the sole is gently stimulated by drawing a stick along the line as in Fig. 8.16. Only increase the strength of the stimulus if no response is obtained, because the plantar response is unpleasant for the patient and if painful the withdrawal response will obscure the physical sign.

The sensory system

The aim of sensory examination is to establish the distribution of any sensory loss in such a way that conclusions may be drawn about the anatomical site of the lesion producing the loss. Where the lesion affects the peripheral nerves the sensory loss is usually of an 'associated type' (Table 8.9), i.e. all modalities tend to be affected in the relevant territory. Pain sense, position sense, light touch and temperature will therefore all be affected where, for example, damage to the brachial plexus leads to sensory loss in the hand. But where the lesion affects the central nervous system the sensory loss is characteristically 'dissociated', i.e. one sensory pathway in the central nervous system will be more affected than the other

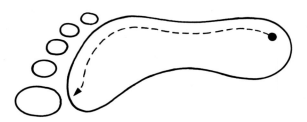

Fig. 8.16 The direction of the stimulus on the sole of the foot to elicit the plantar (Babinski) response.

Table 8.9. Causes of peripheral neuropathy		
Western world	{	Undetermined causes*
		Diabetes*
		Alcoholism*
		B$_{12}$ deficiency
		Drugs
		Paraneoplastic
		Polyarteritis
		Amyloidosis
Tropical disease	{	As above
		Leprosy*
		Pellagra
		Thiamine deficiency

* Common.

by virtue of their anatomical separation. The Brown–Séquard syndrome perhaps best exemplifies this dissociation where hemitransection of the spinal cord gives rise to loss of pain and temperature on one side of the body below the level of the lesion and loss of position and vibration sense on the other side (Fig. 8.17).

Begin your sensory examination with the lower limbs, working upwards over trunk and upper limbs to the neck. This way the highest level of sensory disturbance can most easily be established. The lesion cannot be below this level. Examine first for loss or impairment of light touch, position and vibration; then for pain and temperature so that any dissociation of sensory loss can be immediately identified.

Light touch sensation is tested with cotton wool. Two grades of abnormality are recognized — loss or impairment. Where light touch is 'lost' the patient fails altogether to report the stimulus. Where light touch is 'impaired' the patient recognizes that the perception is less than it should be or when compared with the other side. The over-helpful patient may mislead by reporting spurious impairment of light touch but when such impairment is accompanied by paraesthesia such as tingling it is normally significant.

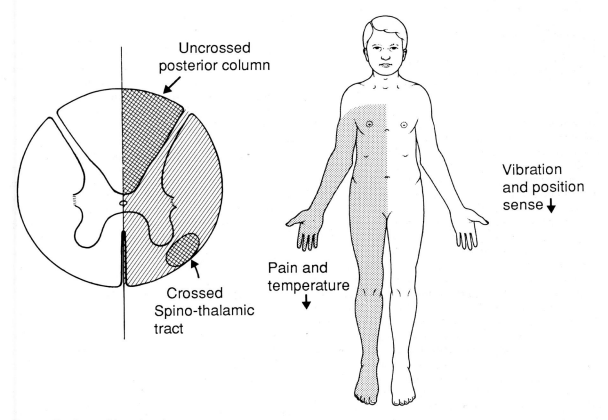

Uncrossed posterior column

Crossed Spino-thalamic tract

Pain and temperature ↓

Vibration and position sense ↓

Fig. 8.17 The Brown–Séquard syndrome.

Test pain sensibility with a pin which should not be sharp enough to penetrate the skin. The distinction the patient is asked to make is whether he can perceive the pricking sensation of the pin point; or whether it feels blunt like a matchstick. Again pain sensation may be lost or impaired thus implying different severities of sensory disturbance. Remember to discard your pin into an appropriate container at the end of the examination; there is always the chance of transmitting hepatitis B or HIV infection, however remote.

Temperature sensation should be tested using warm and cold test tubes. A rapid check of temperature sensation may be made using the cold tuning-fork and the patient asked whether he can feel the cold of the metal.

Position sense should be tested in the big toe and index finger extending the examination to other limb joints when appropriate. Hold the digit near its tip and explain to the patient that he should say 'up' or 'down' according to the direction of movement (not, incidentally, the absolute position in relation to the mean position). The initial displacement of the toe should be fairly gross to train the patient as to what is required. But in the big toe a 5 mm movement at the tip should be easily detectable and a 2 mm movement in the index finger likewise.

Vibration sense is tested using a 128-Hz tuning-fork applied to the malleoli. If the patient cannot feel vibration at the ankle, go on to test for vibration sense at the knees or hips or costal margins as necessary.

In the patient with neither sensory symptoms nor motor signs, sensory examination can be limited to testing for position sense in the upper and lower limbs (because loss of position sense may not be accompanied by any symptoms) and a check that the patient perceives light touch and pin prick normally and symmetrically on the upper and lower limbs.

In some patients the sensory examination may need extending to additional modalities. Two-point discrimination should be tested with blunt dividers specially made for the purpose (but a paper-clip suitably bent may serve as well). The patient is asked to say whether, with his eyes closed, he perceives two or one point of pressure on the skin. The normal threshold of two-point discrimination over the instep is about 2.5 cm whereas on the fingertip less than 5 mm should be detectable. This is a useful test in patients with peripheral or mononeuropathy. It is essential in cases where parietal sensory loss is suspected.

Lesions of the parietal lobe may give rise to an unusual form of sensory dissociation where the patient has preservation of light touch, pain and temperature but loses two-point discrimination and becomes unable to identify objects such as a coin by feel (astereognosis) and cannot identify numbers written by pressure on the palm of the hand (graphaesthesia). Sensory inattention may also be present in such a case. This is demonstrated by touching or pinpricking both arms or legs simultaneously.

In these circumstances, the patient reports the stimulus on the normal side but fails to perceive it on the affected side whereas when the abnormal side is tested alone the sensation is perceived apparently normally. Careful instructions have to be given, e.g. 'please tell me if I touch your right hand, or your left hand, or both hands'.

When you have completed your sensory examination record your findings on a figure chart so that the precise extent of the abnormality on the date has been established.

You should have a fairly clear idea from the history and motor examination what you are looking for, so concentrate on the sensory signs that will confirm or refute your suspicions. Thus where an ulnar nerve lesion is suspected, concentrate on the precise distribution of sensory loss over the ring finger and at the wrist; whereas in a suspected cord lesion the highest dermatome affected will point to the likely spinal segmental level (Fig. 8.18).

General medical examination

Following the neurological examination general physical examination of the patient including blood-pressure measurement and urine testing is essential. Some parts of the general examination are particularly relevant to the nervous system and require special attention. A patient with suspected meningitis or subarachnoid haemorrhage should be examined for neck stiffness on passive neck flexion.

Limitation of straight-leg raising (normally to 90°) may indicate nerve root irritation in the lumbar spinal canal. The patient with signs suggestive of a spinal cord lesion must always have his vertebral column carefully examined for deformity or tenderness to percussion to look for focal skeletal abnormality. The contour of the skull may be a vital sign in a patient with Paget's disease (see Fig. 2.1), meningioma, or

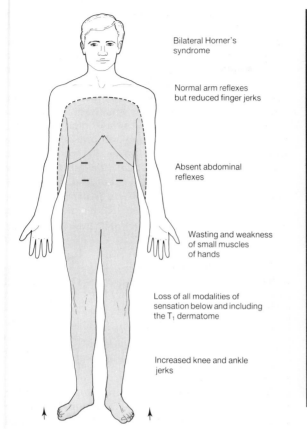

Bilateral Horner's
syndrome

Normal arm reflexes
but reduced finger jerks

Absent abdominal
reflexes

Wasting and weakness
of small muscles
of hands

Loss of all modalities of
sensation below and including
the T₁ dermatome

Increased knee and ankle
jerks

Fig. 8.18 The effects of a cord lesion at T1 level.

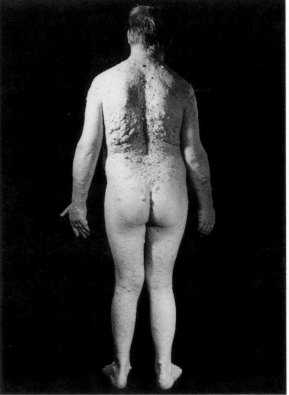

Fig. 8.19 Neurofibromatosis. The patient also had a spastic paraparesis due to multiple neurofibromata compressing the spinal cord.

developmental anomaly in the region of the foramen magnum (Arnold–Chiari malformation). Skin lesions may indicate neurofibromatosis (Fig. 8.19), Sturge–Weber syndrome (Fig. 8.20) or tuberose sclerosis (Fig. 8.21), all of which have important neurological associations. Very occasionally auscultation of the skull or orbits may reveal a bruit denoting arteriovenous malformation, fistula or aneurysm.

In the patient with an acute hemiplegia (Fig. 8.22) possible aetiological factors in the cardiovascular system must be identified including hypertension, carotid bruits, facial plethora and rhythm disturbances (Fig. 8.23).

Any patient with the possibility of raised intracranial pressure such as headache, papilloedema and vomiting, must be examined for evidence of a primary neoplasm, such as bronchus, breast or kidney.

Eye signs may denote thyroid eye disease associated with clinical features indicating thyrotoxicosis. Metabolic disorders may be the cause of epilepsy, or abnormal involuntary movements including tremor.

The unconscious or poorly responsive patient

The examination of the unconscious patient presents an emergency where a clear plan of action is essential. From the outset establish that the airway is clear and that ventilation and circulatory support has been provided where necessary.

Even where the diagnosis seems obvious (for example in severe alcoholic intoxication) possible

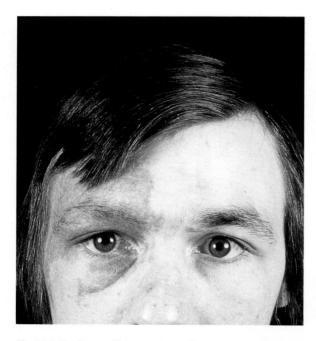

Fig. 8.20 The Sturge—Weber syndrome. The port-wine stain affects the skin innervated by the trigeminal nerve. The vascular network of the orbit and meninges is similarly affected. The patients suffer from epilepsy and glaucoma.

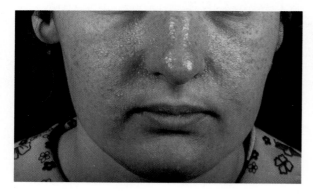

Fig. 8.21 Tuberose sclerosis. This uncommon disease of dominant inheritance is characterized by fits, mental deficiency and adenoma sebaceum. These lesions can be seen on the cheeks.

of these data to a member of the nursing staff or other medical staff.

The examination of the unconscious patient should always start with a general physical examination and venepuncture so that laboratory tests can be set in hand early. The neurological examination should follow these preliminaries. Obviously the management of the patient depends greatly on the circumstances. In the Western world self-poisoning, hypoglycaemia, alcoholic intoxication, head trauma and stroke are common causes for admission to hospital in an unconscious state. In the tropics the association of coma with fever will lead one to consider other diagnoses such as cerebral malaria, meningitis and encephalitis. Some of the more important causes of coma are listed in Table 8.10.

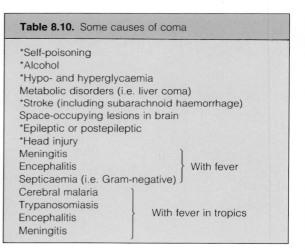

Table 8.10. Some causes of coma

*Self-poisoning
*Alcohol
*Hypo- and hyperglycaemia
Metabolic disorders (i.e. liver coma)
*Stroke (including subarachnoid haemorrhage)
Space-occupying lesions in brain
*Epileptic or postepileptic
*Head injury
Meningitis ⎫
Encephalitis ⎬ With fever
Septicaemia (i.e. Gram-negative) ⎭
Cerebral malaria ⎫
Trypanosomiasis ⎪ With fever in tropics
Encephalitis ⎬
Meningitis ⎭

* Common causes in Western world.

Whether or not the cause of the coma is clearly related to a neurological disorder, an assessment of the level of consciousness, using the Glasgow coma scale, should be made at an early stage (Table 8.11). Observations according to this scale can be repeated later by different observers.

The fundi should be examined for papilloedema, and for haemorrhages — which when subhyaloid in type indicate sudden recent rise of intracranial pressure.

Disturbance of function in the upper brainstem may lead to coma and such disturbance may result from either displacement of the brainstem by a mass lesion above or below the tentorium cerebelli or by a

alternative or contributory causes of coma should always be considered. The history must be obtained from every available source including eye witnesses, family, general practitioner, ambulance personnel and police. Previous hospital records may be invaluable where there is a past history of diabetes or epilepsy. It may be necessary to leave the collection

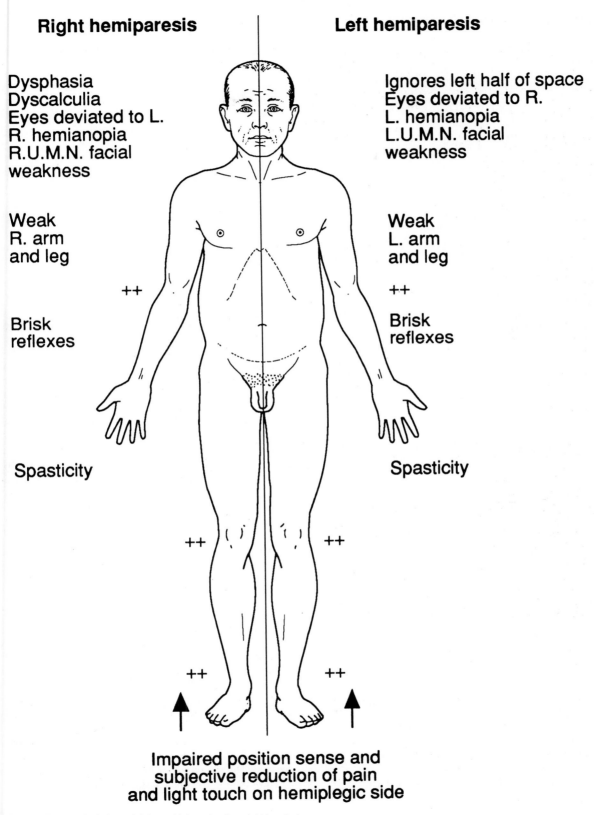

Right hemiparesis

Dysphasia
Dyscalculia
Eyes deviated to L.
R. hemianopia
R.U.M.N. facial
weakness

Weak
R. arm
and leg

++

Brisk
reflexes

Spasticity

Left hemiparesis

Ignores left half of space
Eyes deviated to R.
L. hemianopia
L.U.M.N. facial
weakness

Weak
L. arm
and leg

++

Brisk
reflexes

Spasticity

++   ++

++   ++

Impaired position sense and
subjective reduction of pain
and light touch on hemiplegic side

Fig. 8.22 The physical signs of right and left strokes in a right-handed person.

Table 8.11. The Glasgow coma scale

Eye opening	Spontaneous	4
	To command	3
	To pain	2
	Nil	1
Verbal response	Orientated	5
	Confused conversation	4
	Inappropriate words	3
	Incomprehensible sounds	2
	Nil	1
Best motor response	Obeys commands	6
	Localizes	5
	Withdraws	4
	Abnormal flexion	3
	Extension response	2
	Nil	1

focal lesion in or adjacent to the brainstem. Signs of brainstem dysfunction are:

- asymmetry of the pupils or poor light reaction or dilatation. In drug overdose the pupils typically remain responsive to light although narcotic overdose may lead to pin-point pupils
- tonic deviation of the eyes, or loss of eye movements. Eye movement may be induced by the 'dolls head' manoeuvre where the patient's head is turned quickly to one side with the eyes open. The eyes lag behind the head movement normally but follow passively with head movement if fixation and oculocephalic reflexes are absent
- unilateral ptosis
- corneal reflexes absent or asymmetrical

Physical evidence of hemiplegia should next be sought. Unilateral facial weakness may be evident by one cheek blowing out in expiration or one side of the face failing to grimace as strongly as the other to painful stimuli. The posture of the limbs on one side may suggest hemiparesis and lack of reflex withdrawal to pain, increased (or sometimes absent) reflexes and rarely a unilaterally extensor plantar response may confirm. Test pharyngeal sensation and gag reflex by stimulating the posterior wall of the nasopharynx and test sensation in the limbs by observing the reaction to painful stimuli to the sternum, nasion, hands and feet.

Epileptic status (continuous epileptic discharges in the brain) may give rise to clonic movements that are focal or generalized. The suspicion of epileptic status is an indication for urgent electroencephalography.

Decerebrate extensor spasms of the trunk and limb muscles suggest severe disturbance of function in the upper brainstem or deep cerebral structures. Thus large cerebral haemorrhages compressing thalamus and mid-brain but sparing the pons may present in this way.

It is important to realize that signs of brainstem dysfunction leading to coma may conceal signs of brain disturbance in the hemisphere. In any such case urgent CT scanning is necessary to establish the pathological anatomy of the brain.

The diagnosis of brain death

Modern life-support techniques and the use of organs for transplantation make it essential that rigid criteria exist for the diagnosis of brain death.

To consider the diagnosis of brain death the fol-

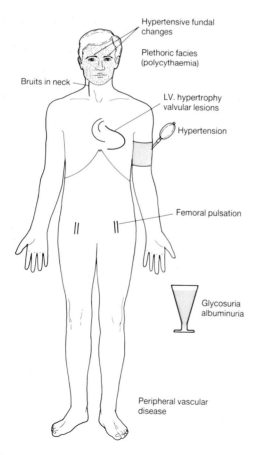

Hypertensive fundal changes

Plethoric facies (polycythaemia)

Bruits in neck

LV. hypertrophy valvular lesions

Hypertension

Femoral pulsation

Glycosuria albuminuria

Peripheral vascular disease

Fig. 8.23 Risk-factors for strokes.

lowing conditions should be fulfilled and should exist concurrently:

1. The patient should be deeply comatose.
   (a) Inherent in this condition is the absence of any depressant drugs in the circulation such as narcotics, tranquillizers and hypnotics.
   (b) Primary hypothermia should be excluded.
   (c) Metabolic and endocrine causes for coma should have been excluded.
2. The patient should be, of necessity, maintained on a ventilator because of previous inadequacy or cessation of respiration.
3. A firm diagnosis of irremedial brain damage should have been established.

Consequent upon these conditions being fulfilled the following tests, which require confirmation after an appropriate interval which might be as long as 24 h, are required for definitive diagnosis of brain death. All brainstem reflexes should be absent. This is accepted if:

1. The pupils are dilated and do not respond to light.
2. Vestibular ocular (calorific) reflexes are absent. These may be tested by irrigating each external auditory meatus in turn with 20 ml of ice-cold water, care having been taken to establish that the tympanic membranes are intact and the external auditory canals are unobstructed. The reflexes are absent when no eye movement occurs.
3. Corneal reflexes are absent.
4. There are no motor responses within the cranial nerve distribution after adequate stimulation.
5. There is loss of gag and bronchial stimulation reflexes.
6. There are no respiratory movements after disconnection from the respirator for a sufficiently long period to allow the $P_{a}CO_2$ to reach 6.7 kPa (50 mmHg).

It is important to remember that spinal reflexes may persist after brain death and that electroencephalography is not necessary to diagnose brain death.

References and further reading

Aids to the examination of the peripheral nervous system. London: Baillière Tindall, 1986.

Elkington AR, Khaw PT. The eye and the nervous system. *British Medical Journal*. 1988; **297**: 59–62.

Godwin-Austen RB, Bendall J. *The neurology of the elderly*. London: Springer, 1990.

Harrison MJG. *Neurological skills*. London: Butterworths, 1986.

Parsons M. *A colour atlas of clinical neurology*. London: Wolfe, 1988.

Wilkinson IMS. *Essential neurology*. Oxford: Blackwell, 1988.

9

Anaemia, blood diseases and enlarged glands

P. J. Toghill and S. S. Jalihal

> Symptoms
> Examination
> References and further reading

This chapter deals with the symptoms and signs in the anaemias, haemorrhagic disorders, haematological malignancies and lymphomas. These are diseases in which a definitive diagnosis requires a blood count, bone marrow examination and/or lymph-node biopsy. Nevertheless, the doctor seeing the patient for the first time should be able to arrive at a realistic diagnosis on basic clinical examination.

Symptoms

Tiredness

Professor Bryan Matthews, the neurologist, complained that 'there can be few physicians so dedicated to their art that they do not experience a slight decline in spirits on hearing that their patient's complaint is that of giddiness'. For many doctors the symptom of tiredness falls into a similar category. Many patients complain of tiredness and suggest that they may be anaemic.

In fact tiredness correlates poorly with anaemia. Most tired patients have normal haemoglobin levels and mild anaemia with levels down to 9.0 g/dl does not usually cause symptoms by itself. Undoubtedly patients with haemoglobin levels below 7.0 g/dl are likely to be tired but they will probably also complain of breathlessness, faintness and pounding headaches. The rate of fall in the haemoglobin level is often the major factor in determining the severity of symptoms. A 50-year-old mother of six may be unaware of her

chronic anaemia of 7.5 g/dl whereas her previously healthy, 20-year-old student son would feel grievously ill if he dropped his haemoglobin to a similar level after a melaena stool.

The point is that with anaemic patients it is of critical importance to measure the haemoglobin level rather than to rely on symptoms. The level of the haemoglobin and the red cell indices define the type of anaemia and the questions that must be asked. The young housewife with an iron-deficiency anaemia needs to be asked about her periods, previous pregnancies and duration of breast-feeding, and dietary habits. A 60-year-old factory worker with a similar blood count needs to be questioned carefully about his indigestion, abdominal pain and rectal bleeding as leads for possible sites of gastrointestinal bleeding.

Bleeding and bruising

In general excessive bleeding and spontaneous bruising are more common with thrombocytopenia than with hereditary defects in the coagulation pathways. In haemophilia, for example, patients bleed spontaneously into muscles and joints.

Much depends on whether the problems are new or old. If an hereditary coagulation defect, like haemophilia, is suspected you need to enquire closely about family history. It is also imperative to ask about blood-loss with operations earlier in life such as circumcision and tonsillectomy. Someone who has coped with surgery of this kind without excessive blood-loss is unlikely to have a significant hereditary coagulation problem. A recent onset of unusual bleeding from mouth and gums with gross bruising after trivial trauma suggests a serious acquired defect. However, easy spontaneous bruising without underlying pathology in middle-aged women (devil's pinches) and in the elderly (senile purpura) are extremely common.

Swollen glands

Swollen lymph glands, unless related to an acute infection such as glandular fever or tonsillitis, have to be taken seriously. It is imperative to find out how long the glands have been swollen and whether or not they have been painful. Pain in enlarged glands after drinking alcohol is suggestive of Hodgkin's disease.

Fever and sweating

These of course are common, non-specific features of disease. However, recurrent or persisting fever in the absence of other pointers may indicate occult lymphoma in the UK or tuberculosis in the undeveloped world. Fever recurring at intervals in Hodgkin's disease is sometimes referred to as Pel–Ebstein fever but it is uncommon.

Night sweats

Drenching night sweats may accompany the fever in the lymphomas or tuberculosis. Ask your patient about the extent of his sweating. If it is sufficient to require a change of pyjamas or the bed-sheets it is highly likely to be due to a serious disorder.

Skin itching (pruritus)

Skin itching without a rash may be the harbinger of serious underlying disease.

It may be a symptom of the lymphomas, usually but not necessarily in those patients with advanced disease. It is often present in polycythaemia when the irritation may become a torment after a hot bath. Patients with other myeloproliferative disorders such as myelosclerosis may suffer pruritus as may those with simple anaemias.

Drugs

Patients with unexplained anaemias must be questioned carefully about drugs. Exposure to some potentially toxic drugs may be obvious as with gold injections for rheumatoid arthritis. What may be less evident is that a patient with aplastic anaemia received chloramphenicol in a proprietary cough medicine bought whilst on a Mediterranean holiday some weeks earlier. Do interrogate patients carefully and firmly about medicines and tablet-taking. It is better not to use the term drug when asking about medications; many patients think you are only referring to addictive substances when you talk about drugs. They may also forget to tell you about substances that are not actually prescribed but which they buy over the counter at the chemists. Patients with glucose 6-phosphate dehydrogenase (G6DP) deficiency from West Africa, the Mediterranean and Asia may develop haemolytic anaemia with certain drugs such as the antimalarials or dapsone. Table 9.1 lists some drugs that have important haematological implications.

Table 9.1. Examples of some drugs that can cause serious haematological reactions

Drug	Use	Possible haematological adverse reactions
Phenylbutazone	Ankylosing spondylitis	Marrow aplasia
Chloramphenicol	Antibiotic	Marrow aplasia
Cotrimoxazole	Antibacterial	Marrow aplasia
Fansidar	Malaria	Agranulocytosis
Carbimazole	Thyrotoxicosis	Agranulocytosis
Gold	Rheumatoid arthritis	Thrombocytopenia
Penicillamine	Rheumatoid arthritis	Thrombocytopenia
Methyldopa	Hypertension	Haemolytic anaemia
Dapsone	Dermatitis herpetiformis	Haemolytic anaemia*

* With G6DP deficiency.

Infection

Many haematological disorders may present with infective episodes, particularly of the respiratory tract. It is not unusual to diagnose chronic lymphatic leukaemia, almost as an incidental finding, in an elderly patient with pneumonia. Neutropenia must be always suspected in a young or middle-aged patient who presents with unusual, florid and ram-paging bacterial infection. Of course, opportunistic infections are common in the immunocompromised haematological patients, such as those receiving chemotherapy.

Pain

Bone pains are common in patients with bone marrow disease, particularly myeloma (see Fig. 17.22) where vertebral collapse is common. A dull, dragging pain over an enlarged spleen, in such diseases as myelo-sclerosis, may be aggravated by episodes of splenic infarction. Remember that sickle-cell crises in the tropics may cause severe abdominal pain simulating surgical emergencies such as acute appendicitis.

Examination

Anaemia

As has been pointed out earlier, clinical assessment of anaemia, particularly in the elderly, can be fraught with difficulties and the only true measure is that of the haemoglobin concentration in the blood. The traditional site used for judging anaemia is the palpebral conjunctiva but this may be reddened unduly by such diverse factors as rubbing, hay-fever and conjunctivitis. The colour of the nail-beds, fingers or tongue may be helpful but it is only when the haemoglobin concentration falls below $7-8$ g/dl that a reasonably confident diagnosis of anaemia can be made clinically. A lemon-yellow tinge of the sclerae with intense pallor of the conjunctiva should suggest the possibility of associated haemolysis. There are, of course, sundry causes of anaemia and indeed multiple aetiologies may be present in any one patient. Nevertheless, there are some discriminatory physical signs. Spoon-shaped, ridged nails (koilony-chia) are frequently associated with long-standing iron-deficiency anaemia with depletion of body iron stores (see Fig. 18.3). Retinal haemorrhages frequently coexist with severe anaemia of B_{12} deficiency and are not necessarily caused by the thrombocytopenia which may also be present. Curiously, retinal haemor-rhages rarely complicate severe iron-deficiency anaemia even at similarly low levels of haemo-globin. Leg ulcers are seen in the chronic haemolytic anaemias, particularly the haemoglobinopathies but less commonly other congenital haemolytic anaemias such as hereditary spherocytosis. A smooth, depapil-lated tongue with angular cheilosis may accompany both chronic iron-deficiency anaemia and the macro-cytic anaemia of B_{12} or folate deficiency (see Figs 5.1 and 5.9). Look for the red spots round the mouth, lips and nose in patients with hereditary haemorrhagic telangiectasia (Osler−Weber−Rendu syndrome) (see Fig. 5.4). Chronic blood loss from these lesions may cause an iron-deficiency anaemia. Physical signs linked with the commoner types of anaemia are shown in Table 9.2.

Excessive bleeding

Spontaneous bleeding into the skin and other organs

Table 9.2. Some physical signs related to the type of anaemia			
	Iron deficiency	Macrocytic anaemia due to B_{12} or folate deficiency	Haemolytic anaemia
Sclerae	White	Faintly icteric	Icteric
Nails	Koilonychia	Normal (clubbed if associated with malabsorption)	Normal
Tongue	Smooth	Smooth and sometimes sore	Normal
Lips	Cheilosis	Cheilosis	Normal
Fundi	Normal	Retinal haemorrhages	Normal
Leg ulcers	Do not occur	Do not occur	Common in haemoglobinopathies
Splenomegaly	Rare	Rare	Common except with sickle-cell disease

Table 9.3. Sites of bleeding with various haemorrhagic disorders

Basis for bleeding	Usual causes	Common sites of bleeding
Thrombocytopenia	Infiltrative bone marrow disease Idiopathic thrombocytopenic purpura Drugs (including chemotherapy) Hypersplenism	Skin (purpura and ecchymoses) (if severe — nose, gastrointestinal tract, CNS, fundi)
Vascular defects	Henoch–Schönlein purpura Infections (i.e. meningococcal septicaemia) Drugs Vasculitis Scurvy	Skin (purpura), gut, kidneys Skin (purpura) Skin (purpura) Skin, gut, kidneys Skin and gums
Coagulation defects	(a) Hereditary defects of clotting (b) Excessive anticoagulation (c) Disseminated intravascular coagulation (d) Liver disease	(a) Soft tissues Joints (b) Retroperitoneal spaces, skin, gut and other sites (c) Various sites (d) Various sites
Hyperviscosity	Macroglobulinaemia Myeloma	Fundi, nose and skin

constitutes a common clinical problem. Such excessive bleeding may be the result of thrombocytopenia, disorders of the small blood vessels, coagulation defects or dysproteinaemia. In general the bleeding due to thrombocytopenia and small vessel defects is initially into the skin (purpura and ecchymosis) whereas with the commoner hereditary coagulation defects it is into muscles and joints. Sites of bleeding in the various haemorrhagic disorders are summarized in Table 9.3.

Purpura is the extravasation of blood from small vessels into the skin and mucous membranes (Fig. 9.1(a) and (b)). The lesions which are usually a few mm in diameter, do not blanch on pressure and fade to a brownish colour after a few days. Purpura may be due to thrombocytopenia or defects of the blood vessels as in anaphylactoid or Henoch–Schönlein purpura. Skin haemorrhages which coalesce are termed ecchymoses (bruises) (Fig. 9.2). Purpura develop first in dependent areas such as shins and ankles because of increased venous pressure. With severe thrombocytopenia, bleeding develops from sites other than the skin such as orifices, gastrointestinal tract and central nervous system. It is important to search for retinal haemorrhages in severe thrombocytopenia as they may be the harbinger of life-threatening intracerebral haemorrhage.

The bleeding of the hereditary coagulation defects is episodic, often unpredictable but frequently provoked by trauma. The commonest of these diseases is haemophilia which is a sex-linked, recessive dis-

order associated with deficiency of the procoagulant activity of factor VIII. The less common Christmas disease is inherited in precisely the same way but is associated with factor IX deficiency. Von Willebrand's disease is transmitted as an autosomal dominant trait and is characterized by a prolonged bleeding time and an abnormality of factor VIII carrier protein. Bleeding in these coagulation disorders is mainly into deep tissues, muscles and joints. Recurrent joint bleeds result in a chronic arthropathy. Bleeding due to excess anticoagulant therapy as with warfarin is frequently retroperitoneal. Such bleeding may cause skin-staining in the loins, psoas irritation and spasm with flexion and internal rotation of the thigh, and nerve palsies such as of the iliofemoral nerve (Fig. 9.3).

Though strictly not a defect of haemostasis, senile purpura should also be mentioned in this section. Characteristically dark red patches appear on the extensor surfaces of the forearms with minimal or even no preceding trauma (Fig. 9.4). Similar lesions may be seen in the tissue-paper skin of those patients on long-term steroid therapy. The basic defect is thought to be defective collagen formation allowing shearing strains to tear small blood vessels.

Excessive and spontaneous bleeding may be seen in the dysproteinaemias, particularly in such high-viscosity states as macroglobulinaemia. The chronic periorbital haematomas seen occasionally in amyloidosis constitute a rare but striking and diagnostic physical sign (Fig. 9.5).

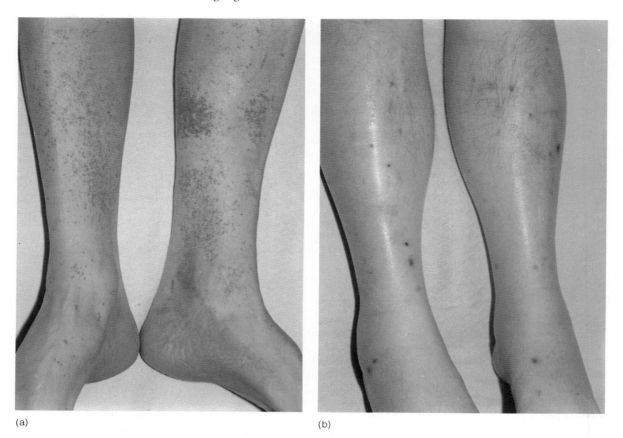

(a)   (b)

Fig. 9.1 Purpura in patients with (a) Henoch—Schönlein disease and (b) meningococcal septicaemia — note that in this disease the purpura are often sparse and need to be looked for carefully.

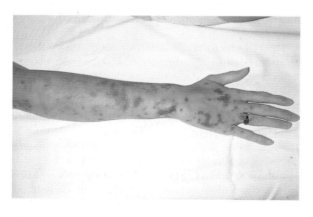

Fig. 9.2 Bruises (ecchymoses) in a patient with coagulation defects due to acute hepatic necrosis.

Splenomegaly

Assessment of spenic size is critical in patients with haematological disorders and has already been discussed in Chapter 6 (see Figs 6.24 and 6.25; Table 6.4). It is not enough to comment on spleen size in finger-breadths below the left costal margin. Measure and record the maximum distance of the medial and lower border at right angles from the costal margin.

Lymph-node enlargement

A question that the doctor often has to answer is 'Does this patient have significant lymphadenopathy?'. Many normal people have palpable lymph nodes in neck, axillae and groins and careful examination and much experience are necessary to select those patients who require further investigation and

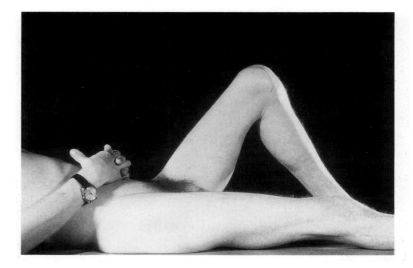

Fig. 9.3 Psoas spasm causing hip-flexion in a haemophiliac with a retroperitoneal bleed.

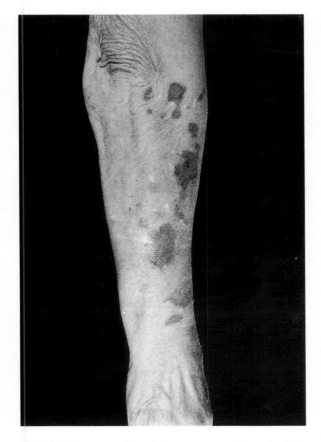

Fig. 9.4 Senile purpura. These lesions are commonly seen in elderly women with thin skin but identical appearances are seen after long-term steroid therapy.

possible biopsy. Some simple points have to be remembered. Lymphoid tissue tends to atrophy with age and therefore the young tend to have larger nodes than the elderly. Certain lymph nodes, notably the tonsillar glands at the angle of the mandible, may remain enlarged and palpable throughout life as a result of recurrent tonsillar infections. Manual workers such as bricklayers and farmers frequently traumatize their hands and arms and may have easily palpable axillary nodes. Inguinal glands are usually palpable in healthy persons but palpable nodes extending down the femoral chain on both sides are a good deal less common. Epitrochlear glands are normally never palpable in health but they enlarge early in diseases such as glandular fever, syphilis, and the progressive generalized lymphadenopathy of HIV infection. They are often easily palpable in rheumatoid arthritis.

Palpation of enlarged glands should be performed with meticulous care. Nodes in the neck are best felt from behind the patient with particular attention paid to the region behind the lower end of the sternomastoid muscle where enlarged glands may be missed. Axillary nodes are best felt with the examiner sitting facing the patient and sliding his left hand into the patient's right axilla and vice versa for the other side. For adequate visualization and palpation of the inguinal nodes the patient is best in a supine position.

The principal causes of generalized lymphadeno-pathy in young adults and older patients are shown in Table 9.4. In attempting to establish a diagnosis on clinical grounds much depends on the age of the

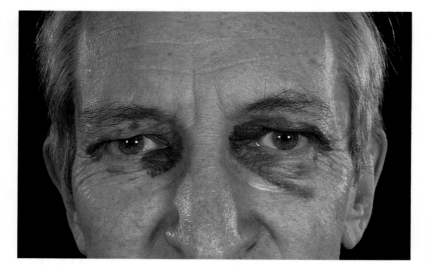

Fig. 9.5 Chronic periorbital haematomas in a patient with amyloidosis — a very rare physical sign, but almost pathognomonic when seen!

Table 9.4. Causes of generalized lymphadenopathy

		Children and young adults	Older patients
Infections	Glandular fever	Common	
	CMV	Common	
	Rubella	Common	Most becoming less
	Toxoplasmosis	Occasional	frequent with
	Brucellosis	Occasional	increasing age
	Secondary syphilis	Occasional	
	PGL	See Chapter 21	
	Non-specific response to viral infection	Common	
Leukaemia	Acute	Occasional	Occasional
	Chronic lymphatic	Does not occur	Fairly common
Lymphoma	Hodgkin's disease	Generalized lymphadenopathy only late in disease	Only late in disease
	Non-Hodgkin's lymphoma	Occasional	Common
Sarcoidosis		Occasional	Occasional
Tuberculosis		In tropics	In tropics
Metastatic disease		Occasional	Fairly common

patient, the duration and severity of his illness, and his racial and social background. Nevertheless, some basic principles hold good. The glands in infective disorders, exemplified by glandular fever, are usually discrete and less than 2 cm in diameter. In infective lymphadenopathy of this type the presence of enlarged epitrochlear nodes may be of particular help. Traditionally, secondary syphilis was stigmatized by the presence of enlarged epitrochlear nodes and the 'sailor's handshake' entailed a surreptitious clasp of the elbow to note their size! Now worries

about progressive generalized lymphadenopathy (PGL) related to HIV infection would be more appropriate. Enlarged glands in the posterior triangles along the posterior border of the sternomastoid may characterize the infective lymphadenopathies; in rubella the occipital nodes are particularly prominent. Tuberculosis is one of the few causes of infective lymphadenopathy in which nodes coalesce. It may be present in more than one lymph-node group.

Massive rubbery-firm lymphadenopathy is a feature of the lymphomas (Figs 9.6 and 9.7(a) and (b)).

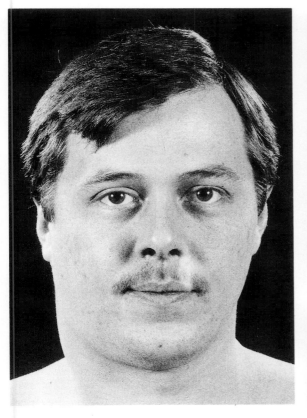

Fig. 9.6 Cervical lymphadenopathy in a patient with Hodgkin's disease. Enlargement of a single group of glands in the neck is the commonest mode of presentation of Hodgkin's disease.

The glands frequently form confluent masses and may involve overlying skin. The differences between the Hodgkin's and non-Hodgkin's lymphoma (NHL) are shown in Figure 9.8. Broadly speaking, in Hodgkin's disease the glands are initially restricted to the neck whereas in the non-Hodgkin's lymphomas the lymphadenopathy is diffuse at an early stage in the disease. Evidence of earlier treatment by radiotherapy may be evident by the tell-tale tattoo marks used by radiotherapists to define the treatment fields. In any patient with lymphadenopathy a careful search must be made for an enlarged spleen. The spleen is unlikely to be more than 2 or 3 cm below the left costal margin in the infective lymphadeno-pathies whereas it may be massively enlarged in the lymphoproliferative diseases.

Metastatic lymphadenopathy is marked by hard, irregular fixed glands in the drainage area of the primary tumour. Nevertheless, with some tumours,

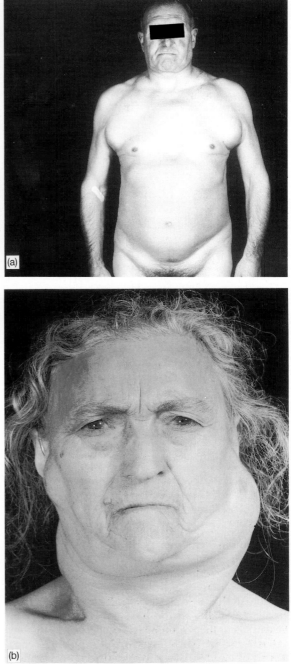

Fig. 9.7 (a) Generalized lymphadenopathy in a middle-age man with non-Hodgkin's lymphoma. Enlarged glands are seen in the neck, axillae and groins. (b) Massive cervical lymphadenopathy in non-Hodgkin's lymphoma.

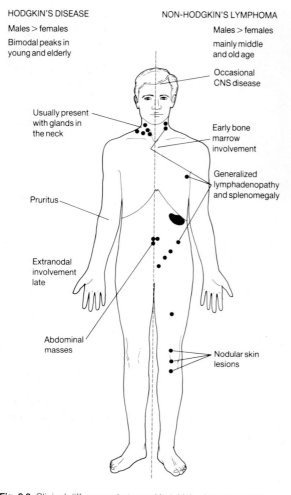

HODGKIN'S DISEASE

Males > females

Bimodal peaks in young and elderly

Usually present with glands in the neck

Pruritus

Extranodal involvement late

Abdominal masses

NON-HODGKIN'S LYMPHOMA

Males > females mainly middle and old age

Occasional CNS disease

Early bone marrow involvement

Generalized lymphadenopathy and splenomegaly

Nodular skin lesions

Fig. 9.8 Clinical differences between Hodgkin's disease and the non-Hodgkin's lymphomas.

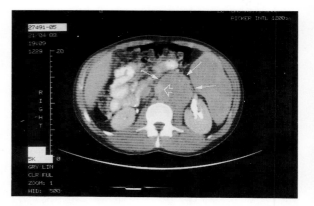

Fig. 9.9 Abdominal CT scan showing gross lymphadenopathy which was not palpable clinically. Note the 'floating aorta' lifted away from the bodies of the vertebrae (open arrow).

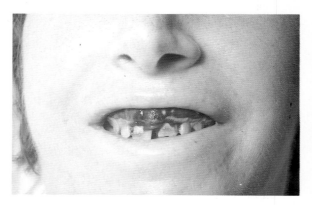

Fig. 9.10 Infected swollen gums in a patient with acute monoblastic leukaemia.

e.g. seminomas, there may be a widespread lymphadenopathy simulating lymphoma. The spleen is not usually enlarged in carcinomatosis.

Whereas enlarged glands are easily accessible and palpable in the neck, axillae and groins, considerable lymphadenopathy in the para-aortic region may be present, as in the lymphomas, which is not palpable. Figure 9.9 shows such an example; the patient complained of night sweats and loss of weight, yet there were no abnormal physical signs.

Acute and chronic leukaemia

Although the diagnosis of leukaemia requires careful blood and bone-marrow examination, certain physical signs point strongly to a suspected diagnosis.

In acute lymphoblastic and myeloblastic leukaemia the association of anaemia with sepsis, haemorrhages and lymphadenopathy are sinister findings. Many patients present at an early stage of the disease with bleeding manifestations due to thrombocytopenia. Bleeding, swollen infected gums are common signs in acute leukaemia. Gum hypertrophy, particularly in acute monoblastic leukaemia, may be so gross as to partly cover the teeth (Fig. 9.10). Haemorrhages and exudates may be seen in the fundi. Various skin manifestations as well as those due to excessive bleeding, include itchy, indurated papules and ulcerated nodules. Any indurated papular lesions must

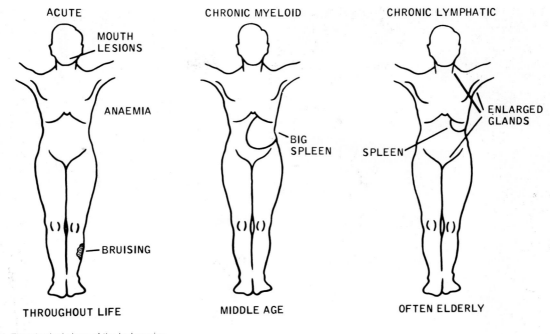

Fig. 9.11 The physical signs of the leukaemias.

always be regarded with suspicion and skin rashes of this type are a feature of chronic and subacute myelomonocytic leukaemia.

The chronic leukaemias may often be differentiated clinically by their physical signs (Fig. 9.11). Chronic granulocytic leukaemia often presents in middle-age with malaise, anaemia and massive splenomegaly, whereas chronic lymphatic leukaemia occurs in middle-aged or elderly folk, who have lymphadenopathy and splenomegaly. In chronic lymphatic leukaemia the enlarged glands may be quite soft and squashy. Generalized redness of the skin, the 'homme-rouge', may be a rare association with chronic lymphatic leukaemia.

Skin lesions of haematological and lymphoid malignancy

As well as the dermatological markers in the acute leukaemias that have been mentioned above, other rashes may supervene. Generalized ichthyosis may be a feature of Hodgkin's disease and nodules of lymphoma may appear on the skin in non-Hodgkin's lymphoma particularly of T-cell type. Probably the commonest skin rashes in haematological malignancy

are the opportunistic infections due to herpes simplex (Fig. 9.12(a)) and herpes zoster (Fig. 9.12(b)). Chickenpox may become a life-threatening disorder in immunosuppressed patients (Fig. 9.13).

The myeloproliferative syndromes

These haematological syndromes are characterized by proliferation of one or more of the elements of the bone marrow. The commonest disorders that form this group are polycythaemia rubra vera (PRV), chronic granulocytic leukaemia, myelosclerosis or myeloid metaplasia and essential thrombocythaemia. A common feature is splenomegaly which is often gross in myelosclerosis and chronic granulocytic leukaemia. The hyperviscosity of PRV and the massive splenomegaly of myelosclerosis may lead to constellations of physical signs that are shown in Figs 9.14 and 9.15. Secondary gout may complicate this group of diseases.

Haemoglobinopathies

These are disorders characterized by either the production of an atypical haemoglobin or by the

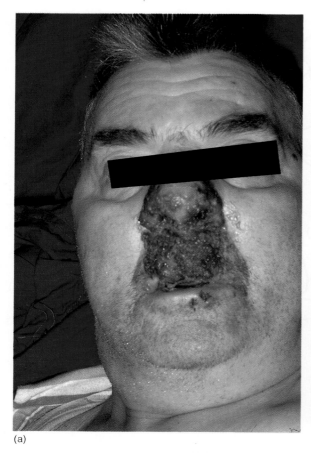

(a)

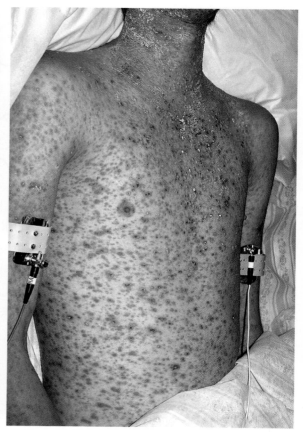

Fig. 9.13 Chickenpox in a young man undergoing chemotherapy for Hodgkin's disease. In this patient the lesions were originally haemorrhagic because of an associated thrombocytopenia.

(b)

Fig. 9.12 (a) Severe spreading herpes simplex in an immunosuppressed patient with chronic lymphatic leukaemia. (b) Herpes zoster in a patient with non-Hodgkin's leukaemia; note the root distribution of the vesicular lesions.

suppression of normal haemoglobin formation. The two most important haemoglobinopathies are sickle-cell disease and thalassaemia.

Sickle-cell disease, the homozygous state, is common in Negroes both in Africa and the Americas and the presence of West Indian migrants has increased the prevalence of the diease in the UK. It carries an appreciable morbidity and mortality. Children are usually small and slim and thrive poorly. Their physical signs with appearances are shown in Table 9.5 and Fig. 9.16. The spleen which is enlarged in childhood is the site of recurrent infarction which progresses to a hyposplenic state. Patients with sickle-cell disease are subject to painful infarcts in many sites. Those with sickle-cell trait only (10−20 per cent of Negroes) have few problems except under anoxic conditions.

POLYCYTHAEMIA

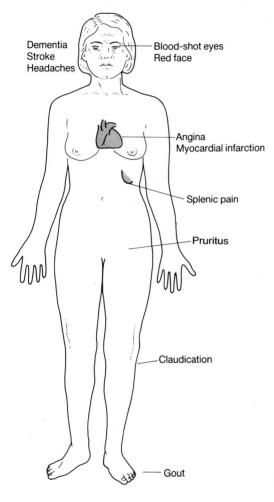

Dementia
Stroke
Headaches

Blood-shot eyes
Red face

Angina
Myocardial infarction

Splenic pain

Pruritus

Claudication

Gout

Fig. 9.14 The physical signs of polycythaemia rubra vera.

CLINICAL FEATURES OF MYELOSCLEROSIS

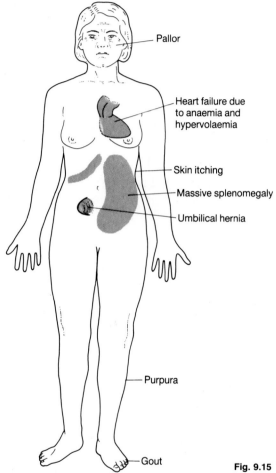

Pallor

Heart failure due
to anaemia and
hypervolaemia

Skin itching

Massive splenomegaly

Umbilical hernia

Purpura

Gout

Fig. 9.15 The physical signs in a patient with myelosclerosis.

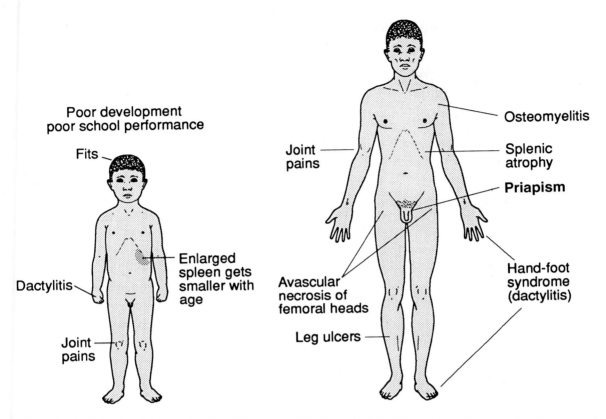

Fig. 9.16 The physical findings in (a) a small child and (b) a young adult with sickle-cell disease HbSS. Physical growth is stunted and mental development impaired. Early in life the spleen is enlarged but it becomes progressively smaller with recurrent infarction. Bactylitis occurs mainly in children and signs of transfusion dependence may be observed in adults.

Table 9.5. Clinical features in patients with haemoglobinopathies

Disease	General appearance	Facies	Spleen	Leg ulcers	Geographical distribution
Sickle-cell disease Hb.SS	Short, slim, narrow hands and feet	Bossing and tower skull	Enlarged in childhood Autoinfarction leads to hyposplenism in adult life	Common, particularly in tropics	Africa West Indies WI immigrants in UK Blacks in USA
Sickle-cell Hb.AS	Appear normal	Normal	Not enlarged	None	India
β-Thalassaemia major	Small, thrive poorly	Gross changes (Mongoloid type)	Grossly enlarged	May be present	Indian subcontinent
β-Thalassaemia minor	Mild anaemia (otherwise well)	Normal	Mildly enlarged in 20%	None	Mediterranean region Africa

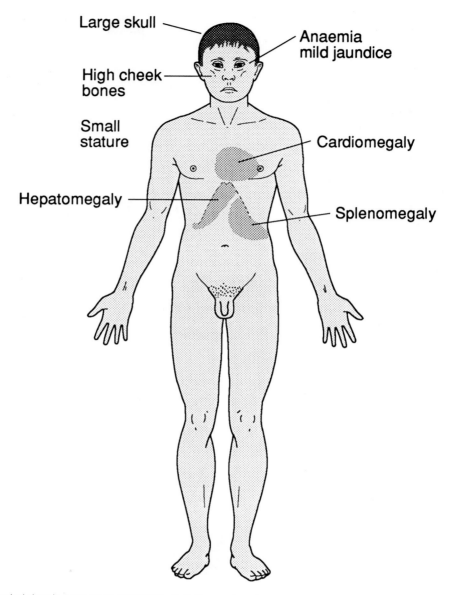

Fig. 9.17 The physical signs in a non-negro adolescent with thalassaemia major.

Thalassaemia is commonly found in a wide area of the world extending as a broad band through the Mediterranean region, into the Middle East, the Indian subcontinent and into South-East Asia. Children with homozygous B chain type disease are stunted with Mongoloid or chipmunk facies due to expansion of the marrow cavity in the skull and malar bones. Hepatomegaly and gross splenomegaly is common and the children do not often survive after early adult life (Fig. 9.17).

References and further reading

Hoffbrand AV, Pettitt JE. *Essential haematology*, 2nd edn. Oxford: Blackwell, 1987.

Hoffbrand AV, Pettitt JE. *Clinical haematology illustrated*. Edinburgh: Churchill Livingstone, 1987.

10

The presentation of psychiatric disorders in medical practice

Margaret Oates and R. Cantwell

Taking a psychiatric history

The psychiatric interview

Mental state examination

Psychological reactions to physical illness

Psychiatric illness in medical practice

Physical disorders of psychological origin

Specific types of psychological or somatoform disorders

References and further reading

This chapter tells you how to approach a patient with a view to taking a psychiatric history and how to complete an examination of the current behaviour and mental state. The psychiatric disorders most commonly encountered in general medical and surgical practice are described and special attention given to two types of disorder in which the relationships between physical and psychological symptoms are particularly close. These are, first, psychological reactions to the presence of physical illness, and second, psychiatric disorders which present with physical symptoms.

Taking a psychiatric history (Table 10.1)

This follows the same basic principles as a medical history. However, certain points are of particular importance. The description of the patient and his or her symptoms should be objective and describe what the doctor actually hears and the patient describes (descriptive), not what the doctor thinks the symptoms and signs mean (interpretive). The history is often the only tool of investigation in psychiatric disorder. It also has, in this situation, an important

function of establishing a working relationship between the doctor and the patient and marks the beginning of the therapeutic process.

The setting

A psychiatric history takes rather longer than a history in medicine and surgery and it is best to allow at least an hour for the first interview.

Many sensitive and private areas of the patient's life may be touched upon and it is therefore essential that the interview takes place in peace and quiet and in privacy. It is difficult to talk intimately about one's life in a curtained-off bed in a busy ward within earshot of other curious patients.

How not to antagonize your patient

It is always important to introduce yourself and explain exactly who you are and why it is that you want to talk to the patient in this way. Many patients in a general medical setting may be upset or even insulted by being asked questions about social and psychological issues and may readily jump to the conclusion that the doctor is implying that they are

Table 10.1. The psychiatric history
Name, age, address, marital status, occupation
Reason for referral
Presenting complaint Problem (or not) as the patient sees it, in his own words
Family history
Personal history
Childhood and adolescence — birth and neonatal health, separations, stability, relationships, unusual or traumatic events
Schooling
Adult life — relationships, occupations and achievements, sex, unusual experiences
Marriage — number, quality, sex, number of children and ages, health
Mental health after childbirth and marital problems
Present social circumstances — housing, members of household, their health and occupation, relationships, finances, problems
Past history Physical and psychiatric illnesses
Premorbid personality Attitudes, character, traits, habits, interests
History of present illness Onset, duration, chronological development, description of symptoms and disability, systemic enquiry. Help and treatment and its effect

'imagining' or 'putting on' their symptoms. They may feel that the doctor thinks that there is nothing wrong with them, that their symptoms are all in their mind. Anger on the part of the patient will not facilitate the flow of information and may well hinder co-operation in the future.

It is, therefore, important that doctors avoid giving this impression and that they should realize that pain of psychological origin hurts just as much as pain of physical origin. A headache that results from tension may be as painful and worrying to the patient as that which results from brain tumour. Breathing difficulties that result from panic and hyperventilation are as frightening and uncomfortable as asthma. Better to introduce the proceedings by saying 'We have been wondering if tension/anxiety/depression/worry has been making you feel ill' or by saying 'You are obviously in a lot of pain but so far we cannot find anything seriously physically wrong to account for it, perhaps we could talk a bit more about what has been happening to you recently'.

The psychiatric interview

The recording of a psychiatric history (Table 10.1) follows somewhat different pattern from that used for medical illness.

Longitudinal approach

If circumstances allow, it is probably better not only to record the information in this longitudinal way but also to take the history in this manner. Taking a longitudinal history involves beginning with the patient's parents and birth and then systematically gathering information about the patient's childhood and teenage years, schooling, independent adult life, marriage, jobs, etc., working gradually towards the present illness. It gives a much clearer idea of patients' usual levels of functioning, their strengths as well as their vulnerabilities, and their coping mechanisms and previous reactions to stress. It allows you to see how and when the current problems arose and in what context. Patients themselves do not always see the link between cause and effect. If you ask a patient after having taken an account of her/his present problems, 'Was anything upsetting you before this illness started' the answer may be 'No, not really'. If, however, you take a longitudinal history it may become apparent to you and to the patient that moving house, a parent dying, a daughter's marriage and a promotion, all occurring in the three months before the onset of the chest pain are indeed very relevant.

Presenting complaint

Start off the history by finding out briefly how the patient feels now and what they see as the problem.

Background

If circumstances allow, say to your patient 'perhaps we can go into this in more detail later, but first of all tell me more about yourself and your family. Are your mother and father still alive? How old are they? What do they do for a living? Have you got any brothers and sisters? Are they in good health? Whereabouts do you come in the family?' and so on. Then proceed through childhood, adolescence and adult life until the present time.

Past history

If the patient has had a lot of illnesses, be they physical or psychiatric, and a lot of unusual or stressful life-experiences, it is often worthwhile charting these by date in columns, with separate columns for events and physical illnesses, when a link in time may become evident. It is also important to ask patients how long it took them completely to recover from illnesses. Do not be embarrassed or reticent about asking patients about past psychiatric problems, e.g. 'Have you ever had problems in the past with depression/anxiety/nerves?'.

Previous personality

It is important to elicit information about the patient's normal personality. Try asking him how he would describe himself and then help him with suggestions such as 'Are you quiet, calm, anxious, shy, friendly, a worrier?'. It is often useful to ask a close relative or spouse to describe the patient as well but always record with 'informant' when information comes from another source. It is usual under the heading of 'previous personality' to include information on habits such as alcohol, tobacco and drugs and also on activities and interests which give an impression of how varied the patient's life is. Always ask patients how much they drink and whether they do so every day and whether they feel that their drinking is a problem to them either socially or physically. If there are features of the patient's drinking habits, for example excessive intake or drinking at unusual times (e.g. in the morning), it is essential to go into the drinking history in detail.

Present illness

The last part of the psychiatric history should be the detailed account of symptoms and functioning during this current episode. We call this the 'history of the present illness'. Use open-ended questions in the beginning; for example 'Tell me how you have been feeling lately'. If the patient does not spontaneously mention them, always ask questions of every patient about sleeping, eating, concentration, ability to cope

with work, irritability, anxiety and depression (the systemic enquiry). If the answers to any of these questions are in the affirmative then the next questions should include options, for example 'Have you had difficulty getting off to sleep, or is it waking early or through the night?'. If you ask questions in these ways, then a negative answer at any stage means that you can discontinue the line of enquiry, whereas a positive answer means that you can proceed further.

Questions about symptoms such as depression and anxiety that are part of ordinary life and experience should be couched in such a way as to ask the patient whether they have been feeling more of these symptoms than usual or more than other people, and whether they have interfered with their functioning or prevented them from doing things. Questions about experiences such as hallucinations and delusions that are not part of ordinary experience can be asked in the following way — 'Have you ever had any unusual or frightening experiences? Have you ever felt that things around you seemed frightening or ominous?' and if the answers to these questions are positive, ask the patient to give you an example of these experiences.

For older patients, or for any patient in whom there is a question of organic cerebral impairment or suspicion of excessive drinking, it is important to ask about memory. If you ask a patient whether they have a good memory they often think that you are talking about memory of the past. It is, therefore, better to ask them if they have had difficulty remembering things from day to day or whether they have forgotten where they have put something or forgotten to keep appointments. Also remember to ask about lapses of memory, black-outs or amnesia by saying 'Have you ever lost a period of time and could not remember what you did, or found yourself in a situation and were unable to remember how you got there?'.

Mental state examination

Throughout the history-taking the patient gives information about his perceptions and experiences. His behaviour and mood during the interview will also reveal aspects of his mental state. Those aspects not fully covered should be enquired into at this stage. You should describe, as clearly and objectively as possible, how the patient was behaving and seemed to you when you saw him. This should not include pejorative or interpretive statements as far as is possible. Statements such as 'provocative or disinhibited' mean little compared to the description 'patient is dressed in white lace negligée, kissed the doctor three times during the interview and attempted to sit on doctor's knee'. A statement that the patient was suspicious and hostile means little compared to the description 'the patient demanded to see what I had written and required reassurance that the room was not bugged with listening devices, insisting on examining the telephone to confirm this'.

Tests of concentration and memory and an evaluation of the patient's intellectual functioning should also be performed and all the information recorded in the order shown in Table 10.2. Great care much be exercised to distinguish between the description of observation (preferably with examples) and the interpretation of them.

Table 10.2. The mental state examination

General appearance and behaviour
Talk (form of thought)
Mood Observed mood: fluctuation, appropriateness, includes distress, fear and perplexity. Patient's subjective account of mood
Ideation (thought content) Preoccupation, abnormal or unusual beliefs, suicidal ideas, possession of thought
Perception Illusions, hallucinations, depersonalization/derealization
Orientation
Concentration and attention
Registration
Short-term memory
Long-term memory
Intelligence
Insight Patient's understanding of his condition

For older patients, patients with alcohol or drug problems and those patients suspected of organic brain disease, a more exhaustive examination of memory and specific cerebral functioning will be necessary, together with a full neurological examination (see Chapter 8).

General appearance and behaviour

Dress Note whether the patient's clothing is appropriate to his age, cultural background and the situation and weather. Does his appearance denote care and interest in himself or not? Is there evidence of self-neglect and if so is it long-standing (ingrained dirt, threadbare clothing, etc.)?

Level of consciousness Is the patient alert or drowsy, does he pay attention to the interview?
Reaction to interviewer Does the patient engage in eye contact or avert his gaze, is he normally courteous and responsive, or over-friendly, or suspicious and reserved?
Motor activity Does the patient sit still in his chair or move around the room, is there generalized excessive movement (over-activity) or restless movements of parts of the body which may be an expression of agitation or have the quality of involuntary movements. Is there diminished movement — little or no spontaneous movement which may be retardation or result from akinesis such as is found in Parkinsonism. Facial expression is an important aspect of motor activity.

Talk

Understanding of the thoughts of patients is only possible by communicating — usually speech (or writing). Abnormalities of the way in which people think (the form or structure of their thought processes) will be evident when they talk. Neurological disorders of speech (dysarthrias and dysphasias) are not necessarily accompanied by disorders of thinking and will need to be separately examined during a neurological examination (see Chapter 8).

Note the rate and quantity of talk. Is the patient talking excessively fast and at length so that it is difficult to interrupt and ask questions (pressure of speech), or slowly with pauses and incomplete sentences (retardation)? Is the flow spontaneous and self-perpetuating or monosyllabic and needing prompting? Is there richness or poverty of detail? These changes are often associated with severe elation or depression of mood. Are the answers to questions appropriate or beside the point; does the flow proceed logically or are the associations between one topic and another lost, so that the conversation is fragmented and difficult to follow? This kind of thought disorder is often found in schizophrenic illnesses and should be distinguished from the rapid progress from one topic to another with logical connections, the 'flight of ideas' found in mania.

Note the use of language: colourful superlatives may be used in mania and the employment of new, strange terms during the interview with personal meaning (neologisms) or idiosyncratic language (malapropisms) may be found in schizophrenia.

Disorders of thinking and the ability to think abstractly (often lost in schizophrenia) may be demonstrated by asking the patient to explain, in his own words, a common proverb, e.g. a rolling stone gathers no moss.

Mood A patient's subjective experience of his mood may be at variance with the doctor's observations. Manic patients, for example, may be obviously elated and euphoric yet say they feel normal or even sad. Depressed patients looking sad and tearful may deny they feel depressed and say they feel nothing or that they deserve to feel like this. There are other kinds of mood disorder; emotional lability, i.e. changing from cheerfulness and normality to tearful distress, may be found with organic brain disease. Occasionally tearful distress may be present in a patient who is reacting to unpleasant circumstances. Suspiciousness, fearfulness, anxiety or perplexity should be noted here.

In some patients their mood appears flat or diminished 'blunted' or inappropriate to the content of the conversation. When it is inappropriate they may laugh or smile (incongruity) for no apparent reason. Such a mood disorder is sometimes associated with schizophrenia.

Ideation This is a description of what the patient is thinking about (thought content). He may be preoccupied with distressing or unpleasant themes. The ideas may be reasonable or overvalued: patients may reflect upon themes of undue attention by others (ideas of reference) or they may feel they are unduly affecting others (ideas of influence). The ideas may be false and unreasonable, out of keeping with cultural values (delusions). These may be fleeting and ill-sustained as in acute illnesses and confusional states, or fixed and more detailed (systematized), as in more long-standing illnesses. The origins of the delusion idea are important diagnostically.

The primary delusion is the sudden attribution of a new meaning to a normal percept and, in the absence of clouding of consciousness, strongly suggests schizophrenia. For example the doctor may ask 'When did you first realize you were under surveillance?' To this the patient might answer 'I saw in gold letters over a shop — Jones the Baker — and realized they were signalling to each other'. The commoner secondary delusion develops as the patient's way of explaining other abnormalities such as of mood, perception, memory of unusual circumstances and may be found in a wide variety of mental disorders.

Perception It should have become obvious by now if patients are subject to hallucinations (abnormal perceptions of objects) or illusions (perception in the absence of a stimulus). If not, ask if things seem as they should be or if the patients have heard people

talking when nobody is there. Note the modality. Auditory hallucinations ('voices') are common in a variety of mental disorders whereas visual, tactile and olfactory hallucinations are commoner in organic and drug-related disorders.

Further enquiry about auditory hallucinations will be necessary. In clear consciousness, voices discussing the patient in the third person or influencing thoughts, emotions and actions are strongly suggestive of schizophrenia.

Orientation, concentration and attention, registration, short-term memory, long-term memory, intelligence See Chapter 14.

Insight It is not sufficient to note whether the patient's insight into his condition is full, limited or absent. It is much more important to record his understanding of his own condition, which may vary from fully agreeing with the understanding of his doctor to completely disagreeing with it. He may partially agree. He may be prepared to accept that an alternative understanding to his own is possible. For example, a patient with very severe pain with no identifiable physical cause may be angrily adamant that it could not possibly be of psychological origin and that the doctors have missed a vital diagnosis. A patient with the same problem could on the other hand be quite prepared to accept that this pain could be related to stress or worry or he might be able to accept a partial solution in that the pain may not be due to life-threatening pathology made worse by stress and worry. The patient's understanding of his own condition therefore has important implications for his future management.

Psychological reactions to physical illness

Patients who are physically ill, whether seriously or not, acutely or chronically, will have an emotional reaction to their illness. They will also have valid psychological needs, which for their proper recovery must be met. For many patients an episode of illness represents a major disruption to their life, work and care of children. It brings about fears for the future and doubts about their ability to care for their responsibilities. Not least there may be fears for their own mortality. Such patients may present with symptoms of fearfulness, anxiety and worry. Others may react by becoming depressed, feeling sad, low-spirited and despairing. A further group may become angry and resentful, particularly about the intrusion upon their privacy and loss of control over their lives.

All of these are essentially normal and understandable responses to an illness and the context in which they occur. The correct attribution of distress as a normal, understandable, valid and healthy response to illness, as opposed to signs of a primary psychiatric disorder is very important in medicine. Effectively to deal with essentially normal distress should be within the coping skills of all doctors. Such states will usually only require from the doctor sympathy, understanding and time to listen. They need to be validated not attributed to a pathological process 'It's alright. I understand how you feel. It is quite usual to feel like this after you have been through such an operation, etc.'. Only in exceptional circumstances, if the distress is particularly intense and prolonged, or the situation particularly unusual would such patients require the help of a specialist, although sometimes the symptoms may require palliative medication.

Acute reactions to stress

These may present in the accident and emergency department, in relatives on general wards or in patients themselves following an accident, violent crime, bad news or unpleasant and unexpected events. The person's behaviour is acutely disorganized and purposeless with tearfulness and distress. He or she may be unable to comprehend what has happened, even denying it, and appearing unable to speak or move ('shock'). Given appropriate comfort and safe containment these states should settle within 24–48 h. Following bereavement they may give way to the syndrome of grief and following traumatic situations there may follow a protracted post-traumatic stress disorder (see below).

Grief reaction

Following the initial phase of denial and distress, the bereaved person will seem depressed for at least six weeks with insomnia, preoccupation with the dead person, a feeling of their presence, even hallucinations of their voice, loss of normal interests and social functioning, loss of appetite and interest in self. For the next six months, even though social functioning may be regained there is often a persistent feeling of loss and sadness and often either feelings of guilt or blame towards others for the circumstances of the death. Between six months and one year new plans will be made, belongings disposed of and new relationships made.

Grief may be prolonged by an inability to grieve initially and may be complicated by the development of a depressive illness.

Psychiatric illness in medical practice

In a psychiatric illness the symptoms are either quantitatively excessive (compared to usual reactions to stress) or qualitatively abnormal (they do not usually occur in health or as understandable reactions to stress). The symptoms are relatively enduring and organized and consistent over time and will result in disability. They interfere with sleep, appetite and concentration as well as diminishing the ability of the patient to carry out normal functioning.

Some patients will present in a general medical setting with psychiatric illnesses. These conditions may have been present before the physical illness, they may have arisen because of the physical illness or its antecedents or as a reaction to the illness.

The psychiatric illness may well intensify existing physical symptoms and may interfere with the patient's ability to co-operate with his treatment. Furthermore the somatic symptoms of the psychiatric disorder may well cause additional physical symptoms and confuse the patient's diagnosis.

Anxiety states

The psychological symptoms of anxiety, fearfulness and worry may be overshadowed by the physical symptoms resulting from autonomic overactivity and muscular tension. Acute anxiety states may present as a medical emergency, often with panic attacks and hyperventilation. This may be alarming to the patient who will find it difficult to believe that his tachycardia, breathlessness and paraesthesia result from overbreathing and do not signal imminent death. Panic attacks may complicate frightening medical emergencies such as a myocardial infarct, left ventricular failure or asthma.

More long-standing anxiety states may present to the physician with problems caused by muscular tension (headache, chest pain, facial pain) tachycardia, gastrointestinal symptoms or anxious scrutiny of normal physiological phenomena (vigilant over-focusing).

Obsessional compulsive disorders

These will rarely arise for the first time in a general hospital but the patient who has had a pre-existing problem or a previous episode may develop such a disorder following an illness or operation. This is particularly so if the illness involves uncertainty about the future or requires the patient's rigorous attention to detail in the management of the illness, for example in diabetes, renal dialysis and colostomy. The patient may be obviously disabled by repeatedly checking and seeking reassurance, driven to repetitive actions (compulsions) typically to do with hygiene and troubled by unpleasant intrusive thoughts or images which cannot be resisted (obsessions). Such patients should be referred to a psychiatrist.

Post-traumatic stress disorder

This condition, which has only recently attracted a specific diagnostic label and public attention as the result of major disasters, has almost certainly been in existence for a long time. Clearly documented descriptions of it go back at least to the time of survivors of the First World War. Whereas post-traumatic stress disorder has a high public profile as one of the consequences of major disasters it should be remembered that less dramatic disasters occur at a personal level every day in a hospital. It is therefore not only patients rescued from aeroplane and railway crashes, or from sportsground disasters, who may develop post-traumatic stress disorder. Equally, patients who have been in road-traffic accidents, raped or indeed who have been through a very traumatic medical procedure may suffer from it. It may be that some people are more predisposed to develop post-traumatic stress disorder than others by virtue of their previous personality or a previous history of psychiatric disorder. However, it must be remembered that even people with normal and robust personality functioning can develop this condition.

The essential feature is the development of characteristic symptoms following a traumatic event that is generally outside the range of usual human experience. The symptoms involve re-experiencing traumatic events spontaneously or as the result of a relatively minor prompt (flashback) accompanied by great distress, the physical symptoms of anxiety, sleep disturbance and nightmares. The patient is often irritable, has diminished social and family interests, difficult to live with, morose and moody. They may become generally fearful and anxious, even developing social phobias and may find it difficult to work and concentrate. This condition, typically, emerges some months after the traumatic event and may persist for a long time with the possibility of being complicated by the development of a depressive illness. The original event usually involves a major threat to the life of the person and the feeling on the part of the victim that death was imminent. It

is less likely to happen if the patient was not conscious at the time. It may be that appropriate psychological handling of the victims of trauma in the immediate aftermath would diminish the possibility of this happening, but in the event of the development of the post-traumatic stress disorder specialist help is usually required. It is not only the victims of trauma who may suffer from this condition but sometimes members of the emergency services involved in their rescue as well. If others in the situation died the problem may be compounded by a considerable amount of guilt (survivor guilt).

Depressive illness

Depressive reactions to ill-health, unpleasant procedures and as part of the adjustment to disability are very common. Those characterized by a variable mood, tearfulness, anxiety, initial insomnia, who respond to opportunity to talk and company will not often require specialist help and treatment.

However, severe depressive illness may occur in older patients, women in the immediate postnatal period and those who are vulnerable by virtue of a past or family history. These are characterized by slowing of thought processes and motor activity, retardation, impaired concentration and interests, apathy, anergia, malaise, late insomnia (waking early in the morning) and a worsening of symptoms in the morning (diurnal variation of mood). There is usually anorexia and weight loss. Some patients may have psychotic symptoms, delusional ideas that they are dying, guilty, being punished and older patients may have delusional ideas that they have venereal disease, cancer or that their bowels are blocked and rotting. Suicidal risk in such patients is high, particularly if they are hopeless and despairing and all patients suspected of a severe depressive illness should be referred to a psychiatrist.

Mania

This condition may present acutely in a predisposed individual following an operation or illness. It is hallmarked by noisy, restless overactivity, insomnia, pressure of talk and flight of ideas. The patient's perception of the world is coloured by his mood. He may be grandiose and interfering, overconfident in his own abilities and judgement and his manner may be either humorous and friendly or irritable and patronizing. Obviously, such a mental state seriously interferes with his medical management and merits urgent referral to a psychiatrist.

Schizophrenia

Again these illnesses may present acutely in casualty or to a family doctor in a predisposed individual after an illness. The acute illnesses present with disorganized and bizarre behaviour, suspiciousness and perplexity. Examination of the mental state may reveal hallucinations, delusions and thought disorder. Urgent referral to a psychiatrist is necessary.

Symptomatic psychoses

Depressive psychosis, mania and schizophrenia-like illness indistinguishable from those described above can be associated with both illicit and prescribed drugs, amphetamines, LSD, corticosteroids, antituberculous drugs, L-dopa, atropine-like drugs, analgesics and anaesthetic agents. They can also occur in both hypo- and hyperthyroidism and Cushing's disease.

Acute confusional states

These may occur in a wide variety of conditions (Table 10.3). They are characterized by fear, bewilder-ment, restlessness, insomnia, fluctuating levels of consciousness, drowsiness, attention and concentration and defective orientation for time, place and person. Recent memory functioning will be impaired. There may be fluctuating and fleeting delusional ideas and hallucinatory experiences, often visual, and mistaken identities. The underlying cause should be identified as soon as possible and treated but symptomatic treatment will often be needed as well.

Alcohol abuse

This may present acutely in casualty with intoxication, injury or disturbed behaviour. Alternatively, withdrawal symptoms may complicate other medical problems in a patient already in hospital. Lastly, long-term abuse has a variety of physical consequences. The features of alcoholism and its physical sequelae are shown in Tables 10.4 and 10.5.

If alcohol abuse is suspected a detailed history is required. You should enquire about the amount and pattern of drinking, features of physical and psychological dependence on alcohol and the consequences (social, financial, legal, physical and psychological) of excessive drinking.

There are two occasions in particular in the hospital setting where alcohol abuse may cause problems in diagnosis. The first may occur in casualty where confusion and disturbed behaviour caused by serious physical illness such as head injury is attributed to intoxication (often also present) with potentially fatal consequences. The second occurs when a patient with unknown alcohol dependence is admitted to hospital. Withdrawal symptoms such as shakes and sweats may go unnoticed and the patient can develop

Table 10.3. Causes of acute confusional state

Head trauma
Degenerative Acute illnesses, superimposed on dementia of any cause
Epileptic Postictal
Vascular Cerebral thrombosis, embolism or haemorrhage, subarachnoid haemorrhage, transient ischaemic episode, hypertensive encephalopathy, hypotensive episode
Infections
  Systemic, i.e. pneumonia or septicaemia
  Cerebral, i.e. meningitis, encephalitis
Endocrine Hypo- or hyperglycaemia, hypercalcaemia. Hypo- or hyperthyroidism
Neoplastic Primary or secondary intracranial tumours
Toxic drugs
  Alcohol
  Barbiturates
  Benzodiazepines
  Antidepressants, anti-Parkinsonian agents, anticonvulsants, analgesics, anaesthetic agents, opiates
  Adverse drug reactions
  Drugs of abuse — cannabis, LSD, heroin
Toxic poisons e.g. Lead
Vitamin deficiencies e.g. Thiamine (Wernicke's encephalopathy)

Table 10.4. Features of alcohol abuse and dependence

Excessive intake
Regular drinking
Secret drinking
Drinking to 'steady nerves'
Social problems (marital and occupational)
Legal and financial problems (e.g. drunken driving)
Physical and psychological problems (see Table 10.5)

Features of dependence in addition to above:
Compulsion to drink (cravings)
Tolerance (increased quantities needed for same effect)
Withdrawal symptoms (e.g. tremor, sweating, nausea usually in the mornings)

Table 10.5. Physical sequelae of alcohol abuse

Cardiovascular	Hypertension
	Cardiomyopathy
	Atrial fibrillation
Gastrointestinal	Oesophagitis
	Gastritis
	Diarrhoea
	Pancreatitis
	Malnutrition
Liver	Acute alcoholic hepatitis
	Fatty liver
	Cirrhosis
Nervous system	Early morning shakes
	Delirium tremens on withdrawal
	Acute intoxication — coma
	Amnesic episodes
	Wernicke's encephalopathy (an acute confusional state with external ophthalmoplegia, nystagmus and ataxia)
	Cortical atrophy (dementia)
	Korsakoff psychosis (an amnesic syndrome with impairment of recent memory and learning, confabulation and neuropathy)
	Retrobulbar neuritis
	Central pontine myelosis
	Peripheral neuropathy
Bones	Unexplained injuries (i.e. old fractured ribs)

delirium tremens with confusion, disorientation, hallucinations, disturbed behaviour and fitting. Delirium tremens often only develops 2–4 days after stopping or cutting down drinking.

Simple advice about how to cut down on heavy drinking *does* prevent greater problems. All doctors should be able to give this. 'Striking while the iron is hot' is likely to be most effective and the casualty or inpatient setting, where the patient may already be coming to terms with the consequences of his or her drinking, provides an ideal opportunity. If the patient has signs of alcohol dependence they may require further specialist help from a psychiatrist.

Drug abuse

Like alcoholism, this may present in casualty or an inpatient setting. Many drugs have a characteristic intoxication and (for some) withdrawal syndrome and you should familiarize yourself with each of these groups, such as the opioids, cocaine, stimulants, hallucinogens, cannabis and solvents. Taking a history follows the same lines as that of alcoholism. You may need to warn patients of the particular risks associated with intravenous drug use including the risk of HIV infection.

Deliberate self-harm

This behaviour results in up to 25 per cent of all medical emergencies. It is commonest in young women following shortly after an acute crisis, usually in a relationship. In such circumstances it may occur impulsively and without premeditation. However, in a significant minority it occurs in older people and in those with psychiatric disorders. Here it often involves premeditation and continuing suicidal risk.

All self-harm must be taken seriously and treated effectively and with compassion. Remember that patients may have taken more than one drug and may not be aware of the medical seriousness of their action. Some of the most serious complications of drug overdose (e.g. liver failure with paracetamol) may occur over 48 hours after ingestion. All patients who self-harm should be seen by a person skilled in the interviewing and assessment of deliberate self-harm (not necessarily a psychiatrist). This interview has two functions: first the detection of psychiatric disorder and assessment of continuing suicidal risk (Table 10.6), and secondly a therapeutic function. The opportunity given to the patient to describe his distress and problems and to receive appropriate advice and help has important effects on improving

Table 10.6. Factors associated with increased suicidal risk after deliberate self-harm

Previous attempt
Continuing suicidal ideation
Evidence of planning and avoiding discovery
Violent method — poisons, hanging, stabbing, railways
Current depressive or schizophrenic illness
Past history of psychiatric disorder
Family history of suicide
Alcoholism, drug abuse
Antisocial personality
Older age group, over 40
Recent bereavement
Divorced, single, widowed
Living alone
Chronic or painful physical illness
Male sex

his or her mental health and reducing risk of further episodes of self-harm.

Eating disorders

These should be considered when investigating a patient, typically a young woman, with severe weight-loss and amenorrhoea. Careful observation may reveal excessive exercising, aversion to a normal diet, secretive disposal of food, artificially increasing weight at weighing; questioning may reveal phobia of normal weight and abnormal attitudes to food. Secretive purging and vomiting may also occur and may follow 'binge' eating.

Physical disorders of psychological origin

The problem with words

There are some physical syndromes and many physical symptoms which can be entirely accounted for by psychological and behavioural processes. The correct term for such conditions and symptoms is 'psychogenic'. The following terms, although commonly used, are best avoided. Their meaning is unclear, their definition variable, the evidence for their existence scanty and most importantly they are often insulting to the patient and have pejorative connotations. Such words are — 'functional overlay', 'hysterical', 'hypochondriacal', 'neurotic' and 'psychosomatic'.

Psychosomatic   Historically this term was used to describe conditions in which the macroscopic and microscopic pathology present was entirely attributable to psychological processes. Indeed it was thought that specific psychological processes were involved in specific disease production. In the past, before the identification of the tuberculosis bacillus it was thought that consumption was a psychosomatic illness and before the discovery of insulin that diabetes mellitus was psychosomatic. In the more recent past ulcerative colitis, asthma and Crohn's disease have been thought to be psychosomatic. Scientific advances in medicine have now disproved this, although some may still feel that psychological processes are important in mediating the outcome to these conditions. It is for this reason that the term 'psychosomatic' is old fashioned conceptually and its use is no longer of relevance to modern medicine. We now know that stress and psychological factors (life events) have an important association with a wide variety of physical illnesses and that psychological factors can influence prognosis and outcome in most conditions.

Hypochondriasis   Hypochondriasis is best defined as the persistent belief by a patient that they have a serious physical illness, despite reasonable evidence to the contrary. It is not so much a diagnosis as a description of a mental attitude. A patient may be a hypochondriac and not be psychiatrically ill, another patient may have physical symptoms of psychological origin and yet not have a persistent and intransigent belief that they are physically ill. The term therefore has little use and should be discarded.

Functional overlay   This is an entirely pejorative term never used by psychiatrists, which has no standard or accepted meaning and should be discarded. Every patient will have an emotional reaction to their illness and every patient is likely to behave when ill in a way that he does not behave when well.

The proper terms to use are as follows:

Illness behaviour and the sick role

When people are ill they behave in a particular manner appropriate to their social and cultural setting. It is by this means that the patient adopts the sick role, identifying to others that he is ill, facilitating treatment and care and increasing the chances of recovery. The behaviour of the average man when inflicted by the common cold is a good example of illness behaviour with a condition that is far from life threatening!

In most societies a patient who adopts the sick role is excused normal family, social and work responsibilities temporarily, is expected to seek appropriate care for his illness and is expected to co-operate with whatever investigations or treatments are advised. This inevitably involves becoming somewhat passive and putting yourself in the hands of others. Somebody who adopts the sick role is also expected to express a wish to recover.

It is only when the illness behaviour or the sick role becomes prolonged or out of proportion to the physical disability, or when the illness behaviour is unfamiliar to the doctor because the patient comes from a different culture that such behaviour becomes a problem. The most common reasons for this are when a patient cannot cope with the anxiety about unpleasant or unfamiliar physical symptoms. For example, the patient may feel that a potentially serious state is not being given enough attention or that pain is being treated inadequately. In this type of situation exaggeration of the physical symptoms may occur together with other types of attention-seeking behaviour. The term 'hysterical' should not be used simply for puzzling or attention-seeking behaviour but should be reserved for the much rarer or complicated behavioural syndrome described below as 'conversion hysteria'. Another common problem area is when a patient cannot understand his physical symptoms or is frightened that he may die or develop permanent disability. In such circumstances an emotional reaction often develops. The commonest one is fear or anxiety or the symptoms of depression (see above). The personality of the patient and the nature and circumstances of their physical illness will determine which reaction develops, if any. It is important to remember that a patient from another culture may be particularly vulnerable to such reactions. They may not share a common language or understanding either of the disease process or the treatment techniques and may be very frightened and bewildered. The illness behaviour and sick role manifestations, which may be quite normal in their own country may seem unfamiliar to the doctor who is treating them.

Psychogenic disorders

This is the generic term for all those physical conditions or symptoms in which psychological mechanisms are necessary and sufficient to explain the production of the symptoms.

Physical symptoms of psychological origin are part of everyday life and everyday reactions to stress. Almost everybody will have experienced churning in the stomach, frequency of micturition or palpitations when frightened. These physical symptoms, although experienced bodily are almost immediately correctly attributed to the fear and not to the primary physical disease process.

In order for a patient to develop a psychogenic disorder this basic mechanism of recognizing the psychological origin of physical symptoms is lost.

Reasons for failure in recognizing the psychological origin of physical symptoms

Education, culture, upbringing and maturity   Children commonly do not recognize the psychological origin of physical symptoms, nor may people who have learning disability or who are very immature. People who have been brought up in an atmosphere of ill-health or preoccupation with bodily function may again attribute physical symptoms to physical disease. It is often said that people from other cultures, particularly rural and undeveloped countries, may attribute physical symptoms of distress to physical disease rather than psychological processes.

The symptoms may be unfamiliar   The first experience of difficulty in swallowing when distressed, or of a tachycardia never experienced before, may not be seen by the patient as a rational consequence of stress.

There may be a delay between cause and effect   It is relatively easy to attribute the physical symptoms of anxiety to fear, if they follow immediately upon a frightening situation. However, if the patient does not experience any symptoms at the time and develops the symptoms some days later the association may be lost to him.

Pathological mental mechanisms may become involved   If the cause of the distress is so upsetting that it cannot be tolerated by the patient, they may convert the psychic energy into physical symptoms (conversion hysteria). This process is known as 'splitting' or 'dissociation' and 'conversion'. They may deny that anything upsetting has happened (denial) or accept that something has happened but not accept the intensity of the distress, attributing it rather to concern about the physical consequences (displacement).

The reaction of others may be important   This is particularly true in children. If a child is upset by something that has happened at school and complains to his mother of stomach-ache, most mothers would focus on the problems at school rather than the stomach-ache. However, if the mother does not and reacts to the physical symptoms, this may lead to repeated reinforcement of physical symptoms rather than the discovery of the psychological causes.

Reasons for the symptom production

When a patient is suffering from psychogenic disorder there must be a reason for the symptom production. These can be most commonly

The somatic symptoms of anxiety   These symptoms are all mediated by autonomic overarousal and include dry mouth, sweating, fine tremor, sensation of lump in the throat and difficulty swallowing, tachycardia (palpitations), gut hypermotility (butterflies in the stomach), diarrhoea, frequency of micturition, hyperventilation and sensation of tightness in the chest, dizziness and light-headedness and various manifestations of muscle tension, including headache and backache and muscular fatigue.

The physical symptoms of depression   Apart from sleep disturbance (typically early morning wakening and waking through the night), appetite loss and weight loss, loss of energy, motivation and extreme fatigue are common symptoms. A patient may have difficulty in concentrating and remembering which may lead him to worry about cerebral pathology. He may have constipation, loss of libido, which together with loss of energy and loss of weight may make him concerned that he has cancer or some other debilitating illness. These symptoms are often known as the biological symptoms of depression.

The behavioural responses to distress When people are distressed they are frequently agitated, do not eat or drink, weep a great deal and may smoke and drink coffee to excess. These may cause physical symptoms. Other common physical responses to distress are loss of appetite, air swallowing, hyperventilation and muscle tension. If the cause for the distress is long-standing the symptoms themselves may become chronic.

Vigilant focusing and selective attention are common causes of symptom production when patients are chronically distressed or anxious. The patient may become aware of minor physical symptoms or indeed of normal physiology, e.g. specks of dust before their eyes, the sound of their heart beating in their ears or normal bodily sensations. The process of vigilantly focusing on these symptoms magnifies them and the patient becomes increasingly preoccupied.

More rarely the pathogenic idea may be the cause of symptom production. This may happen in profoundly depressed people who may believe guiltily that they have an illness such as venereal disease, which is the result of minor past peccadilloes, or that they smell. It may be bizarre or delusional and very idiosyncratic as in monosymptomatic delusional hypochondriasis and other rare variants of schizophrenia. The pathogenic idea in severe depressive illnesses is often symbolic of the way that the patient feels about themselves.

In order to be certain that a syndrome or a symptom is psychogenic the patient should fulfil the criteria outlined in Table 10.7.

Somatoform disorders

This is the modern term for psychogenic disorder, i.e. conditions which present with physical symptoms but for which there are no demonstrable organic findings and there is a strong presumption of psychological mechanisms in their production. It was an American term but has been introduced into European nomenclature for the classification of diseases (ICD-10).

Table 10.7. Criteria for the diagnosis of psychogenic symptoms

The symptom should not be typical of physical disease
There should be associated symptoms of anxiety or depression
Evidence of symptom increase under stress and reduction when the stress is relieved
There should be a personal history or a family history of psychiatric disorder
There should be no demonstrable physical pathology
The mechanism for symptom production should be understood by the doctor
The reason for the patient's failure to recognize the psychogenesis should be understood by the doctor
Physical treatments should be shown to have failed
Psychological treatments should be shown to succeed

Specific types of psychogenic or somatoform disorders

Somatization disorder

This is a relatively common and chronic polysymptomatic disorder that tends to begin before the age of 30 and has in the past attracted different epithets. One of which familiar to physicians is 'thick-file patient' and another more familiar to psychiatrists 'Briquet's syndrome'. The essential features are recurrent and multiple physical complaints of several years' duration for which a great deal of medical attention has been sought but which are not due to any physical disorder. It pursues a chronic and fluctuating course. The complaints are often presented in a dramatic or exaggerated way and typically the medical history is complicated and many diagnoses and multiple investigations have been considered, often involving many different specialities. The symptoms may commonly be pseudoneurological or conversion symptoms, difficulty swallowing, loss of speech, deafness, blindness, loss of consciousness, pseudoseizures, paralysis, etc., gastrointestinal or cardiovascular symptoms. The patients may be very distressed and disabled by their symptoms and fearful of their health. However, they appear to enjoy hospitalization and medical attention.

Conversion hysteria

In the Western world this is a relatively rare condition and most commonly the symptoms are those which suggest neurological disease — blindness, deafness, loss of speech, seizures, paralysis, etc. However, they are usually not neurologically sophisticated and do not follow the distribution of the pyramidal tracts nor of the distribution of peripheral nerves. The symptoms are usually those of organs served by the voluntary nervous system but are not under conscious control. The mechanism is that described above, usually of the splitting of an unusual degree of stress and the subsequent conversion of the psychological energy into physical symptoms. Frequently this leads to the suppression of the original cause to its denial and an apparent indifference to the symptoms that result ('la belle indifference'). Up to the time of the First World War conversion hysteria was common in Great Britain and still remains a common neurotic condition in the Third World. However, its rarity in modern-day medicine should lead to great caution in making a diagnosis and it should not be used merely when a physical explanation for a symptom cannot be found. The mechanisms found in conversion hysteria are primitive and in the absence of a major psychological trauma the possibility of the patient having a profound depressive illness should be considered. Another possible facilitating mechanism for this process could be the presence of undetected organic cerebral pathology. This may not be directly related to the symptom production but may merely act in a non-specific way.

Psychogenic pain

This is a condition in which the predominant feature is the complaint of severe and debilitating pain in the absence of any physical disease and the presence of the obvious aetiological role of psychological fac-

tors. It is usually inconsistent with the anatomic distribution of the nervous system and may involve the excessive use of analgesics. Without pain relief, requests for surgery and frequent visits to different doctors (doctor shopping) occur. In some cases the pain may have an obvious psychological significance, such as pain mimicking angina in an individual who has had recent experience of a relative with such a problem.

Factitious disorder

Patients with this condition differ from those with somatoform disorders in that they feign symptoms and signs of physical illness, often with considerable skill. They may travel from doctor to doctor and undergo many unnecessary investigations and operations. They do not gain any external rewards (such as financial compensation) from their behaviour, distinguishing them from malingerers. Instead, they appear to have a psychological need to adopt the sick role and derive some comfort from the attentions of hospital staff. Doctors and nurses often feel very angry at being 'out-witted' by such patients and a direct challenge to the patient often results in his disappearance and later reappearance in another setting. The condition is difficult to treat and a psychiatrist should be involved if it is suspected. Factitious disorder is also known as Munchausen's syndrome.

References and further reading

Bird J, Harrison G. *Examination notes in psychiatry*, 2nd edn. Bristol: Wright, 1987.
Gelder M, Gath D, Mayou R. *Concise Oxford Textbook of Psychiatry*. Oxford: Oxford University Press, 1994.
Goldberg D, Benjamin S, Creed F. *Psychiatry in medical practice*, 2nd edn. London: Routledge, 1994.

11

Medical symptoms and signs in pregnancy

P. C. Rubin

History
Examination

Pregnancy is not the exclusive domain of the obstetrician and doctors in most areas of medicine will from time to time be called upon to see a pregnant woman. There are numerous changes in anatomy, physiology and biochemistry during a normal pregnancy and these can produce traps for the unwary. The purpose of this chapter is to highlight the ways in which normal pregnancy can produce symptoms, signs or changes which in other circumstances would be considered abnormal.

History

Most pregnant women will have at least one of the following symptoms:

Breathlessness

Three-quarters of pregnant women experience shortness of breath. Around half of them will become breathless on climbing more than one flight of stairs while the remainder are symptomatic on mild exertion such as walking on level ground.

The cause is unknown. It is not a simple mechanical matter of the gravid uterus pressing on the diaphragm, since most women become breathless before (and some well before) 20 weeks gestation and symptoms reach their peak around 30 weeks.

Mild breathlessness by itself, coming on progressively in a previously healthy woman, does not require investigation.

In contrast, breathlessness is likely to be a manifestation of disease if any of the following apply:

- it comes on suddenly
- it is accompanied by chest pain and/or haemoptysis
- there is wheezing
- there is a history of heart or lung disease
- the patient comes from a developing country where congenital or rheumatic heart disease may have gone undiagnosed

Palpitations

Heart rate increases during pregnancy but not in a way which is noticed by the patient. Where an increased heart rate is remarked on by a pregnant woman, hyperthyroidism should be considered.

Occasional ectopic beats, both atrial and ventricular, are common and may well be noticed by the patient but are of no importance.

Sustained palpitations, particularly if accompanied by light-headedness or syncope, are usually caused by supraventricular tachycardia. This condition is more common in pregnancy than in young women who are not pregnant and may recur in successive pregnancies while being quiescent between times.

Ankle swelling

Pitting oedema of the lower limbs occurs in 80 per cent of pregnant women and is a normal finding. The oedema increases with gestation and also gets worse towards the end of each day. The cause of this oedema is mainly a combination of the uterus obstructing venous return and reduced colloid osmotic pressure (resulting from falling albumin concentration).

Ankle swelling may be important if:

- there is a history of renal or cardiac disease
- it is unilateral (suggesting possibility of venous thrombosis)

Indigestion

Dyspepsia and heartburn occur in up to 70 per cent of pregnant women with most suffering their worst symptoms in the third trimester. The cause is gastro-oesophageal reflux resulting from a reduction in lower oesophageal sphincter pressure. Peptic ulcer in pregnancy is rare.

Nausea and vomiting

Morning sickness in a young woman is virtually diagnostic of pregnancy. Eighty-five per cent of women will experience nausea or vomiting during pregnancy and while for most the symptoms are confined to the first trimester, around 20 per cent are troubled throughout pregnancy. Sometimes the symptoms are so severe (hyperemesis gravidarum) that parenteral feeding is necessary.

Constipation

Constipation of sufficient severity to cause abdominal discomfort is a frequent accompaniment of pregnancy and is often made worse by iron tablets. Haemorrhoids are often an unwelcome accompaniment.

Urinary frequency

Symptoms of urgency, frequency or nocturia are experienced by many pregnant women. In some cases the symptoms are caused by a urinary tract infection and in others they are not, but the only way to find out is to culture the urine. This must be done in all women complaining of such symptoms because it is important that urinary infections are treated.

Examination (Fig. 11.1)

The physical changes which occur as the result of pregnancy are usually self-evident, but some features which would ordinarily indicate disease do occur.

The skin

During pregnancy the skin undergoes several changes, most notably hyperpigmentation, but only two physical signs could be mistaken as suggesting underlying pathology, namely liver disease.

Spider naevi

These appear in over 50 per cent of pregnant women, appearing between eight and 20 weeks gestation. Both in appearance and distribution they are the same as spider naevi of chronic liver disease. They increase in number, as pregnancy progresses and have largely disappeared by eight weeks following delivery. Some may persist.

Palmar erythema

This appears in the first trimester and becomes more marked as the pregnancy proceeds. Around 70 per cent of pregnant women develop palmar erythema, usually over the entire surface of the palm but sometimes affecting only the thenar and hypothenar eminences. The erythema has resolved in most women by eight weeks post partum.

Spider naevi and palmar erythema in the absence of any other features of liver disease can be safely regarded as normal.

The cardiovascular system

The circulation becomes hyperdynamic in pregnancy and the heart is rotated about its anteroposterior axis as the uterus enlarges. Several physical signs result from these changes:

- the peripheral pulse is of large volume in a manner which could suggest aortic valve disease and the heart rate is increased
- the apex beat is progressively displaced and by the third trimester can be up to 2 cm from the mid-clavicular line in the fourth intercostal space
- a third heart sound, resulting from rapid ventricular filling, is audible in well over 50 per cent of pregnant women and can be mistaken for an opening snap or a diastolic murmur
- an ejection systolic murmur, arising either from the pulmonary or tricuspid valve, can be heard in virtually all normal pregnant women: phonocardiographic studies put the figure at 96 per cent. The murmur may be heard widely over the precordium but is never particularly loud
- in addition to murmurs of valvular origin, systolic or continuous murmurs may be heard in the right or left intercostal space, around 2 cm from the sternal edge. Their source is thought to be

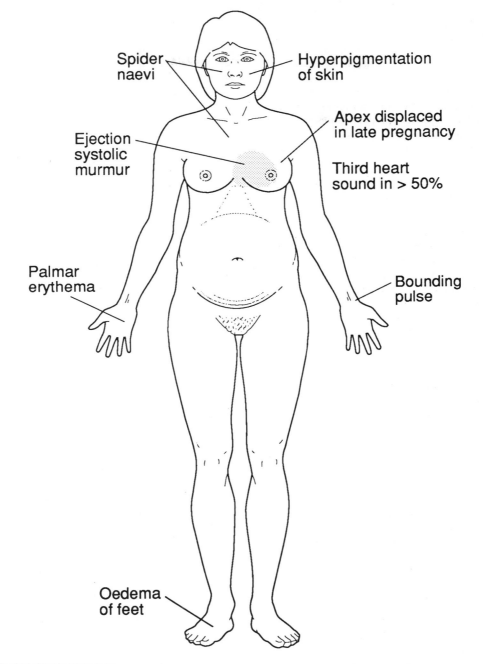

Spider naevi

Hyperpigmentation of skin

Apex displaced in late pregnancy

Ejection systolic murmur

Third heart sound in > 50%

Palmar erythema

Bounding pulse

Oedema of feet

Fig. 11.1 Physical signs in pregnancy.

increased blood flow in the mammary vessels and they can be abolished by pressing with the stethoscope

- in contrast, a murmur is likely to be important if it is pansystolic, late systolic, loud or varies with respiration

As mentioned above, peripheral oedema is very common in pregnancy and should not be interpreted as a manifestation of heart failure unless there are other diagnostic features.

Renal glycosuria is common during pregnancy.

ECG

Q waves and T wave inversion may be seen in lead III in normal pregnancies. This could clearly be misleading — for example as being part of the $S_1Q_3T_3$ pattern seen in some cases of pulmonary embolus — and the ECG must be interpreted as part of the overall clinical picture.

12

Endocrine system and metabolism

S. P. Allison and R. B. Tattersall

> The thyroid gland
> Disorders of body weight
> Growth and development
> The pituitary
> The adrenals
> Diabetes mellitus
> References and further reading

Endocrinology and metabolism may be divided into the conditions which present frequently and are of regular concern to most doctors, and those which are rare and the province of highly specialized clinics. Among the former are diabetes, thyroid disease, obesity, disorders of growth and development, gynaecological problems including the menopause and bone disorders such as osteoporosis. Among the latter are pituitary and adrenal diseases and the many and bizarre disorders which illumine the life of the specialist endocrinologist. This chapter focuses on the clinical presentation of the common disorders, but also refers to the more important of the rare conditions.

The thyroid gland

Thyroid disease is often suggested as an explanation for many non-specific symptoms. Patients appear with psychological ills and mildly abnormal or mis-interpreted thyroid function tests, in the hope that thyroid treatment will be a cure. Both doctors and patients are usually disappointed. It is, therefore, most important to define accurately those symptoms and signs which are ascribable solely to thyroid disease. The gland may present abnormalities of function or of size, although there is no correlation between the two. The grossly thyrotoxic patient may

have a small gland and a large gland may be under-active. There may be associated disorders of other organs, for example those affecting the eyes and muscles. The symptoms of an over- or underactive thyroid may be so insidious that the patient or the close family fail to notice them. It is to be hoped that an alert doctor who maintains a low threshold of suspicion will pick them up before the grosser features of thyrotoxicosis or myxoedema manifest themselves. Leading questions are often needed to elicit the full history.

The gland secretes thyroxine (T4) and triiodo-thyronine (T3) which circulate largely bound to proteins, mainly thyroid-binding globulin and pre-albumin. T4 is converted in peripheral tissues to the more active T3. Overactivity of the thyroid is confirmed by the finding of high levels of free and bound T4 and T3 with low levels of thyroid stimulating hormone (TSH) (measured by sensitive assay). Primary hypothyroidism is confirmed by high TSH levels, since abnormally low T4 and T3 levels fail to suppress pituitary TSH secretion.

Symptoms

Beware of diagnostic greed and do not be put off by the many variants of thyroid symptoms.
Swelling in the neck Enlargement of the thyroid gland is commonly described as a goitre. The patient or the

family may have noticed a swelling in the neck and fear malignancy. Pain is common only in subacute (de Quervain's) thyroiditis or in the case of haemorrhage into a cyst. Constant discomfort sometimes occurs in Hashimoto's thyroiditis. Some anxious patients also complain of discomfort on swallowing with other types of goitre.

Appetite and weight Thyroid overactivity in younger patients is classically associated with increased appetite and weight loss, although occasionally the hyperphagia is such as to cause weight gain, or appetite is actually diminished. Conversely, hypothyroidism may cause weight gain. Try to record precise values of past and present weights. These data are invaluable in future management.

Intolerance of heat and cold Intolerance of heat and night sweats 'having to throw the bedclothes off at night' are common but not invariable features of thyrotoxicosis. 'Feeling the cold' is associated with hypothyroidism.

Neuropsychiatric symptoms Thyroid overactivity causes tremor, irritability, restlessness, overactivity and insomnia. It may exacerbate underlying psychiatric disorders and in severe cases, hallucinations and psychosis are described. Differentiation of mild thyrotoxicosis from anxiety state can be difficult without supportive evidence from thyroid function tests.

Conversely the hypothyroid patient may be slowed and dull and occasionally depressed but sometimes quite cheerful with the so-called 'myxoedema wit'. In extreme cases, psychosis may occur. Common neurological symptoms of hypothyroidism include deafness, carpal tunnel syndrome due to compression of the median nerve by myxoedema at the wrist, and a deep, slow voice like a record being played too slowly. Hoarseness may occur in myxoedema or when the recurrent largyngeal nerve has been affected by malignancy.

Cardiovascular and respiratory symptoms Atrial fibrillation, palpitations or shortness of breath are commonly associated with toxic nodular goitre in the older patient, but may be a feature of thyrotoxicosis at any age. Shortness of breath may also occur in myxoedema in which pericardial effusion, myocardial degeneration and coronary artery disease are not infrequent. A large retrosternal goitre may compress the trachea and cause stridor and dyspnoea.

Gastrointestinal symptoms In thyrotoxicosis intestinal hurry may be such as to cause diarrhoea and, in extreme cases, steatorrhoea. In hypothyroidism there is usually constipation.

Menstruation Oligomenorrhoea is typical of thyrotoxicosis and menorrhagia of hypothyroidism.

Muscles Myopathy particularly of the proximal and girdle muscles is a common feature of Graves' disease. In one of our patients who was a weight-lifter, it was the presenting symptom. Fleeting pains in the muscles are common in the early stages following successful treatment of thyrotoxicosis.

Skin and hair With hypothyroidism the patient may complain of dry skin and thinning hair; increased sweating is characteristic of the thyrotoxic patient, who may also complain of hair loss, particularly early after treatment. The hair returns to normal 6−9 months later.

Examination

The gland itself

The normal gland consists of two lateral lobes extending from the thyroid cartilage to the sixth tracheal ring and connected by an isthmus. It relates posteriorly to the carotid artery and recurrent laryngeal nerves. The four parathyroid glands usually lie within its fascia posteriorly.

Look for swelling or asymmetry from the front and side. Palpation is best carried out from behind the seated patient with the fingers over the anterior triangle of the neck pointing downwards towards the suprasternal notch. Ask the patient to take a sip of water into the mouth and then to swallow. Swellings of the thyroid usually move freely on swallowing, and even a retrosternal goitre may be detected in the suprasternal notch. The various types of goitres are listed in Table 12.1. In Graves' disease (exophthalmic goitre), the thyroid is diffusely and symmetrically enlarged, with a softish consistency and a systolic bruit on auscultation. The gland of Hashimoto's disease is of similar appearance, but is often firmer and may be slightly tender. In subacute or de Quervain's thyroiditis the gland is very tender.

Diffuse enlargement is seen with many non-toxic and iodine-deficient goitres, although, as the years pass and the processes of atrophy and hypertrophy proceed such glands may become nodular or become over- or underactive. The nodular goitre (Fig. 12.1) is frequently asymmetrical and firm, with, as the name suggests, one or more nodules. Palpation may be deceptive; in that what seems to be a single nodule often turns out, on further investigation, to be just part of a multinodular goitre.

Single nodules may represent functional adenomas associated with thyroid overactivity. Non-functioning single nodules should always be viewed with suspicion and investigated further to exclude malignancy (see Table 12.2). An isotope scan will differentiate single from multiple nodules and a 'hot' from a 'cold' single nodule. Ultrasound differentiates

Table 12.1. Types of goitres

Causes	Clinical features
Iodine deficiency	Endemic. Usually non-toxic
Unknown*	
Autoimmune*	(a) Stimulating antibodies Graves' disease (hyperthyroidism + exophthalmos
	(b) Destructive antibodies Hashimoto's thyroiditis Hypothyroidism
Viral	Subacute thyroiditis (de Quervain's) Painful Transiently hyperthyroid
Solitary nodules*	See Table 12.2
Hereditary enzyme deficiency	Rare. Diffuse goitre Hypothyroid
Physiological*	During puberty and pregnancy
Malignant	Usually carcinoma, occasionally lymphoma

* Common

Table 12.2. Apparent solitary nodules in the thyroid

Toxic solitary nodule
Adenoma
Cyst
Nodule in a multinodular gland*
Carcinoma
    Follicular
    Medullary (rare)
    Papillary

* Accounts for about half of the so-called solitary nodules.

a cystic nodule, which is nearly always benign, from a solid one which may be malignant and require biopsy. Undifferentiated carcinoma of the thyroid may present as diffuse enlargement of the thyroid which is fixed and fails to move on swallowing. Palpate carefully for enlarged local lymph glands which may be the site of secondary spread.

Very large goitres may embrace the whole neck (Fig. 12.2) or cause superior vena canal obstruction

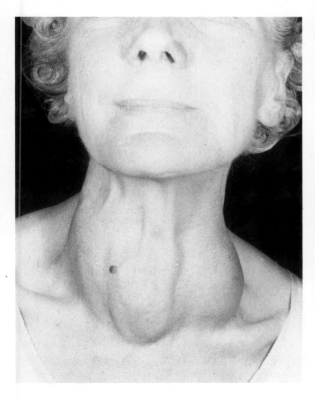

Fig. 12.1 An asymmetrical, multinodular goitre in a euthyroid patient.

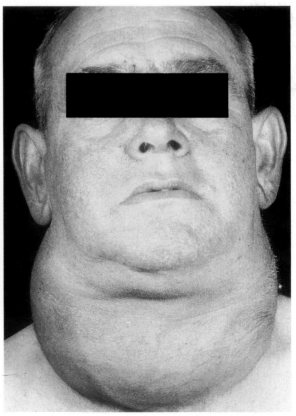

Fig. 12.2 A very large goitre embracing the whole of the neck.

(Fig. 12.3). When the goitre is completely substernal the clinical diagnosis is often difficult.

Signs of thyrotoxicosis

As well as being an act of courtesy, rising to greet your patient to shake hands offers important clues straightaway. The patient with an anxiety state not only appears anxious, but may be pale, with cold moist hands. The thyrotoxic patient will also be agitated but the face is flushed and shiny and the hands are warm and sweaty. Even when seated, the patient is restless and hyperkinetic. There is a fine tremor of the outstretched hands. Finger clubbing occurs but is rare. There is a tachycardia and atrial fibrillation may be present. The systolic blood pressure is raised and the pulse pressure increased with a collapsing quality. The apex beat is forceful and a functional systolic bruit may be heard over the precordium as well as over the thyroid. In severe cases, there may be high-output heart failure.

Upper lid retraction due to overactivity of the levator palpebrae superioris is the most common eye sign in thyrotoxicosis (Table 12.3). The white sclera is constantly exposed between the upper lid and the iris (Fig. 12.4) and is most apparent when the patient's gaze follows the examiner's finger upwards. As the finger is lowered the upper lid lags behind the movement of the eye in a series of jerky movements. The sign often disappears following treatment.

Associated features of Graves' disease

Graves' eye disease Exophthalmos is caused by

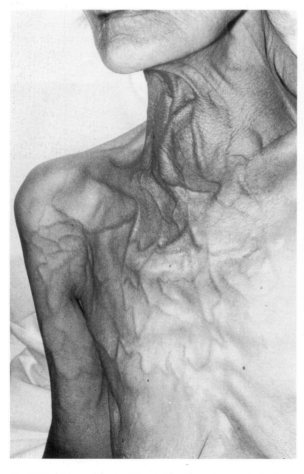

Fig. 12.3 A large goitre, mainly substernal, causing mediastinal obstruction; note the presence of distended veins over the chest wall.

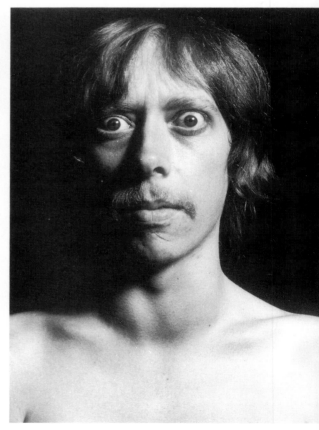

Fig. 12.4 Lid retraction. Note the exposure of the white sclera between the upper lid and iris. The thyroid gland is diffusely and symmetrically enlarged.

Table 12.3. Eye signs in thyrotoxicosis

Lid retraction
Lid lag
Exophthalmos
Chemosis
Periorbital oedema
Ophthalmoplegia

an autoimmune myopathy of the external ocular muscles, causing swelling and weakness. The condition is associated with, but not caused by, Graves' thyrotoxicosis and may precede it by many years or occur independently. It takes many years to improve and may even worsen following thyroid treatment. Fortunately it is only found in a minority of patients. The exophthalmos is frequently asymmetrical being more marked in one eye. From the front, protrusion of the eyeball is apparent and the sclera is visible between iris and lower lid as well as between iris and upper lid (Fig. 12.5). The degree of proptosis and its asymmetry can best be appreciated if the examiner stands behind the sitting patient, looking down the plane of the forehead.

There are several other features which may present in isolation or in any combination:

- *periorbital oedema*: the upper and lower lids and periorbital tissues appear swollen and oedematous, particularly first thing in the morning (Fig. 12.6(a))
- *chemosis*: the patient complains of sore, gritty eyes which appear red and infected. In severe cases the conjunctiva may become oedematous. If exophthalmos is sufficiently severe as to prevent the eyelids meeting, the eyes become additionally dry, infected and sore (Fig. 12.6(b))
- *ophthalmoplegia*: minor degrees of weakness of any of the eye muscles may occur independently and give rise to diplopia (Fig. 12.6(c)). In severe exophthalmos, however, paralysis particularly of upward and outward gaze may be gross since the superior rectus and inferior oblique muscles are predominantly affected

Pretibial myxoedema (Fig. 12.7) Infrequently, severe Graves' disease is associated with raised purplish-brown blotches over the shins, which persist despite cure of thyrotoxicosis.

Myopathy Look for wasting and weakness of muscles, particularly in the scapular and shoulder regions. Some patients with myopathy of the buttocks

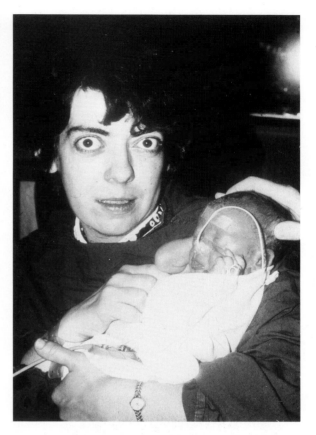

Fig. 12.5 Bilateral exophthalmos. Note the asymmetry and the exposure of the sclera above and below the iris. This lady's newborn baby also had thyrotoxicosis.

and thighs may have problems climbing stairs or rising from a squatting position.

Signs of hypothyroidism

Hypothyroidism is surely one of the most over-diagnosed diseases in medicine. Yet early cases are still regularly missed. Even in severe hypothyroidism facial changes may be minimal particularly in the young (Fig. 12.8). Gross myxoedema should be unmistakeable (Fig. 12.9) with the overweight, dry scaly skin, thinning hair and eyebrows, the puffiness of the features, low-pitched slow voice, slow movements and bradycardia. The tongue is enlarged and the hands puffy. The slow relaxation of the tendon reflexes characteristic of hypothyroidism is best demonstrated by eliciting the ankle-jerks with the patient kneeling in a chair and gripping the back. If in doubt, make comparison with a control subject.

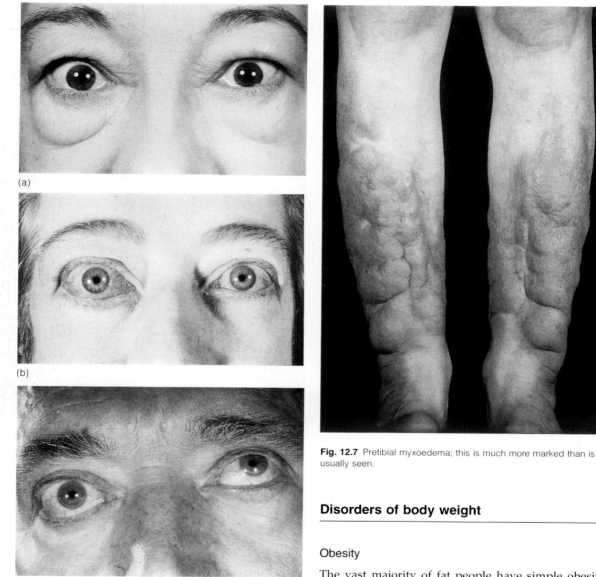

(a)

(b)

(c)

Fig. 12.6 Other features of Graves' eye disease: (a) periorbital oedema; (b) injection of the conjunctivae with chemosis; (c) ophthalmoplegia.

Fig. 12.7 Pretibial myxoedema; this is much more marked than is usually seen.

Disorders of body weight

Obesity

The vast majority of fat people have simple obesity (Fig. 12.10) and an endocrine cause is found in less than 2 per cent. Cushing's syndrome is rare, whereas overweight associated with hirsutism, oligomenorrhoea and hypertension is common. Weight gain in most hypothyroid patients is modest. Rarely, as a result of head injury or tumour damaging the hypothalamic region, a pathological appetite may develop. In the absence of a history or examination suggesting these conditions, overweight may be assumed to be unrelated to any disease process and to be caused by an imbalance between energy intake and expenditure over years. Take a careful history, including data

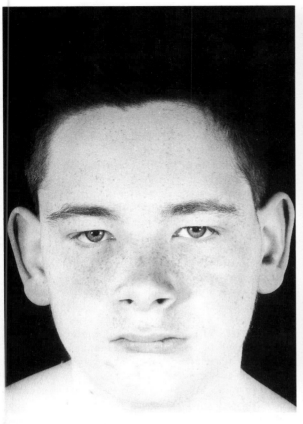

Fig. 12.8 Myxoedema in a young adult; a sleepy appearance in a sleepy patient!

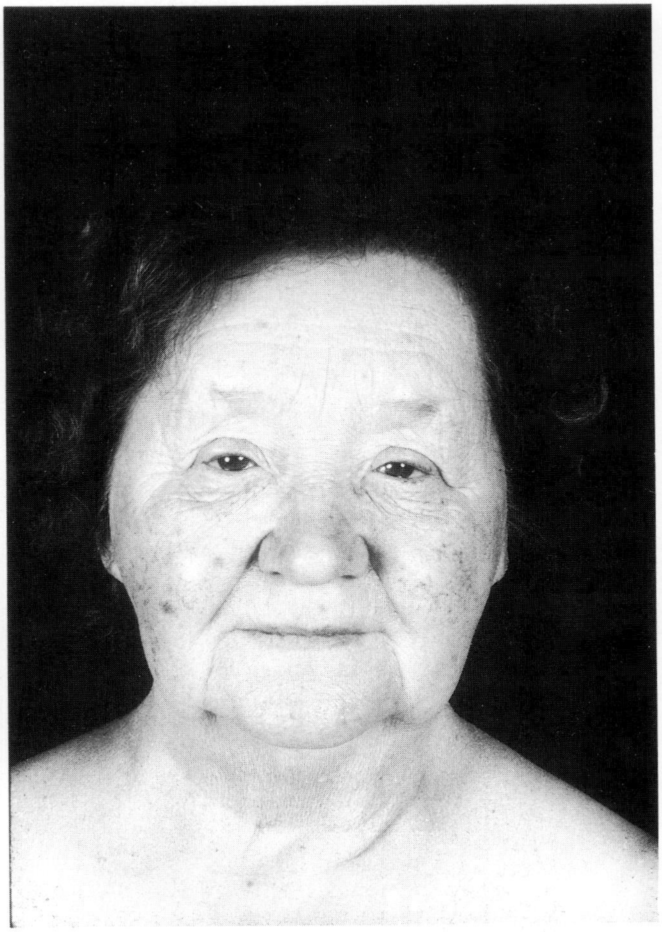

Fig. 12.9 Myxoedema in the adult.

on weights of parents and siblings. Does obesity date from childhood or is it of recent origin? Make some estimate of daily energy intake and of exercise. Oligomenorrhoea is caused by overweight as well as underweight. Excessive adipose tissue alters tissue metabolism of androgens, giving rise to hirsutism.

In your examination, record height and weight and compare the patients' weight for height with standard tables and calculate the BMI (see Chapter 2). Is the patient 10 per cent or more overweight and if so is it due purely to adipose tissue or associated with a large bone and muscle mass? Some idea of the relative proportions of fat and lean mass can be gained by measuring the circumference of the upper arm with a tape-measure mid-way between the acromion and the olecranon and the triceps skin and fat fold at the same level with skin calipers. Record the blood pressure with a special large cuff since obesity of the arm causes falsely high readings using the standard

cuff. Make sure that you test the urine, or preferably the blood, for glucose to exclude diabetes as a consequence of obesity.

Anorexia nervosa

Non-specific anorexia and cachexia may result from serious organic disease or from depressive illness. The more specific condition of anorexia nervosa is usually seen in young women and associated with disordered body image which leads them to eschew carbohydrate and to some extent fat. There may be a history of self-induced vomiting. Secondary to weight loss, there is depression of hypothalamic function with amenorrhoea. Despite evidence to the contrary the patient persists with the delusion of being too heavy.

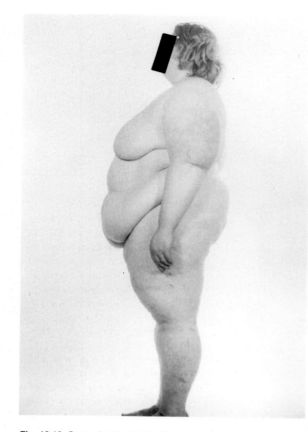

Fig. 12.10 Gross simple obesity. There is generalized distribution of fat with a pendulous apron and much deposition of fat over the buttocks and thighs. CT scanning has shown us that in obese men, in contrast to women, much of the fat is within the abdominal cavity.

Growth and development

Short stature and delayed development for age may be picked up by efficient health screening of school-children but often the doctor is asked for advice because of parental anxiety and teasing at school. A full history and careful examination is usually sufficient to decide whether the symptoms are pathological and if so whether they have an endocrine or other cause.

History

Obtain data on birth weight and subsequent height and weight measurements. Ask about maternal health during pregnancy and intercurrent illnesses and drug treatment during infancy and childhood. Asthma,

renal disease, heart disease, nutritional deficiency and steroid treatment may all impair growth. The family history is crucial, since the average of the parents' height is a guide to that expected in the child. Plot serial data for height and weight on Tanner's growth charts. If the patient is below the third centile, can this be explained by hereditary factors? Ask for the age at which puberty took place in the parents, since delay in puberty and the growth spurt associated with it is often inherited. Also plot serial height data on a growth velocity chart. A growth rate of more than 4–5 cm per annum virtually excludes any disease process.

In the very small number of patients in whom growth velocity is lower than this, the child is small in relation to the rest of the family and there is no history of disease, consider other pathology and carry out appropriate investigations. Growth hormone, thyroxine and sex hormones all contribute to growth and specific deficiencies should be sought. Look for chromosomal abnormalities, e.g. Turner's syndrome (see Fig. 2.14) with its short stature, neck-webbing and increased carrying angle of the arm. The stages of puberty in girls are assessed according to breast development, body hair and the menarche (onset of periods). Failure of any signs of puberty to appear by the age of 14 years warrants concern. In boys, onset of puberty is rarely delayed beyond the age of 17 years and is staged by changes in penile and testicular size, voice changes and body-hair development. If the testes appear undescended, palpate again after the patient has had a warm bath. Retraction should not be mistaken for maldescent. Testicular size should be measured in ml by comparison with standard Prader beads.

Adult male hypogonadism

This is associated with absent or small, soft testes which are non-tender to pressure. You need to ask about relative or complete failure of erection and/or ejaculation: do not forget about undescended testes or mumps orchitis in childhood. Consider chromosomal abnormalities such as Klinefelter's syndrome or hypogonadism secondary to pituitary disease (Fig. 12.11).

The pituitary

Like the thyroid, the pituitary may cause disease either because of enlargement or change in function,

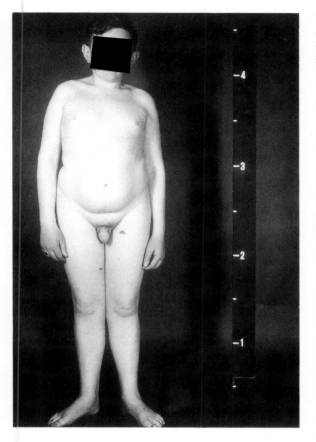

Fig. 12.11 Hypogonadism in the adult man. Note small stature (152 cm), absent body hair and infantile testes.

or both. Non-functioning tumours may arise within the pituitary or outside it, e.g. craniopharyngioma, and cause disease by pressure on surrounding parts, particularly the optic chiasma causing bitemporal hemianopia (Table 12.4). Lateral extension into the cavernous sinus may give rise to ophthalmoplegia, extension may occur downwards into the sphenoid bone. Pressure from functioning or non-functioning tumours may encroach upon normal pituitary tissue,

Table 12.4. Effects of pituitary tumours

Local effects of tumour (i.e. bitemporal hemianopia)
Raised intracranial pressure
Hormone production, e.g. acromegaly
Destruction of remaining functioning pituitary, i.e. to
  give hypopituitarism

the pituitary stalk, and the hypothalamus, causing anterior pituitary damage with defect in secretion of gonadotrophins, growth hormone, thyroid-stimulating hormone or ACTH. Damage to the posterior pituitary gives rise to diabetes insipidus. All these aspects should be addressed by the history and examination.

History and examination

Local effects of an enlarged pituitary   The patient may complain of recent deterioration in vision, particularly of the lateral part of the visual fields. Such a patient not only demands a detailed history and examination but also the formal examination of the optic discs and visual fields (see Chapter 22). Do not expect always to find a well-defined bitemporal hemianopia; pituitary tumours rarely grow symmetrically. Infarction and haemorrhage into a tumour is described as pituitary apoplexy and presents with the sudden onset of severe headache and visual failure, constituting a neurosurgical emergency.

Hypopituitarism   An expanding tumour or other destructive process first damages gonadotrophin and growth hormone secretion with failure of growth and development in childhood and adolescence, impotence in the male, amenorrhoea and infertility in the female and loss of body hair with regression of secondary sexual characteristics in both sexes. Further destruction results in TSH and ACTH failure with secondary hypothyroidism and failure of glucocorticoid secretion. In contrast to Addison's disease, mineralocorticoid secretion is maintained. Panhypopituitarism causes lethargy, tiredness and lack of energy with anorexia, weight loss and general debility. Acute intercurrent illness may precipitate a hypopituitary crisis characterized by coma, hypothermia, hypoglycaemia and hypotension.

Examination shows the patient to be pale. The scalp hair is thin, the eyebrows sparse and the body hair absent. The skin is thin and often smooth. In the male muscle mass is lost and the testes are small and soft. Blood pressure may be low. Sheehan's syndrome refers to a form of hypopituitarism which is caused by pituitary infarction associated with severe postpartum haemorrhage. The patients fail to lactate or to re-establish menstruation. At a later date, sometimes years afterwards, other effects of anterior pituitary failure occur.

Functioning tumours

Prolactinoma   Although manifestations of hypogonadism may represent damage to gonadotrophin-producing cells, it may also be caused by excess prolactin secretion, prolactinoma. Hyperprolactinaemia not only causes galactorrhoea, but inhibits the pituitary—gonadal axis causing amenorrhoea and infertility in the female and diminished androgen secretion in the male. Measurement of serum prolactin levels will confirm the diagnosis.

Acromegaly Tumours secreting growth hormone may cause damage by space occupancy but also give rise to the characteristic symptoms and signs of growth-hormone excess. Before epiphyseal closure this results in gigantism, but once the epiphyses have closed the effect is to cause the thickening of tissues known as acromegaly (see Fig. 2.11). This is so insidious that the patient and relatives may fail to notice it until the changes have been present for some years. The patient may notice an increase in the size of the hands and feet (Fig. 12.12) and require to take larger gloves and shoes. Many complain of headaches and sweating. There is coarsening and thickening of the skin and features with increased hirsuitism in the female; prognathos develops and the tongue enlarges. Overgrowth of bone results in osteoarthritis with joint pains, carpal tunnel syndrome, myelopathy and nerve-route compression. It is these neurological and musculoskeletal abnormalities which can make the acromegalic life so miserable. Many patients have a tendency to hypertension and early cardiovascular disease as well as to diabetes. Although the diagnosis in many patients can be made at a glance (see Fig. 2.11) some younger patients with large tumours may have relatively subtle physical changes (Fig. 12.13).

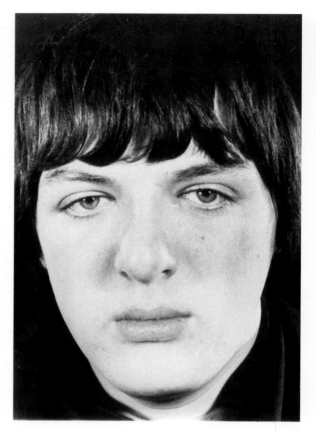

Fig. 12.13 A young man with a large pituitary tumour but with minor signs of acromegaly.

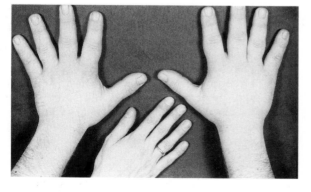

Fig. 12.12 Compare the huge hands of the acromegalic with the hand of the photographer.

In early cases where there may be doubt the most striking physical sign is in the thickness of the skin. Pick up a fold of skin on the back of the acromegalic's hand and compare it with your own or preferably someone of the same age and sex as the patient; the gross thickening of the skin is usually obvious.

Cushing's syndrome (Fig. 12.14)

This syndrome results from prolonged exposure to glucocorticoid excess and falls into four categories:

- iatrogenic due to prolonged high-dose steroid treatment
- a benign or malignant tumour of the adrenal in which one adrenal is enlarged and hypersecreting. There is feedback suppression of the pituitary with low secretion of ACTH and atrophy of the opposite adrenal
- ectopic ACTH production from a secreting tumour

Cushing's syndrome are associated with low serum potassium levels adding to the muscle weakness associated with the wasting effect of cortisol.

Nelson's syndrome When the adrenals have been removed for the treatment of Cushing's disease the ACTH-secreting tumour continues to enlarge and secrete ACTH and allied compounds such as melanocyte-stimulating hormone (MSH) resulting in intense progressive pigmentation as well as the space-occupying effects of the tumour.

The adrenals

Addison's disease Destruction of the adrenal cortices by autoimmune endocrinopathy or by tuberculosis results in failure of both glucocorticoid and mineralocorticoid secretion. Symptoms are of weakness, anorexia and weight loss. The symptoms are so non-specific that the diagnosis may be missed without careful examination. On examination the patient is often thin and wasted. There is pigmentation of the skin (Fig. 12.15) particularly striking in the palmar creases and in areas of pressure from clothing straps. Pigmentation should also be sought in the buccal mucosa. The blood pressure should be taken lying and standing. It is usually low with an excessive postural drop. In the face of intercurrent illness an acute Addisonian crisis may be precipitated because of the inadequate cortisol response to stress. This presents with abdominal pain, vomiting, and collapse mimicking an acute abdomen.

Diabetes mellitus

Symptoms

The presenting symptoms were vividly described by Aretaeus (second century AD) who wrote:

> Diabetes is a wonderful affection, not very frequent among men, being a melting down of the flesh and limbs into urine ... the patients never stop making water, but the flow is incessant as if from the opening of aqueducts ... the thirst is unquenchable and if for a time they abstain from drinking, their mouth becomes parched and their body dry.

This reminds us that the three commonest presenting symptoms are thirst, polyuria and weight loss.

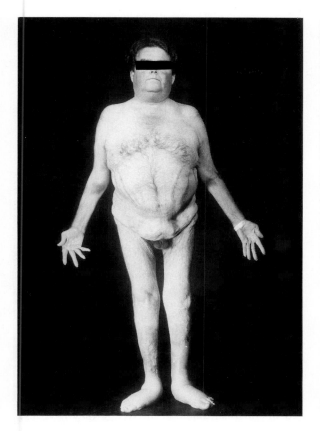

Fig. 12.14 Cushing's syndrome. The characteristic features are the truncal obesity, striae, round 'moon' face, thin limbs and foot oedema.

may occur, e.g. oat-cell carcinoma of lung or carcinoid. Both adrenals are enlarged and hypersecrete
• Cushing's disease due to an adrenocorticotroph hormone (ACTH)-secreting tumour of the pituitary giving rise to bilateral adrenal hyperplasia

Clinical features These are of central obesity and moon face with wasting of limb muscles. Purple striae are seen upon the obese trunk and the face has a high colour. The skin is characteristically thin and fragile. Again test a fold of skin on the back of the patient's hand and see how it compares with someone of the same age and sex. The skin of Cushing's syndrome is as thin and fragile as that of an elderly patient and the same large purpura are seen due to the loss of elastic support fibres surrounding the dermal vessels.

There may be oedema of the legs and also of the conjunctivae. Evidence of hypertension and of hyperglycaemia should also be sought. Malignant causes of

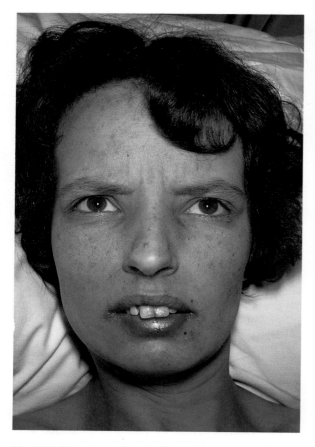

Fig. 12.15 Skin pigmentation in Addison's disease. Though dark-haired, this lady had previously had a delicate complexion.

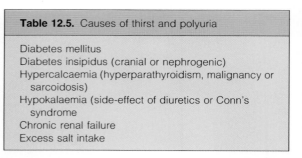

Table 12.5. Causes of thirst and polyuria
Diabetes mellitus
Diabetes insipidus (cranial or nephrogenic)
Hypercalcaemia (hyperparathyroidism, malignancy or sarcoidosis)
Hypokalaemia (side-effect of diuretics or Conn's syndrome
Chronic renal failure
Excess salt intake

Thirst

Establish that the patient has polydipsia not just a dry mouth which might be a side-effect of drugs with anticholinergic actions (such as antidepressants) or due to Sjögren's syndrome (an autoimmune condition in which there is progressive destruction of the salivary and lachrymal glands) (see Table 5.1). The commonest cause of thirst without polyuria is insensible fluid loss from working in an over-heated environment. Diabetes mellitus is the commonest but not the only cause of thirst and polyuria (Table 12.5). In the seventeenth century it was distinguished by Thomas Willis from other causes by tasting the urine; in deficiency of or resistance to antidiuretic hormone (cranial or nephrogenic diabetes insipidus), the urine was tastless or insipid. In diabetes mellitus, where the urine contains glucose, it was sweet, hence the name mellitus or honey-like. In a patient with thirst the simplest screening test for diabetes mellitus (hereafter referred to as just diabetes) is to test the urine for glucose.

Polyuria

Few people know how often they urinate during the day (do you?) and the best indication of polyuria is nocturia. Nocturia in middle-aged men can lead to a suspicion of prostatism and it is not uncommon for patients to be put on the waiting list for a prostatectomy, found to have glycosuria, and have their symptoms cured by being put on a diet!

Weight loss

Patients often assume that the weight they have lost while developing diabetes is entirely due to fluid but Arataeus knew better when he described it as a 'melting down of the flesh and limbs'. We can think of diabetes as being caused by a deficiency of insulin or resistance to its action. The body goes into what has been called 'accelerated starvation' and excessive gluconeogenesis results in production of glucose in the liver using as substrates the carbon skeleton of amino acids from breakdown of muscle and glycerol from fat. Even a modest degree of insulin resistance or deficiency will lead to endogenous glucose production whereas lipolysis and ketonuria indicate more severe insulin deficiency.

The degree of weight loss, if it can be documented, is an important pointer to future treatment. Ask whether your patients weigh themselves regularly or, if they do not, when was the last time they were weighed (perhaps in another department in the hospital?). Also find out their previous maximum weight and the age at which it was reached. Weight is as much a scientific measurement as serum creatinine and there are tables of ideal weight for height.

Other presentations of diabetes (Table 12.6)

Most newly diagnosed diabetic patients will admit to thirst and polyuria if you ask them carefully but sometimes another symptom dominates the clinical picture. Pruritus vulvae (itching in the vagina and vulva) is particularly common in middle-aged women and may lead to referral to a gynaecology clinic. The equivalent in men is balanitis which often leads men to refer themselves to the genitourinary clinic. Poly-phagia (excessive appetite) is very rare and suggests coincidental thyrotoxicosis. In the newly diagnosed, middle-aged diabetic patient, loss of appetite is sinister and suggests carcinoma of the pancreas. It is not unusual for men to realize that they have diabetes when they see spots of crystallized glucose on their shoes and in the tropics it is well known that diabetic urine attracts ants!

Hyperglycaemia can be asymptomatic and screen-ing surveys in the general population always turn up as many previously undiagnosed as already known diabetics. Without screening some of these will be diagnosed at routine medicals (e.g. for work or life insurance) while in others the hyperglycaemia remains undetected for years until the patient presents with a diabetic complication.

Examination of the newly diagnosed diabetic

The purpose of the examination is to confirm the diagnosis, classify the type of diabetes and detect complications.

Confirmation of the diagnosis

In health, blood glucose concentrations are remark-ably constant and rarely outside the range 3.5—8.0 mmol/l. In patients who present with typical diabetic symptoms, a single fasting plasma glucose over 7.8 mmol/l or a random value over 11.1 mmol/l clinch the diagnosis. A glucose-tolerance test is only necess-ary in cases of doubt if blood glucose levels are lower than this. Although we usually talk about blood glucose it is important to note that most labora-tories actually measure plasma glucose, which is slightly higher than whole-blood glucose.

Classification

Most cases of diabetes are idiopathic and are simply classified as:

INSULIN DEPENDENT (IDDM, type 1 or juvenile-onset diabetes)
NON-INSULIN DEPENDENT (NIDDM, type II or maturity-onset diabetes)

However, diabetes, like anaemia and jaundice, is a syndrome with many possible causes (Table 12.7). An important part of the history and examination is to look for these rare causes. Some, such as Cushing's syndrome, acromegaly and thyrotoxicosis, can be recognized from their typical appearance. Most endocrine causes combine hyperglycaemia and hypertension but remember that antihypertensive treatment (especially the combination of a thiazide and beta-blocker) greatly increases the risk of devel-oping ordinary diabetes. Other causes of secondary diabetes can be suspected from physical signs such as the pigmentation of haemochromatosis or unusual features in the history like recurrent abdominal pain which suggests chronic pancreatitis or carcinoma of the pancreas.

The first decision to make is whether your patient has IDDM and needs insulin treatment urgently to prevent ketoacidosis. IDDM is a partly inherited auto-

---

Table 12.6. How diabetes can be discovered

Routine urine test
  e.g. at insurance or employment medical.
  Screening surveys always find as many previously
  unknown as already diagnosed diabetics

Symptoms
  Thirst
  Polyuria
  Weight loss
  Pruritus vulvae
  Balanitis
  Tiredness

Complications
  Complications as the presenting feature of diabetes
  are only found in the middle-aged and elderly.
  They may be
  Microvascular
  Poor eyesight (retinopathy)
  Renal failure (nephropathy)
  Foot ulcers (neuropathy)
  Macrovascular
  Claudication
  Angina
  Heart attack
  Other
  Poor eyesight due to cataracts

Table 12.7. Classification of diabetes

	Suggestive clinical features
1. Insulin dependent (type 1)	Ketonuria Another autoimmune disease (e.g. Addison's or hypothyroidism)
2. Non-insulin dependent (type 2)	
(a) Obese	>120% ideal body weight
(b) Non-obese	<120% ideal body weight
(c) Maturity onset diabetes of the young (MODY)	Family history
3. Pancreatic	
(a) Haemochromatosis	Pigmentation Hepatomegaly Hypogonadism
(b) Chronic pancreatitis	Abdominal pain Previous attacks of acute pancreatitis Alcoholism
(c) Carcinoma of the pancreas	Abdominal pain Disproportionate weight loss
4. Hormonal	
(a) Cushing's syndrome	
(b) Acromegaly	
(c) Thyrotoxicosis	
(d) Phaeochromocytoma	
(e) Hyperaldosteronism (Conn's syndrome)	
(f) Glucagonoma	
5. Drug-induced	
(a) Steroids	
(b) Antihypertensive agents (thiazides and beta-blockers)	
(c) Others	
6. Rare genetic syndromes e.g. DIDMOAD (diabetes insipidus, diabetes mellitus, optic atrophy and deafness)	

immune disease in which people with certain tissue types (HLA DR3 and DR4) destroy their own beta cells, a process which is often marked (but not caused by) islet cell antibodies. HLA typing and measurement of islet cell antibodies are not routinely available and the question of insulin dependence has to be decided clinically. Clues to severe insulin deficiency are shown in Table 12.8. Three points need to be stressed:

- IDDM can occur at any age and is not uncommon in the thin, middle-aged woman with a short history of diabetic symptoms especially if she already has another autoimmune disease (e.g. hypothyroidism)
- traces of ketonuria can be caused by starvation but moderate or heavy ketonuria in a patient with diabetic symptoms indicates IDDM

Table 12.8. Clinical features suggesting severe insulin deficiency (IDDM)

Moderate or heavy ketonuria
A short history of symptoms
Severe symptoms
Marked weight loss (irrespective of absolute weight)
A first-degree relative on insulin
Personal history of autoimmune disease

- the absolute level of blood glucose is a poor guide to the need for insulin. Many maturity-onset (NIDDM) diabetics with a blood glucose of 30 mmol/l can be safely treated with diet alone whereas some young patients with a blood glucose of 20 mmol/l may be severely acidotic and need urgent insulin treatment.

Complications (Table 12.9)

Eyes The main eye complication is retinopathy. Maculopathy (most common in IDDM) produces slow visual loss and is best detected by testing visual acuity using a Snellen's chart. Proliferative retinopathy (most common in IDDM) is often asymptomatic until a vitreous haemorrhage occurs and is detected at a treatable stage by ophthalmoscopy.

Trying to look at the fundi through undilated pupils is like trying to describe the inside of a room through the keyhole. The pupils should be dilated with 0.5 or 1 per cent tropicamide which wears off within a few hours. The features to look for are:

- microaneurysms: small red dots which are the earliest sign of retinopathy and usually occur first around the macula. Larger haemorrhages are called blot haemorrhages (Fig. 12.16)
- irregularity and tortuosity of veins
- hard exudates: creamy white and waxy in appearance. These may occur in plaques or circles (Fig. 12.17)
- cotton wool spots: these are often inaccurately described as soft exudates; they are actually retinal infarcts (Fig. 12.18)
- new vessels: the cardinal sign of proliferative retinopathy may be found peripherally or on the optic disc (Fig. 12.19)

Limbs Necrobiosis lipoidica diabeticorum (Fig. 12.20) is most common on the shins. The lesions are atrophic, shiny and usually crossed by telangiectatic vessels. The cause is unknown.

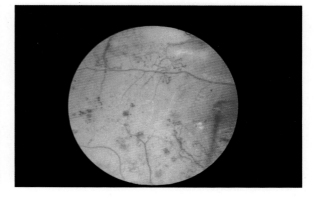

Fig. 12.16 Dot and blot haemorrhages. There is also some proliferative retinopathy in the lower part of the field.

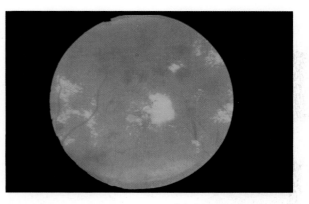

Fig. 12.17 Hard exudates. This is the type of retinopathy typically seen in middle-aged diabetics.

Table 12.9. Diabetic complications

Microvascular	Macrovascular	Miscellaneous

Retinopathy
  Background
  Maculopathy
  Preproliferative
  Proliferative
Nephropathy
  Proteinuria
  Hypertension
Neuropathy
  Sensory
  Motor (amyotrophy)
  Autonomic (postural hypotension, impotence)
  Mononeuropathy (third and sixth nerve palsy, foot drop, etc.)
	Coronary artery disease
	  Angina, previous myocardial infarct, atrial fibrillation, abnormal ECG
	Cerebrovascular
	  Stroke
	Peripheral vascular disease
	  intermittent claudication, absent pulses, rest pain, gangrene
		Necrobiosis lipoidica diabeticorum
		Cataracts
		Psychological problems
		Hyperlipidaemia

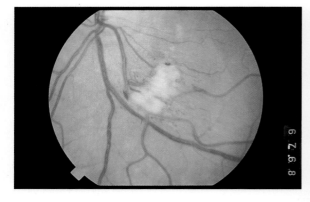

Fig. 12.18 A retinal infarct in diabetes. These appearances are non-specific and may be seen in such disorders as polyarteritis nodosa or subacute bacterial endocarditis.

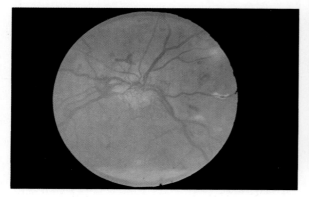

Fig. 12.19 Proliferative retinopathy. In this patient the new vessels are seen on the optic disc.

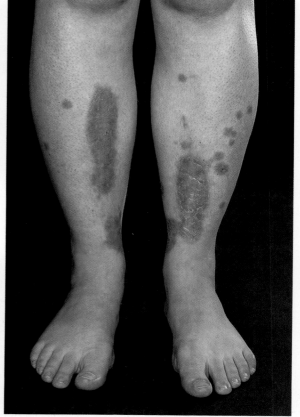

Fig. 12.20 Necrobiosis lipoidica diabeticorum. The site of this relatively unusual complication of diabetes is typical.

Foot lesions are a major cause of morbidity in diabetes and may progress to gangrene and amputation. They may be purely neuropathic, purely ischaemic or most commonly due to a combination of the two. All types of neuropathy make the foot vulnerable.

Sensory neuropathy makes the foot insensitive so that abnormal pressures or injuries, i.e. from a tight shoe or a stone in the shoe are not noticed. Motor neuropathy leads to wasting of the intrinsic muscles of the foot and deformity, especially clawing of the toes and abnormal prominence of the metatarsal heads. Autonomic neuropathy causes loss of sweating and loss of autoregulation of the blood flow to the foot. The former causes dry inelastic skin and the latter arteriovenous shunting so that the foot becomes relatively ischaemic in spite of good peripheral pulses.

Walking on abnormally prominent metatarsal heads leads to callus formation and eventually a painless, punched-out neuropathic ulcer (Fig. 12.21).

The features to note on examination of the feet are shown in Table 12.10.

Signs of neuropathy Look for muscle wasting; in amyotrophy this will be seen in the quadriceps. Wasting of the small muscles of the feet cannot be seen directly but is implied if there is the typical deformity of claw toes and abnormally prominent extensor tendons. Muscle wasting in the hands always indicates severe neuropathy in the feet!

The first sign of neuropathy is absent ankle-jerks. Unfortunately this is a poorly reproducible sign unless you do the test carefully with a relaxed patient. Absent knee-jerks indicate very severe neuropathy.

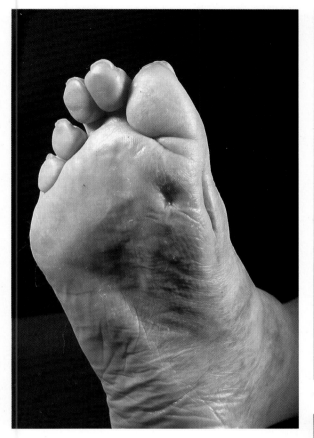

Fig. 12.21 A neuropathic ulcer in a diabetic foot. This is a typical site over the head of the first metatarsal.

Table 12.10. Check list for examination of the diabetic foot

Sensory
  Pinprick
  Vibration sense with a tuning-fork or biothesiometer
  Joint/position sense
Motor
  Wasting
  Deformity
  Weakness
  Ankle- and knee-jerks
Autonomic
  Sweating
  Skin texture
  Abnormally prominent veins on dorsum indicate AV
    shunting
Vascular
  Feel and grade popliteal, posterior tibial and
    dorsalis pedis pulses •
General
  Coldness
  Lack of hairs
  Ingrowing toenails
  Cracks between the toes
  Athlete's foot
  Hallux valgus
  Patches of callus ('corns')

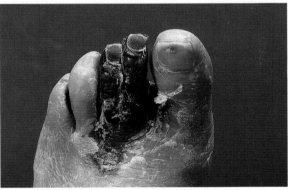

Fig. 12.22 Dry gangrene of toes. Often the arterial disease is so extensive that below-the-knee amputation is required.

Sensory neuropathy is indicated by reduction of pinprick sensation and loss of vibration sense. Like the ankle-jerks these are difficult signs to assess properly and many diabetic clinics use an instrument called a biothesiometer to quantitate vibration sense.

Signs of ischaemia The most reliable signs of peripheral vascular disease are the peripheral pulses. In the diabetic ischaemia is predominantly distal (Fig. 12.22) and the first signs are weakness or absence of the dorsalis pedis and posterior tibial pulses. It is important to remember that 5 per cent of normal people have an aberrant dorsalis pedis. Popliteal pulses can be difficult to feel unless the limb is well relaxed. Finally feel the femoral pulses and auscultate them and the lower abdomen for bruits.

If there are symptoms or signs of ischaemia a more accurate way of assessing the circulation is to use a Doppler probe; if surgery is contemplated an arteriogram will be necessary.

Nephropathy The earliest sign of diabetic nephropathy is microalbuminuria which is not necessarily detected by dipsticks such as Albustix. If albuminuria is present in the newly diagnosed patient, a midstream urine test (MSU) should be done to exclude urinary infection. Albuminuria in a patient with retinopathy is almost always due to diabetic nephropathy. If there is no retinopathy, albuminuria should be investigated as it would in the non-diabetic patient.

Postscript

Diagnosis of diabetes is easy and most newly diagnosed patients will not have any physical signs. However, when you find the raised blood glucose, you are diagnosing an incurable (but controllable) illness the treatment of which requires more patient participation than most other illnesses. The patient's ability to comply with diet, self blood glucose monitoring, insulin injections, etc. depends on many factors including his or her personality, intelligence, social circumstances and understanding of the disease. While taking the history and examining the newly diagnosed diabetic, the experienced physician is trying to get a picture of the patient as a person so that one can anticipate potential stumbling blocks to treatment. When doing the examination he or she will explain the physical findings as the first part of the educational process. For example, if insensitive feet are found he or she will point this out and explain the possible consequences, for example that using a hot-water bottle may lead to severe but painless burns.

References and further reading

Tattersall RB, Gale EAM. *Diabetes: clinical management*. Edinburgh: Churchill Livingstone, 1990.

Tunbridge WM, Home PD. *Diabetes and endocrinology in clinical practice*. London: Edward Arnold, 1991.

Watkins PJ. *ABC of diabetes*, 3rd edn. London; British Medical Association, 1993.

13

The examination of elderly patients

M. J. Bendall

> History-taking and its pitfalls
> The examination
> References and further reading

The elderly are often thought of as a homogeneous group, defined as those of greater than pensionable age (60 years for women and 65 years for men in the UK). In reality, the opposite applies and the elderly, in relation to medicine, are a very heterogeneous group; individuals aged between 65 and 75 years are generally fit and active, whereas those over 75 years may more often have, with increasing age, multiple diseases which present atypically and lead to progressive disability and dependance on the help of others. It is to this second group, usually referred to as the very elderly, that this chapter addresses itself. The majority of people in this group are women and the feminine gender is therefore used throughout.

Much of what applies to the examination of a younger patient applies equally to an elderly one, but, for three main reasons, examining old people is often much more complicated.

First, the elderly tend to suffer from multiple diseases. A young patient is usually sick with one disease or with disease of one organ or organ system and although the elderly patient may present with an acute illness, this is usually superimposed on chronic conditions. Thus the illness bringing the patient to medical attention may be a chest infection, but she may also have arthritis, a stroke and dementia, all of which influence both her response to the chest infection and her subsequent recovery.

Secondly, the acute illness commonly presents atypically, not with classical signs (for example, crushing chest pain due to myocardial infarction) but in the non-specific ways listed in Table 13.1. Any acute illness in an elderly person may present in one of these ways.

Table 13.1. Non-specific presentations of disease in the elderly

1. Falls
2. Immobility — 'gone off her feet'
3. Incontinence
4. Confusion
5. Acute 'acopia' — relatives or other carers can no longer cope
6. Hypothermia — usually secondary to other 'silent' illnesses (infection, myocardial infarction)
7. Iatrogenic illness — as a result of multiple therapy for multiple diseases

Thirdly, the complication rate, after the patient has presented, is much higher than in the young. The old lady admitted with a mild stroke may, in sequence, fall and fracture her femur, develop a bedsore and then become incontinent.

History-taking and its pitfalls

The interview should take place in a quiet, well-lit place. See that the patient and yourself are as relaxed as possible and sit so that the patient can clearly see your face. Listen to the patient carefully; it is often the chance remark that gives the initial clue as to what is going on. Be prepared to take your time. The elderly usually respond more slowly to questions than the young but this does not necessarily indicate mental impairment. In some cases slowing of verbal response may be due to Parkinson's disease, myxoedema or depression. High-tone deafness is common in the elderly and so speak in a clear, low-pitched voice. Failure to appreciate deafness may lead to an incorrect diagnosis of dementia. If the patient has a functioning hearing-aid make sure she uses it during the interview. Some wards, particularly those in departments for the elderly, have specially designed amplifiers for the purpose of interviewing deaf people; ask if such an instrument is available.

Early in the interview try to form some idea of whether the patient is muddled or not. At some stage a formal assessment of cognitive function must be performed. However, if this is done before you have gained her confidence, you run the risk of offending a patient with normal mental function by asking, what to her, are a series of 'simple' questions. Initially look for clues in her replies; for example, a patient who refers to a deceased spouse as if he was still alive. When you have gained the patient's confidence, you may need to introduce questions from the Abbreviated Mental Test (see Chapter 14) with a comment such as 'I'm now going to ask you some questions which may seem very simple to you, but they are an important part of my examining you; I hope you don't mind'.

Sometimes a patient and her relatives say 'she has a marvellous memory' or 'she's as clear as a bell'. These remarks are often based on long-term memory which may be well preserved in the early stages of dementia. The patient may have very clear recollections of her childhood, or the First World War, but on formal questioning be unable to recall what she ate for lunch half an hour previously! Again specific questions about current daily activities are essential: does she leave the gas on, does she burn pots and pans?

Even if the patient has a normal memory she may still be totally unrealistic about her capabilities: few of us readily acknowledge our limitations to a relative stranger. Collateral evidence from relatives, friends, neighbours, home-helps and social workers is important for all patients and vital if a patient is muddled.

Make sure that the points elicited in the history refer to the current illness and not some past event. If the patient is disorientated in time she can easily confuse events that happened last week with those that happened last year. If this possibility is not recognized early on, the doctor may become very confused as well!

As assessment of the time-course of any symptom is very important. A sudden deterioration in health is likely to be due to acute illness (for example myo-cardial infarction, pulmonary embolus, stroke or infection); ask specifically whether the presenting symptom (including falls, incontinence, confusion, or 'acopia'*) is of recent onset or long-standing and gradually getting worse.

If a patient or her relatives say that she is 'doing OK' be wary. Such comments are often based on low expectations of what the elderly are like and can do. Specific questions about activities of daily living (washing, dressing, toileting, shopping and cooking) tell much more about what she is really like: most elderly people are independent in these activities. Another useful marker of dependency is how much outside help (home-help, meals-on-wheels, district nurse, day centre or day hospital attendance) the patient requires: thus a patient receiving home-help once a week is likely to have a minor degree of disability, whereas one having this support five days a week together with daily meals-on-wheels is likely to be heavily dependent.

Some patients and relatives perceive such features of disease as falls, incontinence and confusion as inevitable parts of ageing and fail to mention them spontaneously. Ask about them specifically.

An idea of what the patient was like and what she was doing some weeks before her illness is important, not only in assessing its time course, but also in gaining an idea of the level of function to be anticipated following rehabilitation. If she was out and about shopping, and doing everything for herself until the recent illness, then the likelihood is that her present level of disability is due to the acute illness and is therefore potentially remediable. Setting realistic goals for rehabilitation should begin at the time of the history.

The multiplicity of disease in the very elderly leads to multiple medication. The more drugs that an elderly patient takes, the more likely she is to have side-effects from them; iatrogenic disease is common in the elderly. Even when the patient's general practitioner considers the patient to be taking only one or two drugs, drug hoarding from previous illnesses occurs and the patient may, in fact, be taking many more. Try to find out what drugs the patient has at home. Show them to her; if she is forgetful this may prompt her to give a much more detailed picture of her current medication. Don't forget that she may fail to take some or all of her prescribed drugs!

After the history, examination and some of the initial investigations are completed be prepared to

---

* 'Acopia' — an ugly neologism but a useful abbreviation for 'being unable to cope'.

go back over some of the history again if there appear to be inconsistencies, or if investigations show unexpected results. As always this must be done in a manner which does not upset the patient, but which smooths the relationship.

The examination

A thorough physical examination is essential and most of what applies to younger people applies equally well to the elderly. Certain features are particularly important and it is these which are discussed here.

The environment

If the patient is examined at home the condition of the dwelling not only indicates her previous abilities over a period of time, but also the effectiveness of support being provided. The state of her dress and general level of cleanliness are similarly useful indicators.

Hearing, vision and speech

The elderly often become isolated because of problems with these functions. During the history a simple assessment of hearing can be made by the interviewer varying the volume with which questions are asked. Check the patient's ears for wax. Wax is unlikely significantly to impair hearing in someone with otherwise normal hearing, but may be, so to speak, the last straw when hearing is impaired. Hearing-aids are often not worn even when provided. If she has a hearing-aid make sure that it is working and that the patient knows how to use it. Know yourself how to change a hearing-aid battery and what the switch positions mean (Table 13.2).

If she has poor vision, in addition to ophthalmoscopic examination, test for refractive errors using an ophthalmic 'pin-hole' and a Snellen chart. The pin-hole acts as a perfect lens which corrects any

refractive error; if vision improves significantly using this technique, then a formal check on refraction by an optician is indicated. Poor vision may even be due to such a simple matter as dirty spectacle lenses. Washing the glasses under the tap may improve things considerably!

In addition to the speech disorders related to neurological diseases mentioned in Chapter 8, speech in the elderly may be unclear as a result of ageing processes affecting the speech mechanisms, dental trouble or to ill-fitting dentures. With age, speech tends to become slower, of lower volume and higher pitched. Often the voice becomes querulous, but whether this is due to ageing or to psychological factors is unclear. Dental caries may act as a focus of acute or chronic infection or, by chronic irritation, lead to oral ulcers. Poor-fitting dentures may be associated with oral ulceration and poor nutrition. The 'portcullis' sign (the top denture falling on to the bottom one when the mouth is opened) may be due to poor fitting, but if it arises *de novo* may indicate dehydration or a stroke leading to loss of tone in the buccal musculature (Fig. 13.1). Orofacial dyskinesia (chewing movements of lips and jaws) due to treatment with major tranquillizers and occasionally to other extrapyramidal disorders may also cause dysarthria. An oral lesion often found in the elderly which can cause considerable anxiety to the patient and her relatives is 'caviar tongue' — clusters of sublingual varicosities; these seem to be unrelated to other pathology and reassurance can be given.

The nervous system

The examination of the nervous system in the elderly may be complicated both by difficulties of obtaining a clear history of preceding events and by the effect of age on the normal neurological examination.

A history of a sudden change in behaviour or physical capacities may be all that is available; the patient who has had a stroke may exhibit only minor changes in physical signs — slight facial asymmetry, mild slurring of the speech, slight changes of tone. These changes may be apparent only to a doctor who has known the patient for a long time. Her relatives should be asked 'Has there been any change in speech or walking recently, or does her face look different?'.

Wasting of the small muscles of the hands, in the absence of other evidence of neurological disease, is common in the frail elderly; the cause is unclear, though decreased use of the hands may be a factor. The ankle-jerks may be reduced or absent in other-

Table 13.2. Hearing-aid switch positions

O = Off
M = Microphone — for person-to-person conversation
T = Inductive loop aerial pick-up — used in theatres, cinemas, churches and telephone boxes
M&T = Microphone and inductive loop together — increases flexibility of use in particular situations

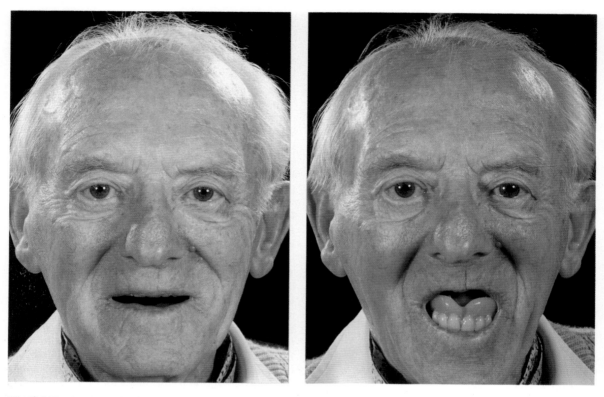

Fig. 13.1 The 'portcullis sign'.

wise normal individuals. The pupils may be small and dilate poorly in a darkened room, making fundal examination very difficult; a pupillary-dilating drug may be necessary to achieve an adequate examination, but the risk, though small, of precipitating glaucoma with such a drug must be remembered. The pupils may be unequal in size or irregular in shape as a result of scarring by previous episodes of iritis.

Feet

Attention should be given to the feet, not only in respect of peripheral vascular disease and peripheral neuropathy, but also of the toe-nails. Any patient who has difficulty in bending, poor vision or clumsy hands will have difficulty in cutting nails properly and this may lead to pain on walking or even immobility. In extremely neglected patients onychogryphosis (overgrown, claw-like toe-nails) may develop, and these require expert chiropody (Fig. 13.2). Footwear also influences mobility; often the patient has an ancient pair of poorly-fitting slippers and needs a

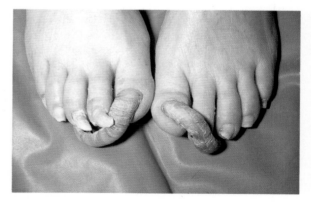

Fig. 13.2 Onychogryphosis. This common disorder, which may be seen in younger folk too, often prevents the wearing of comfortable shoes. It requires skilled chiropody.

well-fitting pair of shoes. Occasionally the pattern of wear on the shoes may give clues; for example, a patient with a foot-drop due to a minor stroke may demonstrate increased wear over the outer, anterior aspect of the sole on the affected side.

Gross swelling of the legs is often due to immobility and postural stasis and does not necessarily imply heart failure. The 'armchair legs' syndrome of the elderly (Fig. 13.3) responds better to mobilization than to diuretics!

Skin

With ageing, skin undergoes a series of changes including thinning, loss of elasticity, increased capillary fragility and, in poorly nourished patients, a decrease in subcutaneous fat and loss of collagen. These changes lead to senile purpura (see Fig. 9.4) and increased looseness of the skin — the latter making detection of dehydration by assessment of skin turgor over the forearm or anterior abdominal wall particularly difficult. Over the forehead the skin is closely anchored to the underlying fascia and this is the best area for assessing dehydration in the elderly.

A variety of skin conditions become more common with age including benign senile angiomas (Campbell de Morgan's spots), seborrhoeic warts and malignant basal-cell and squamous-cell carcinomas. Bullous lesions due to pemphigus, pemphigoid (predominantly a disease of the elderly), Stevens–Johnson syndrome and drugs also occur in old age.

Particular attention should be given to the skin over the 'pressure areas' (the bony protuberances over which pressure sores may develop). Reddening of the skin may be a warning of undue pressure. This redness with surrounding induration indicates pressure necrosis of subcutaneous tissues. The 'iceberg' phenomenon may be present — a small, superficial area of ulceration or necrosis with a much larger underlying area of induration. This is often easily overlooked but may indicate the true extent of dead tissue. Nursing staff may be worried by the ulcer getting bigger and may view this as a failure of nursing care. Usually what is happening is that the ulcer extends as an inevitable part of the evolution of the condition to reveal the full extent of the necrotic tissue.

The development of a pressure sore is a disaster for the patient, for it is a source of sepsis, a metabolic drain and a hindrance to rehabilitation. Prevention is essential and use of a points system, such as that devised by Norton *et al.* (Table 13.3), is a simple and very effective way of identifying those at high risk of developing the condition.

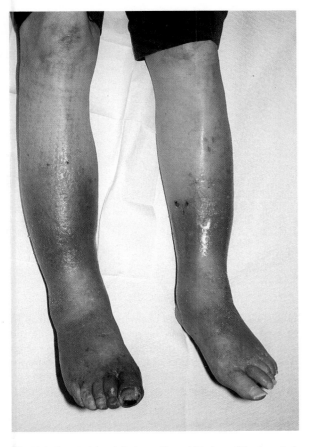

Fig. 13.3 'Armchair legs'. Prolonged immobility from sitting in a chair often results in oedema, cellulitis and ulcers of the skin.

The temperature

A single measurement of the patient's temperature is rarely useful unless the patient is hypothermic (rectal temperature below 35 °C) or pyrexial (temperature above 37.5 °C). Because of the risk of missing hypothermia an elderly patient's rectal temperature should always be taken with a thermometer with a range extending down to at least 30 °C, well below the range of instruments usually provided in hospital wards! Nurses sometimes fail to use a low-reading thermometer because 'there isn't one available'. What they often mean is that there isn't a 'blue bulb' low-reading thermometer available. Certain types of low-reading thermometer are not made with blue bulbs and under these circumstances a thermometer otherwise used orally should be set aside and used solely for rectal thermometry.

'Normal' temperatures vary quite widely even in younger individuals; in the elderly the temperature

Table 13.3. System of scoring the risk of developing pressure sores

Physical state		Mental state		Activity		Mobility		Incontinence	
Good	4	Alert	4	Ambulant	4	Full	4	None including those catheterized	4
Fair	3	Apathetic	3	Walk with help	3	Slightly limited	3	Occasional	3
Poor	2	Confused	2	Chairfast	2	Very limited	2	Usually incontinent of urine or faecally incontinent	2
Very weak	1	Stuporose	1	Bedfast	1	Immobile	1	Double (urine and faeces)	1

A score of 14 points or below indicates a liability of subsequently developing pressure sores; 12 points or less indicates the risk to be very great.

taken six-hourly and plotted for two or three days usually gives much more information than a single reading. Occasionally elderly patients develop systemic infections with the body temperature staying in the normal range. The temperature chart, however, usually shows a rise in the base-line temperature within that range.

Blood pressure

There is evidence that, in patients aged under 80 years who have blood pressures consistently exceeding 160 mmHg systolic and/or 90 mmHg diastolic, antihypertensive therapy offers reduced risk of stroke and cardiac disease. In those over 80 years high blood pressure in itself is rarely of immediate concern. There is little evidence that treatment of hypertension in those over 80 years old is of benefit and in this group high blood pressure may even be associated with increased survival and lower blood pressure with decreased survival. The latter is probably the result of other underlying life-threatening disease. Acute illnesses of many types, particularly left ventricular failure and stroke, lead to a sharp rise in blood pressure but are not indications for antihypertensive therapy, which, in individuals with established cerebrovascular disease may lead to a fall in cerebral bloodflow and to a risk of cerebral thrombosis.

More important, in the elderly, is postural hypotension which is a fall in systolic blood pressure of greater than 20 mmHg when the patient rises from the lying to the standing position. There are many causes of postural hypotension, the condition often being multifactorial in origin (Table 13.4). The characteristic clinical features are complaints of dizziness and faintness, and even when these symptoms are not present, postural unsteadiness and falls

Table 13.4. Causes of postural hypotension in the elderly

1. Autonomic dysfunction due to
   (a) Age-related change in physiological mechanisms
   (b) Disease causing change in physiological mechanisms such as
       Diabetic neuropathy
       Cerebrovascular disease
       Parkinson's disease
       Polyneuropathy
2. Drug-related
       Antihypertensive agents
       Diuretics
       L-dopa
       Phenothiazines
       Tricyclic antidepressants
       Benzodiazepines
       Nitrates
3. Other illnesses
       Myocardial infarction
       Pulmonary embolus
       Dehydration and sodium depletion
       Infections

occur. In the early stages of the condition the drop in blood pressure may only be present first thing in the morning, when the circulating blood volume is at its lowest. In order to be certain that postural hypotension is not present the pressures should be measured when the patient first rises in the morning.

The incontinent patient

Any immobile patient who is unable to ask for help to the toilet, due, for example to dysphasia, fear or dementia, will be incontinent of urine. Regular two-hourly toileting often restores continence in such patients. Persistent incontinence requires further evaluation. A list of the common causes of incontinence is given in Table 13.5.

The size of the bladder should be assessed. The patient may have retention with overflow. This in turn may be due, in men to prostatic disease and, in both sexes, to faecal impaction. Rectal examination will reveal both, but, if the rectum is empty of stool, it is important to exclude 'high constipation' by abdominal palpation and abdominal x-ray. Apart from these conditions, the commonest cause of urinary incontinence is the 'unstable bladder' associated with loss of higher neurological bladder control usually due to cerebrovascular disease or senile dementia. The patient is unpredictably incontinent

Table 13.5. Common causes of incontinence in the elderly

Urinary incontinence
Unstable bladder
Prostatism
Atrophic vaginitis
Pelvic floor disease
Retention with overflow
   Faecal impaction
   Drugs
   Prostatism
   Urethral stricture
   Atonic neurogenic bladder
Acute urinary tract infection — in the presence of one or more of the above factors predisposing a normally continent patient to urinary incontinence
Acute confusional state
Psychological factors — e.g. a 'dirty protest' at a social situation that the patient finds unbearable

Faecal incontinence
Abnormal intestinal activity
   Diarrhoea
   Faecal impaction
Abnormal neurological control
   Dementia — unstable rectum, loss of social awareness, neglect of the call to stool with secondary impaction
Neurological damage to
   Spinal cord
   Cauda equina
   Peripheral nerves
Abnormalities of the pelvic floor
   Stretching of the pelvic floor
   Trauma to the anal sphincter

and usually gets little warning of impending micturition. In multiparous women distinguishing this problem from stress incontinence secondary to pelvic floor weakness can be a difficult problem because the unstable bladder often contracts under the stimulus of coughing or standing up ('pseudo-stress' incontinence). Ask the patient to cough while standing and observe the perineum. In simple stress incontinence urine only leaks for a brief period when the abdominal pressure, and hence the intravesical pressure, exceeds the sphincter closing pressure. The bladder does not contract and the short pressure surge from the cough produces a short spurt of urine. In 'pseudo-stress' incontinence the cough causes the unstable bladder to contract and the stream of urine is prolonged and stops slowly as bladder pressure drops below sphincter pressure.

Faecal incontinence is often a concomitant of the unstable bladder, but comes later in the course of the patient's underlying illness. Any patient with faecal incontinence should be examined for faecal impaction, treatment of which, even in the very demented, may lead to control of the incontinence. Faecal incontinence in the absence of urinary incontinence is almost invariably due to local bowel pathology, most commonly constipation and impaction, but also to acute infective diarrhoea, colonic tumours, diverticular disease, inflammatory bowel disease, anal stricture, anal prolapse and malabsorption.

Mobility and gait

One of the major problems with elderly patients is restoring mobility. An early assessment of gait is invaluable both diagnostically and in defining a baseline against which to measure progress. Many neurological conditions have characteristic gait patterns some of which are described elsewhere. Some of the changes may be very subtle. In an elderly person with a pyramidal lesion, the slight dragging of a foot may be the only obvious sign, sometimes the dragging being heard rather than seen (but check that the noise is not due just to poorly fitting footwear). One of the earliest signs of Parkinson's disease may be a failure to swing the arms when walking.

In planning rehabilitation the amount of help a patient requires to walk is important: how many helpers are needed, are the helpers giving physical or psychological support, what aids are used? If the patient is unable to walk, can she transfer from bed to a chair and back again, from a wheelchair to the toilet and how much help is required?

Activities of daily living (ADL)

A multidisciplinary assessment of whether a patient performs certain tasks essential to independent living is vital to good patient management. A commonly used system of measuring independence is the Barthel ADL Index (Table 13.6) which measures increasing independence on a scale of 0 to 20. The Index can be used to assess premorbid and current function, and also in monitoring progress or otherwise during rehabilitation.

Aids and appliances

No examination of an elderly person is complete without an examination of the aids that they are using. Are the aids suitable, safe and of the correct size?

A walking-stick or frame should come to the level of the ulnar styloid when the patient stands with her arms by her sides and it should have a rubber ferrule on the bottom to prevent slipping on the floor.

Wheelchairs should have adequate brakes and foot-rests. Those with pneumatic tyres should be checked to see if the tyres are fully inflated. Flat tyres can render an otherwise wheelchair-independent person immobile. Wheelchair brakes will not work on flat tyres. The brake requires a fully inflated tyre to obtain sufficient purchase to stop the chair moving. The loss of braking makes the wheelchair unstable

---

Table 13.6. The Barthel ADL Index

Activity	Score	
Bowels	0	Incontinent or needs enema
	1	Occasional accident (once a week or less)
	2	Continent
Bladder	0	Incontinent, or catheterized and unable to manage catheter
	1	Occasional accident (not more than once in 24 hours)
	2	Continent
Grooming	0	Needs help with personal care (face, hair, shaving, teeth)
	1	Independent
Toilet	0	Dependent
	1	Needs some help
	2	Independent (on and off toilet, wiping and dressing)
Feeding	0	Unable
	1	Needs some help (e.g. cutting up, spreading butter)
	2	Independent
Transfers	0	Unable — no sitting balance
	1	Major help (physical from one or two people), can sit
	2	Minor help (verbal or physical)
	3	Independent
Mobility	0	Immobile
	1	Wheelchair independent (able to negotiate corners, doors, etc.)
	2	Walks with help of one person (verbal or physical)
	3	Independent (with or without walking aid)
Dressing	0	Dependent
	1	Needs help (can do about half unaided)
	2	Independent (including buttons and zips)
Stairs	0	Unable
	1	Needs help (verbal, physical, or carrying walking aid)
	2	Independent both up and down
Bathing	0	Dependent
	1	Independent (bath and shower unsupervised)

and liable to tip up when the user tries to get out of it. A bicycle pump is a handy piece of equipment to have around!

Check the height of the patient's chair. She may be immobile because it is a low, sagging armchair which results in her quadriceps femori working at a mechanical disadvantage. Try getting her to stand from a higher armchair or an ordinary dining chair.

Conclusion

The initial examination of a very eldery patient requires great attention to detail and is necessarily time-consuming. Even quite small, simply resolved factors can make the difference between dependance and independence. The time taken is never wasted. Even if the patient does not become independent the information collected at this stage inevitably plays a vital role in planning her on-going care. Additionally the fact that the patient will see that you are interested in practical problems important to her will cement the doctor–patient relationship. There is nothing more destructive of the patient's trust than for her to believe you are not interested in the things that concern her.

References and further reading

Godwin-Austen R, Bendall MJ. *The neurology of the elderly.* London: Springer, 1990.

Jarrett D. Geriatricians examine the parts that other physicians fail to reach. *Geriatric Medicine.* 1987; *Nov*: 29–35.

Norton D, McLaren R, Exton-Smith AN. *An investigation of geriatric nursing problems in hospital.* London: Centre for Policy on Ageing, 1962.

Pathy MSJ. Geriatric medicine. *Hospital Update.* 1982; *Dec*: 1509–18.

Royal College of Physicians of London/British Geriatrics Society. *Standardised assessment scales for elderly people.* London: Royal College of Physicians, 1992.

Ware M. *Medicine in old age*, 2nd edn. London: British Medical Association, 1985.

14

How to examine an old person who seems muddled

T. Arie

First principles
The examination
The history
Further reading

Keep an open mind. When 'confused' old people are referred to hospital, minds snap shut, the main thought often being how to avoid blocking a bed. Yet life and death may depend on careful appraisal. Two points are crucial: transient confusional states (resembling at first sight dementias) may be reversible; old people admitted in such a state have later safely driven themselves home in their own cars. Next, even where dementia is established, much can be achieved by careful analysis of the problems, defining what can be mended, and what cannot — even if the condition is not reversible.

Confusion or delirium is a non-specific reaction of the brain to a wide variety of noxious stimuli. In old age (as in very young children) confusion may develop at a lower threshold than normal; confusional states (along with incontinence, immobility and falls) are common non-specific presentations of almost any disorder, physical or mental. But many old people are slower, mentally as well as physically, may be deaf and occasionally are dysphasic; they may be thought to be 'confused' when they are not.

Most 'confused' old people are very old; most very old people are women — hence the use of the feminine gender.

First principles

Take time. Do not rush your examination, or be greedy for instant information. As people get old,

they find it harder to assimilate new material, though they get there in time; and hospitals are anxious and disorientating places even for younger people. Old people newly admitted to unfamiliar wards or seen in out-patient departments are often perplexed and slowed, along with the normal anxiety generated by such occasions. The following points are therefore important:

- whenever possible, 'confused' old people should be assessed at home, or in their normal setting, though this is not always possible
- see that the patient is comfortable, warm and appropriately positioned (e.g. if orthopnoeic, provide appropriate pillows)
- if she uses spectacles or a hearing-aid, see that she has them (and that the hearing-aid is working, see Table 13.2). If she uses dentures, see that she has them if she wants them
- make sure that urgent needs (e.g. to empty the bladder) have been attended to or the patient's mind will be on them rather than on the interview (just as yours in a busy day may be on the next patient). If the patient has been incontinent, make sure that the mess has been cleaned up. If a bedpan is needed, see that it is provided
- introduce yourself, by name and profession, and be prepared to repeat your introduction. Explain what you are doing, and add a few reassuring comments that help to set the scene
- speak clearly, but don't shout — not all old people

are deaf, and if they are, their deafness is unlikely to be of the sort that responds to shouting

- be prepared to repeat yourself — but not as if you were talking to an idiot; for many old people the penny drops, but not always as rapidly as the harrassed house-physician would like. (Sometimes the doctor is so busy thinking of other things that have got to be done that he doesn't even notice that the penny has already dropped!) Don't be shy to hold the patient's hand or give other forms of reassurance
- address the patient correctly by name — a muddled person often has the feeling of being in the wrong place, that there's been some mistake; hearing one's own name surely helps to reassure. Don't call old people 'Mum' or 'Pop', or use first names — it is not only discourteous, but may actually disorientate someone of a generation not used to familiarity.

The examination

Take a moment to set the scene by appropriate conversation, which itself will often give much information that you are seeking; chat and you can learn whether the patient knows where she is, the name of the hospital, where she lives, what children she has and so on. Information on the cognitive state is often best acquired in the course of such conversation, though standard questions are desirable, especially for monitoring change over time.

Assess whether the patient is delirious. In mild and subacute forms this may be difficult. Delirium, or acute confusion, is a level of awareness, sometimes called 'clouding of consciousness', which fluctuates to and fro along a spectrum which lies between the two extremes of full awareness and coma. It is often easier to recognize than describe: clouds seem to float across the patient's thinking and awareness, so that one minute she is with you, the next not. The patient may be restless. There may in severe form be illusions, delusions and hallucinations. Acute confusional states are almost always due to specific, most commonly physical, derangements, often reversible.

Assess the patient's comprehension. Note any evidence of dysphasia or deafness (and give a thought to language problems where local dialect or foreign origin is a factor).

Assess cognitive function by a series of focused questions. Some of these will naturally seem artificial

and even absurd, so introduce them by words such as 'I am going to ask you some questions that may sound silly, but I want to check how good your memory is'. A short list of standard questions is given in Table 14.1. A widely used and simple, but fuller, test is the 'mini-mental state' questionnaire (Table 14.2(a) and (b)). Always pay attention to the way in which the patient tackles the tasks, just as you do to the final score; look, for instance, for perseveration; for very easy distractability (?confusional state); for the patient who seems to concentrate carefully but makes fundamental mistakes (?dementia); or for the very slowed response (?depression) — though none of these of course are specific. Don't forget the possible influence of sedating or befuddling drugs.

Examine for dyspraxias. Ask the patient to perform simple tasks which you illustrate — e.g. simple folding of a piece of paper.

In addition to the standard tests for dysphasia and dyspraxia, consider also those disorders of body and space-image which originate from lesions in the non-dominant parietal lobe — e.g. dressing apraxias, or anosognosia or hemiagnosia. Look for visual-field defects and for hemi-inattention.

Clock drawing A useful test of visuospatial function as well as of general cognitive status, is the clock test. Present the patient with a plain piece of paper with a circle on it (at least 5 cm in diameter). Then ask her to 'put in the face of a clock'. Sometimes this needs repeating once or twice, for it is an odd request. Tell the patient you want her to 'put in the numbers just as if it were a clock face'. This test can detect subtle and specific impairments (e.g. hemi-inattention). Again, the manner in which the task is approached is often as significant as the finished product. If a patient makes a good clock face (always allow for poor eyesight), go on to ask her to put the

Table 14.1. Ten simple questions

Age
Time (hour)
Year
Name of place
Recognition of two people
Date of birth
Date of Second World War
Monarch
Counting backwards from 20 to 1
Five-minute recall — 42 West Street

Table 14.2. Mini-mental state examination
(*a*)

'MINI-MENTAL STATE'

Patient . . . .
Examiner . . . .
Date . . . .

Maximum
Score   Score

ORIENTATION

Max	Score	
5	( )	What is the (year) (season) (date) (day) (month)?
5	( )	Where are we: (country) (county) (town) (hospital) (ward)?

REGISTRATION

3 ( ) Name 3 objects: 1 second to say each. Then ask the patient all 3 after you have said them. Give 1 point for each correct answer. Then repeat them until he learns all 3. Count trials and record.

Trials . . . .

ATTENTION AND CALCULATION

5 ( ) Serial 7s. 1 point for each correct. Stop after 5 answers. Alternatively spell 'world' backwards.

RECALL

3 ( ) Ask for the 3 objects repeated above. Give 1 point for each correct.

LANGUAGE AND COPYING

9 ( ) Name a pencil, and watch. (2 points)
( ) Repeat the following: 'No ifs, ands or buts'. (1 point)
( ) Follow a 3-stage command: 'Pick up a paper with your right hand, fold it half, and put it in on the floor'. (3 points)
( ) Read and obey the following: 'Close your eyes'. (1 point)
( ) Write a sentence. (1 point)
( ) Copy design. (1 point)

30 . . . . Total Score
ASSESS level of consciousness along a continuum

Alert   Drowsy   Stupor   Coma

* A score of 20 or less strongly suggests dementia or other significant impairment.

hands at a fixed time — e.g. 'twenty to three'. Samples of clocks drawn by patients are in Fig. 14.1.

Confusion and cognitive impairment may seem the chief point at issue, but do not neglect the other aspects of a mental state examination, such as whether the patient is depressed, elated, anxious, agitated, obsessional, deluded or hallucinated. The mental state examination has already been dealt with in Chapter 10. Taken for granted too is that the patient will be fully examined physically and appropriate laboratory tests performed.

The history

This comes before the examination, but it is sometimes useful to do a quick examination of the patient first, so as to get an approximate frame of reference against which to gather the history. The patient may give a good history (a fact which is itself significant diagnostically), but in apparently confused old people it is the history from another informant that is paramount. If the patient has just been brought into hospital, make sure you catch any accompanying people, such as friends, neighbours, or policemen — they may disappear and never be seen again. Getting

Table 14.2.
(b)

INSTRUCTIONS FOR ADMINISTRATION OF
MINI-MENTAL STATE EXAMINATION

ORIENTATION

(1) Ask for the date. Then ask specifically for parts omitted, e.g. 'Can you also tell me what season it is? 'One point for each correct.

(2) Ask in turn 'Can you tell me the name of this hospital?' (town, county, etc.). One point for each correct.

REGISTRATION

Ask the patient if you may test his memory. Then say the names of 3 unrelated objects, clearly and slowly, about one second for each. After you have said all 3, ask him to repeat them. This first repetition determines his score (0−3) but keep saying them until he can repeat all 3, up to 6 trials. If he does not eventually learn all 3, recall cannot be meaningfully tested.

ATTENTION AND CALCULATION

Ask the patient to begin with 100 and count backwards by 7. Stop after 5 subtractions (93, 86, 79, 72, 65). Score the total number of correct answers.

If the patient cannot or will not perform this task, ask him to spell the word 'world' backwards. The score is the number of letters in correct order, e.g. dlrow = 5, dlorw = 3.

RECALL

Ask the patient if he can recall the 3 words you previously asked him to remember. Score 0−3.

LANGUAGE AND COPYING

Naming: Show the patient a wrist watch and ask him what it is. Repeat for pencil. Score 0−2.

Repetition: Ask the patient to repeat the sentence after you. Allow only one trial. Score 0 or 1.

3-Stage commands: Give the patient a piece of plain blank paper and repeat the command. Score 1 point for each part correctly executed.

* Reproduced with permission from Folstein *et al.* (1975).

a history from an available informant is a matter of emergency and may be life-saving. Key points (listed as 'hows') are as follows:

- how long has the patient been like this? — i.e. when was the patient last 'normal'? If the history is short — days, weeks or even months — the patient is unlikely, in the absence of an obvious physical cause, to be demented; one is probably dealing with an acute confusional state, or perhaps a depressive 'pseudodementia'. Often informants have difficulty in giving an exact time, so ask about specific occasions — e.g. was she like this last Christmas; how did this compare with the Christmas before?

- how did it begin? Suddenly or gradually? Was it associated with some potentially relevant event? — an illness? an injury? a fall? or a bereavement, actual (e.g. of a loved person or even a pet), or symbolic (e.g. loss of function, or of the patient's home)? Did it relate to a sudden change of sur-

roundings? Remember that major 'life-events' in health or social circumstances, and most particularly bereavements, are potent precipitants of depressive states, which commonly in very old people present as 'confusion'

- how often? — i.e. has it happened before, in what circumstances and what was the outcome? To what treatment did it respond before?

- how has it progressed? — has the patient been steadily in the same condition, or has the course fluctuated?

- how has she been treated? — i.e. what drugs has she been taking? Medicines, particularly prescribed medicines, are among the commonest causes of confusional states; especial culprits are those drugs which are anticholinergic. Take a careful drug history and ask to inspect containers. Speak to the general practitioner on the 'phone if in doubt. Don't forget to enquire into alcohol consumption and diet

- how bright? — poor performance on mental status

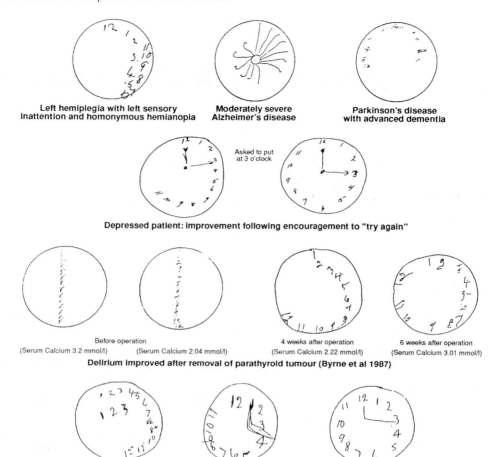

Left hemiplegia with left sensory inattention and homonymous hemianopia

Moderately severe Alzheimer's disease

Parkinson's disease with advanced dementia

Asked to put at 3 o'clock

Depressed patient: improvement following encouragement to "try again"

Before operation
(Serum Calcium 3.2 mmol/l)

(Serum Calcium 2.04 mmol/l)

4 weeks after operation
(Serum Calcium 2.22 mmol/l)

6 weeks after operation
(Serum Calcium 3.01 mmol/l)

Delirium improved after removal of parathyroid tumour (Byrne et al 1987)

Day one

Two weeks later

Five weeks later

Improvement following toxic delirium (Shulman et al 1986)

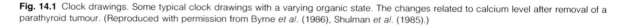

Fig. 14.1 Clock drawings. Some typical clock drawings with a varying organic state. The changes related to calcium level after removal of a parathyroid tumour. (Reproduced with permission from Byrne *et al.* (1986), Shulman *et al.* (1985).)

questioning may be due to borderline intelligence; there are many people who have never known the name of the Monarch! Always look for evidence of previous capacity, e.g. type of job, reputation among neighbours

Finally — not all muddled old people are demented. To give them the benefit of meticulous appraisal is not only their right, but makes work with this growing group of almost all doctors' patients more interesting and more satisfying.

Further reading

Byrne EJ *et al*. General assessment of serum calcium corre-

lates with mental state. *International Journal of Geriatric Psychiatry*. 1987; **2**: 163–8.

Folstein MF, Folstein SE, McHugh PR. 'Mini-Mental State'. A practical method for grading the cognitive state of patients for the clinician. *Journal of Psychiatric Research*. 1975; **12**: 189–98.

Jones RG, Arie T. The acutely confused patient. In *Practical geriatric medicine* (eds Exton-Smith AN, Weksler M). Edinburgh: Churchill Livingstone, 1985.

Mulley GP. Differential diagnosis of dementia. *British Medical Journal*. 1986; **292**: 1416–18.

Shulman KI, Shedletsky R, Silver IL. The challenge of time: clock-drawing and cognitive function in the elderly. *International Journal of Geriatric Psychiatry*. 1986; **1**: 135–40.

15

Black-outs, collapses and shock

P. J. Toghill

> What exactly happened?
> Sudden loss of consciousness with spontaneous
> recovery
> Collapse and continuing coma
> Collapse with shock

Doctors are often called to see patients who have been brought to hospital in shocked and collapsed states. Others may have lost consciousness but will have recovered by the time they arrive. 'Collapse ?cause' is the usual description on the casualty admission card. Not every such patient can give a lucid history and co-operate in a clinical examination but the initial assessment is critical as the underlying condition may be life-threatening. Further investigations are usually necessary and a call for help is obligatory if the diagnosis is not clear. Nevertheless, a working diagnosis can usually be reached quickly by an appraisal of the circumstances and a search for relevant physical signs. If the patient is shocked, resuscitation needs to be underway quickly even before the patient is moved on for definitive treatment. This short chapter offers a scheme for dealing with the common problem of 'collapse ?cause'.

What exactly happened?

Much depends on an accurate account of what exactly happened. For example, did the patient collapse suddenly after being entirely well previously? What was he or she doing at the time? Was there loss of consciousness and if so for how long? Has complete recovery of consciousness occurred? Some of these points may be answered by the patient but more usually they are given by friends or relatives, witnesses, or ambulance personnel.

In every case of collapse certain ground rules are essential:

- don't let witnesses, friends or relatives disappear until you have interrogated them fully and recorded their observations
- if the patient is unaccompanied, ask others to ferret out as much as they can of the circumstances of the episode
- look for clues of present or past illnesses whilst clothes are being removed. There may be hospital out-patient cards in pockets or medi-alert badges
- keep any tablets or empty bottles that may have been near the patient
- find the name of the patient's family doctor and try to determine if there have been any other recent medical contacts

Sudden loss of consciousness with spontaneous recovery

Sudden loss of consciousness with relatively swift recovery, frequently termed 'black-outs' or 'funny turns' in the UK, 'spells' in North America and 'le petit mort' in France, may pose perplexing diagnostic problems (Table 15.1). Time must be found to tease-out descriptions of attacks from patient and witnesses. In making a diagnosis much depends on the age of the patient, previous similar episodes and the circumstances of the attack. There are often no helpful physical signs (see Chapter 8). In the young most

Table 15.1. Sudden loss of consciousness with spontaneous recovery

	Type of attack	Circumstances	Possible findings
Young	Syncope	Anxiety	Pale, clammy, nausea
	Vasovagal	Prolonged standing in hot, stuffy surroundings	Rapid recovery when recumbent
	Hypoglycaemia	Diabetic on insulin	Sweating; dilated pupils Quick recovery with glucose (orally or i.v.) or glucagon
	Epilepsy	Most attacks occur without obvious triggers	Dependent on type of epilepsy
	Hyperventilation	Anxiety or excitement	Tingling in extremities Carpopedal spasm
	Dysrhythmias*	Cardiomyopathies	Those related to the primary cardiac condition
Middle-aged or old	As in young		
	Postural hypotension	Drugs. Autonomic neuropathy (see Table 13.4)	Fall in systolic pressure >20 mmHg on standing
	Dysrhythmias	At any time	See Fig. 15.1
	Aortic stenosis	With exertion	LV+ loud systolic murmur at base of heart
	Cough or micturition syncope	Collapse after prolonged coughing or collapse in middle-aged or elderly men whilst micturating	Nil
	Drop attacks	Often in middle-aged women	'Legs give way'. Often no loss of consciousness

* Rare cause.

sudden losses of consciousness are due to syncope (vasovagal attacks) or epilepsy.

Vasovagal syncope

This almost always occurs in the standing position, in response to fear, anxiety, acute stress or prolonged immobility; the resulting collapse ensures that a horizontal position is quickly reached and adequate cerebral perfusion restored. Complete recovery takes only a minute or two but there may be sweating and bradycardia during this time. Young people tend to 'grow-out' of syncopal attacks but the middle-aged and elderly are not immune.

Epilepsy

Those suffering from epileptic fits may carry appropriate indentification but this is a group where the accounts of witnesses are critical. Tonic–clonic seizures are usually easily recognized by lay people. Complete recovery is delayed for a few minutes by confusion. Where no background information is

available a bitten tongue, muscular pains or urinary incontinence may suggest that a fit has occurred. Extensor plantar responses may be found in the postictal state but resolve with recovery. Other forms of epilepsy such as complex partial seizures (see Chapter 8) are much more difficult to diagnose but a description of similar episodes may be obtained from relatives or friends.

Hyperventilation

Overbreathing due to excitement or anxiety causes tingling in the limbs and around the mouth and sometimes carpopedal spasm. It is unusual for consciousness to be lost entirely though some patients claim to do so transiently.

Hypoglycaemia

Never forget the possibility of hypoglycaemia in an unknown patient; increasing confusion and sweating before loss of consciousness should alert one to this possibility.

As well as being vulnerable to the sorts of episodes seen in the young the middle-aged and elderly are more likely to suffer other more serious causes of sudden loss of consciousness.

Cardiac rhythm disorders

Of these, perhaps the most dramatic is the Stokes–Adams attack due to complete heart block. Here the collapse is sudden, catastrophic and without warning. Fig. 15.1 shows an elderly lady who collapsed suddenly with such an attack, falling forward and sustaining extensive facial injuries.

Other cardiac causes of collapse

These have been discussed in Chapter 3 and include aortic stenosis, micturition and cough syncope and postural hypotension (see Table 13.4). In the elderly episodes of postural hypotension are extremely common, often being provoked by drugs; in younger patients they may be a disturbing symptom during convalescence from debilitating illnesses.

Cerebrovascular disease

Transient ischaemic attacks (TIAs) are common in elderly arteriopathic subjects. By definition neurological recovery occurs within 24 hours. In such patients, whilst disturbed consciousness may be a feature at the onset, the developing neurological signs clarify the diagnosis. Basilar insufficiency is an unlikely cause of transient loss of consciousness in the absence of other brainstem symptoms. Basilar migraine, which usually affects young women, is an unusual cause of black-outs. The sequence of prodromal symptoms with dysarthria, ataxia, confusion and visual disturbances may be followed by gradual loss of consciousness over several minutes; on recovery there is a throbbing, migrainous headache.

Collapse and continuing coma

The important causes of coma are listed in Table 8.10. Only two of these start with catastrophic suddenness — stroke and subarachnoid haemorrhage. However, when the mode of onset is unknown consideration of self-poisoning, alcohol intoxication and hypo- and hyperglycaemia should figure highly in the differential diagnosis of the comatose patient. Where a patient has suffered severe shock with profound cerebral anoxia there may be continuing coma. The examination of the unconscious patient has already been dealt with in Chapter 8.

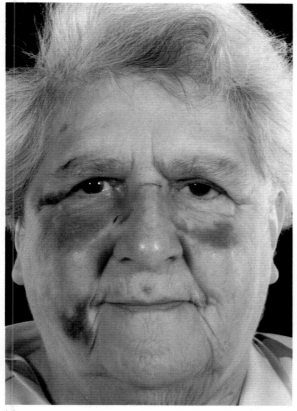

(a)

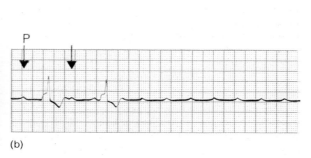

(b)

Fig. 15.1 (a) This lady suddenly collapsed, falling forwards and injuring her face. There was no warning. (b) The cause is shown on the ECG tracing — a Stokes–Adams attack.

Collapse with shock

If the patient has collapsed and remains in a shocked state there is no time to waste and a diagnosis must be achieved as quickly as possible. Gather all the background information and try to identify the probable type of shock. This will then generate further questions but there is rarely time for a fully comprehensive history.

Typically we see a distressed, restless, anxious patient with cold, clammy skin, a fast thready pulse, impaired peripheral perfusion and hypotension.

Cardiogenic shock

In a middle-aged or elderly person the most common cause is likely to be cardiogenic shock caused by some form of 'pump failure' such as myocardial infarction or cardiac tamponade. Chest pain may not necessarily be a feature of myocardial infarction, particularly in the elderly.

Hypovolaemic shock

Loss of blood volume due to haemorrhage is usually easy to recognize. Intense pallor, hypotension and tachycardia are evident to all. Although usually due to acute gastrointestinal haemorrhage, the cause may not be immediately obvious; a large bleed from a duodenal ulcer may not necessarily cause haematemesis and may take time to pass through the gastrointestinal tract before appearing as melaena.

Hypovolaemic shock may also be due to salt and

Table 15.2. Common causes of shock

Mechanism	Possible diagnosis	Important points to ask about	Physical signs to look for
Cardiogenic shock	Myocardial infarction	Previous 'heart problems' particularly angina	Low output state LVF
	Rhythm disturbances	Smoking Diabetes Hypertension	Triple rhythm Tachy- or bradycardia
	Dissecting or ruptured aneurysms	As above but consider aneurysm particularly when much back or abdominal pain	Absent or variable carotid, brachial or femoral pulses
Hypovolaemic shock blood	Bleeding from gastrointestinal tract	History of dyspepsia or ulcers Alcoholism or history of liver problems	Melaena on PR Hepatosplenomegaly or stigmata of CLD
water and electrolytes	Gastroenteritis Vomiting Diarrhoea Addisonian crisis	Sites of fluid loss Tiredness, pigmentation	Dehydration Lax skin Soft eyeballs Dry tongue
Septic shock	Gram-negative septicaemia	Usually associated with recent gut or urinary tract surgery	Fever Flushed Bright-eyed Bounding pulse } in the early stages
Anaphylactic shock	Injections Wasp-stings, etc.	Associated with specific incident	Vasodilatation Wheezing Urticaria
Surgical shock	Rupture of viscus Pancreatitis, etc.	Character of abdominal pain	Rigid abdomen Release pain Absent bowel sounds

water loss in a wide range of clinical disorders including gastroenteritis, intestinal obstruction, cholera in the tropics and Addisonian crisis. Here the patient's appearance is primarily one of dehydration with loss of skin turgor and a dry tongue.

Septic shock

In septic shock a different appearance may be seen in the early stages with a bright-eyed patient who is flushed and warm; the pulse may be full and the blood pressure well maintained. This pattern is often associated with Gram-negative septicaemia following bowel surgery, biliary obstruction or urinary infection and is more often encountered in patients who collapse on surgical wards than in those who are brought into Accident and Emergency Departments.

Anaphylactic shock

The release of histamine and other compounds result in marked vasodilation. Though the blood volume is unchanged there is a functional hypovolaemia with poor peripheral perfusion. The causal factor is usually obvious, as with the injection of a drug such as penicillin, or a bee- or wasp-sting.

Surgical shock

Under these circumstances the features of the primary condition, i.e. pain from a perforated viscus, usually overwhelm the accompanying shock which is a secondary phenomenon.

Table 15.2 shows some of the commoner patterns of shock.

16

Physical signs in clinical dermatology

B. R. Allen

Introduction
The history
Examination
References and further reading

Introduction

The skin is important, not only as an organ with vital physiological functions but also as a flag by which we communicate with the outside world. Problems with internal organs can be concealed from those we meet but our skin is clearly visible and everyone wishes theirs to be perfect. The multi-million pound cosmetics industry is based upon this understandable and inherent desire for perfection so it is easy to appreciate that skin disease places a psychological strain on sufferers out of proportion to the disturbances in function which the pathology produces. Stigmatization frequently results in embarassment and consequent avoidance of social and sexual contact. Perhaps it is not surprising, therefore, that patients with psoriasis, a persistent and often lifelong condition, show an increased incidence of alcoholism and psychiatric disturbances.

Like most other organs the skin has a limited repertoire of reactions but these can occur combined together in an almost infinite number of permutations. The result is, to a dermatologist, an organ of fascinating variety and complexity. The contribution that cutaneous physical signs make towards diagnoses which, at first, seem to be purely internal in their manifestations is often overlooked. For example the pallor of anaemia, the excessive sweating of phaeochromocytoma, the malar flush of mitral valve disease (Fig. 16.1), the icterus of billiary obstruction or, quite simply, the age and sex of the patient are all conveyed at a glance by visible cutaneous signs. In addition there are specific reactions in the skin which may indicate an internal disorder some of which are given in Table 16.1.

If by careful history-taking and examination, the changes which have taken place can be identified, logical thought and deduction will, in most cases, enable a reasonable list of differential diagnoses to be drawn up.

The purpose of this chapter is not to describe in

Table 16.1. Skin reactions indicating internal disorders

Eruption	Cause or systemic association
Acanthosis nigricans	Malignancy (usually of stomach)
Dermatomyositis	Malignancy (ovary, bronchus)
Erythema nodosum	See Table 16.11 and Fig. 16.7
Icthyosis (acquired)	Malignancy
Nailfold telangiectasia	Connective tissue diseases
Necrobiosis lipoidica	Diabetes mellitus (see Fig. 12.20)
Nodules	Rheumatoid disease (see Fig. 17.13)
	Gout (see Fig. 17.16(b))
Pretibial myxoedema	Thyrotoxicosis (see Fig. 12.7)
Pyoderma gangrenosa	Ulcerative colitis (Fig. 16.2)
Livedo reticularis	Polyarteritis nodosa
Xanthelasma	Hypercholesterolaemia (Fig. 2.6)

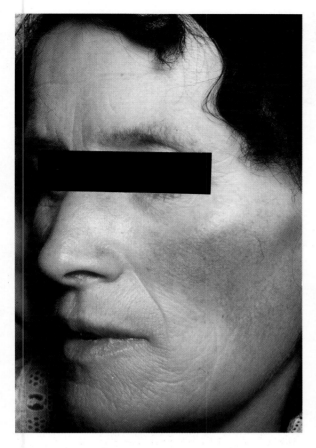

Fig. 16.1 The malar flush in mitral valve disease. The cause of this physical sign is poorly understood.

elaborate detail individual dermatological diseases but to draw attention to the patterns of cutaneous reactions and outline the steps whereby a sensible approach can be made.

The history

Sir William Osler claimed that in 80 per cent of patients a correct diagnosis could be made on the history alone. This is no less true in dermatology than in other branches of medicine, but, dermatology being such a visual subject, there is a great temptation to skimp the history in order to have a quick look at the skin and reach a speedy, if inadequate, diagnosis; this should be avoided.

Never pre-judge what the patient is going to tell you. A teenager with quite prominent facial acne may actually have come about his athlete's foot or an elderly lady with a visible rodent ulcer, her intertrigo; gentle questioning about any additional abnormalities you have noticed can come later.

Generally the types of skin problem which cause a patient to seek advice can be classified into two broad groups:

- localized blemishes and abnormalities which, although minor, may loom very large in the patient's mind, together with skin tumours both benign and malignant
- more generalized eruptions and also problems with the skin appendages such as sweat glands, hair (Table 16.2) or nails (Table 16.3 and Fig. 16.3)

It is not appropriate to discuss here the former group in detail. It is of course, important to be able to

Table 16.2. Abnormalities of hair

(a) Hair loss

Generalized
  Severe illness
  Hypothyroidism
  Hypopituitarism
  Iron deficiency
  Drugs   (Particularly cytotoxic drugs)
Localized
  Male pattern   Characteristic
    baldness   distribution
  Alopecia areata   Normal scalp surface
  Scarring   Loss of follicles
  Infection   Bacterial and fungal
  Traumatic   Habit, hair style
  Lichen planus
  Lupus erythematosus

(b) Hypertrichosis (excessive hair growth)

Generalized
  Racial   Indian subcontinent
  Familial
  Polycystic ovaries   Sometimes sole symptom
  Anorexia nervosa   Vellus or lanugo hair
  Drugs   e.g. phenytoin
  Androgens   Adrenal tumour, congenital
                                   adrenal hyperplasia
Localized
  Naevoid
  Inflammatory skin
    disease
  Occlusion   e.g. plaster of Paris

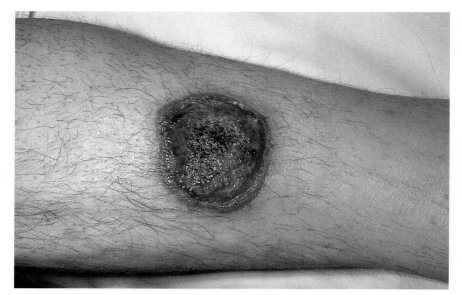

Fig. 16.2 Pyoderma gangrenosa. This rare skin lesion is the classic example of a skin condition associated with internal disease. The necrotic ulcers, most often on the legs, are usually associated with ulcerative colitis. Total proctocolectomy almost always results in rapid healing.

distinguish a pigmented naevus from a malignant melanoma and to recognize Kaposi's sarcoma; the general rules of examination to be outlined below apply no less to small individual lesions than to more extensive eruptions.

Presenting complaint

What caused the patient to seek advice? Was it just the appearance of the rash or lesion which was not approved of or were there symptoms as well? Was the condition spreading rapidly? Did a friend say that it looked like skin cancer and say she knew someone with a rash like it who was dead in six months? Lesions which are out of sight, behind an ear or on the back, may be noticed first by others if they are asymptomatic.

Duration

It can be surprisingly difficult to get an accurate idea of the duration of skin conditions. This is particularly true of skin tumours and other readily visible conditions. As a general rule patients tend to underestimate the length of time such lesions have been present. This is probably based on embarassment and the expectation of a hostile reaction at having delayed seeking advice.

Nature of the lesion

What exactly did the patient notice first? Was it something visible that was noted by chance when the patient undressed? Or did symptoms such as itching or soreness develop before there was anything visible? What did the original lesion look like? This is something worth enquiring about in some detail since subsequent change and treatment, both appropriate and inappropriate might have greatly altered the appearances.

Subsequent change

What has happened to the lesions since they started? Have the original ones disappeared and been replaced by others or has there been relentless spread? Do the lesions come in crops? Is there a pattern to their spread? Do they, for example, show a tendency to spread from the centre to the periphery or did they have an acral distribution to start with and now show signs of moving more centrally?

Associated symptoms

The presence of pain, weeping, bleeding, and, above all itching should be noted. If present, the periodicity of the itching and exacerbating and relieving factors

Table 16.3. Nail abnormalities

Abnormality	Common cause
Clubbing	Respiratory disease (see Fig. 4.1 and Table 4.7)
Onycholysis (lifting free margin)	Psoriasis. Fungal infection
Koilonychia (spoon shape)	Iron deficiency (see Fig. 18.3)
Pitting	Psoriasis (Fig. 16.3)
Longitudinal ridging	Age
Transverse ridging ('Beau's lines')	Systemic illness (see Fig. 18.4)
Onychogryphosis thickening and twisting)	Trauma. Ageing (see Fig. 13.2)
White streaks	Fungal infection
Yellow nails	Slow growth

Table 16.4. Causes of pruritus

Generalized

Due to skin disease
  (i) Infections and infestations, e.g. tinea, scabies, pediculosis, insect bites
  (ii) Eczema all types
  (iii) Miscellaneous, e.g. lichen planus, prickly heat (miliaria), urticaria, dermatitis herpetiformis, pityriasis rosea
  (iv) Idiopathic, e.g. 'senile' pruritus

Due to internal disorders

  (i) Cholestasis
  (ii) Renal failure
  (iii) Polycythaemia (see Fig. 9.14)
  (iv) Iron deficiency
  (v) Lymphoma (see Fig. 9.8)

Localized

Some illustrative examples are:
  (i) Eyelids (allergic eczema due to make-up)
  (ii) Perianal region (idiopathic, haemorrhoids)
  (iii) Legs (asteatotic eczema)
  (iv) Vulva (diabetes)
  (v) Scalp (in children) (pediculosis)

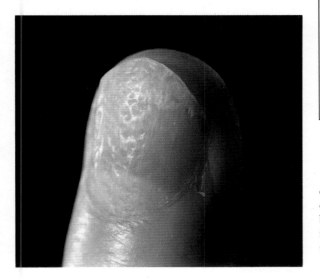

Fig. 16.3 Pitted nails in psoriasis.

noted. The major causes of generalized pruritus and some illustrative examples of local pruritus are given in Table 16.4.

Topical applications

Ask what has the patient been applying to the skin; be reluctant to take 'nothing' for an answer. Irrespective of what may have been prescribed, rare indeed is the patient who has used nothing on a rash before seeking a medical opinion. Often protestations of denial are belied by the odour of proprietary medicines. What is actually visible at present might easily be the result of self-medication, or inappropriate therapy; the original condition may have long since undergone spontaneous resolution.

General history

Taking a dermatological history is not the orderly procedure that formal lists in textbooks would have us believe.

Previous skin disease This can take you right back to birth so it is not inappropriate to ask 'Did your mother ever say that there was anything the matter with your skin as a baby?'. Infantile eczema for example, may clear in a year or two and be overlooked. Seborrhoeic eczema of infancy, believed by some to be an early manifestation of psoriasis, clears even earlier, usually by the age of six months. Certain ichthyoses may present at birth as a so-called 'Collodion baby'.

Physical signs in clinical dermatology

Other illnesses both past and present Not only the illness itself but also the medication which is being given might be important. Some disorders recognizably due to internal diseases have already been listed in Table 16.1 and some distinctive drug eruptions are shown in Table 16.5.

Occupation Skin disease is one of the major reasons why industrial injury benefit is claimed. Many hundreds of the chemicals used in industry can irritate the skin or give rise to an allergy, so precise details of work and working conditions are well worth determining. Anyone with an interest in skin problems should also never miss an opportunity to visit local factories to see at first hand what is happening; a certain knowledge of working practices and colloquial terms can also greatly aid rapport in history-taking.

Hobbies These, not work, may be the source of trouble.

Geographical factors Great Britain is a multiracial society and travel abroad is easy. Unusual tropical infections, including HIV infection, can be acquired from even the shortest of stays in endemic areas. For those with fair skins living for long periods in sunny climates can bring its own problems. Many of the skin changes attributed to ageing (Table 16.6) are in fact brought about by solar damage, although this is not a popular gospel to preach on the beaches of the Mediterranean. The effects are cumulative and it is believed that exposure in childhood might be more damaging than in adult life.

Table 16.6. Effects of age on the skin

(a) General reduction in	
Epidermal thickness	
Scalp hair density	
Pigmentation	Especially hair
Sweat gland function	Irreversible
Sebaceous gland activity	
Elastic tissue	Especially in sun-exposed areas
(b) Local lesions	
Purpura	On minor trauma (see Fig. 9.4)
Telangiectasia	On light-exposed areas
Benign tumours	
Campbell de Morgan's spots	After age of 20
Seborrhoeic keratoses	
Lentigines	On light-exposed skin
Premalignant tumours	
Solar keratoses	Particularly tropical sun
Lentigo maligna	Very slow growing
Malignant tumours	
Basal cell carcinomata	On light-exposed areas
Squamous cell carcinomata	On light-exposed areas
(c) General non-specific changes with age	
Dry skin	
Pruritus	
Eczema of the lower legs	
Gravitational diseases	

Table 16.5. Distinctive drug eruptions

Type of eruption	Common cause
Acneiform	Androgens
Alopecia	Cyclophosphamide and other cytotoxics
	Sodium valproate
Erythema multiforme	Non-steroidal antiflammatory agents
	Suphonamides
Fixed drug eruptions	Phenolphthalein
	Sulphonamides
Lichenoid	Gold
	Antimalarials
Photosensitivity	Tetracyclines
	Phenothiazines
Urticaria	Penicillin

Examination

The main aspects of examination are inspection and palpation and whilst inspection must have pride of place palpation is also important not only to aid diagnosis but also to reassure the patient that you do not fear their skin disease.

Inspection

Distribution of lesions

In order to carry out a proper examination of the skin the patient should be fully undressed. Obviously common sense must prevail and eyebrows might be raised if every patient with a wart on the thumb was asked to strip, but do not be put off by a declaration that 'it only affects my hands and lower legs'. This usually just indicates a disinclination to undress and vital clues as to the diagnosis might be concealed.

Inspection of the skin really starts from the other side of the room. Is the general skin colour normal or is it hypopigmented (Table 16.7) or hyperpigmented (Table 16.8) or generally red (erythrodermic) (Table 16.9). What is the pattern of the lesions on the skin surface? Are they, for example symmetrical, or just affecting exposed areas? If so does the distribution suggest photosensitivity (Table 16.10) or a reaction to external factors.

Be sure that the whole of the skin has been examined. Part the hair and, however elegant the hair style, examine the surface of the scalp. Look behind the ears and into the external auditory meati. Include an inspection of the mouth (see Chapter 5). Raise the arms and inspect the axillae, look at the nails and nailfolds, look under breasts, gaze into the depths of the umbilicus and examine closely the genitalia and perianal area. Finally, however reluctant the patient is, remove the socks and look at the feet and between the toes.

Morphology

Having determined the overall pattern of the lesions it is necessary to look closely at them individually and a nomenclature has been developed in order to simplify description.

A macule is a lesion which can be seen easily but is impalpable, for example, a freckle. Where the lesion can be felt as well as seen it may be described as a papule or, if more extensive, a plaque or deeper, a nodule. Dermal oedema with no overlying epidermal change, such as is seen in urticaria, produces a weal.

Table 16.8. Causes of hyperpigmentation

(a) **Generalized**	
Racial	
Tanning	
Pregnancy	Particularly around mouth (See Fig. 11.1)
Addison's disease	Generalized pigmentation particularly in exposed areas (See Fig. 12.15). Brown patches on buccal mucosa
Renal failure	
Cachexia	
Haemochromatosis	
Drug induced	e.g. busulphan
(b) **Localized**	
Freckles	On light-exposed areas
Lentigines	In elderly
Café-au-lait patches	Consider neurofibromatosis when more than six patches.
Peutz–Jeghers	Perioral (see Fig. 5.5)
Post-inflammatory	A common cause
Acanthosis nigricans	With hyperkeratosis in axilla and other flexures

Table 16.7. Causes of hypopigmentation

(a) *Generalized*	
Albinism	Complete
Hypopituitarism	Relative
Vitiligo	With end-stage confluent disease
(b) *Localized*	
Piebaldism	Congenital
Tuberose sclerosis	Congenital
Vitiligo	Acquired
Post-traumatic	Scarring, any cause
Leprosy	(With local anaesthesia)
Morphoea (localized scleroderma)	(+ thickening)

Table 16.9. Causes of erythroderma

Psoriasis	Commonest
Eczema	All types
Toxic erythema	e.g. viral infections
Drug allergy	
Lymphoma + chronic lymphatic leukaemia	Rare
Unknown	Seen occasionally in elderly men

Table 16.10. Causes of photosensitivity

(a) *Genetic*
    Albinism   Total lack of melanin
(b) *Metabolic and nutritional*
    The porphyrias   (Except acute
                                     intermittent)
    Disorders of tryptophan   e.g. pellagra
    metabolism
(c) *Drug-induced*
    Phenothiazines
    Tetracyclines   And derivatives
    Thiazide diuretics
    Piroxicam   And other NSAIDs
    Chlorpropramide
(d) *Idiopathic*
    Polymorphic light   Especially young
    eruption   women
    Solar urticaria
(e) *Topical photosensitization*
    Chemical   e.g. perfumes
(f) *Conditions worsened by light*
    SLE
    Discoid LE
    Psoriasis   (in active phase)

Fluid-filled blisters on the skin are arbitrarily divided on the basis of size into smaller vesicles and larger bullae. Beware of patients who talk of 'blisters' in the skin; the term is often used by lay people to mean a weal not a fluid-filled lesion so it is necessary to clarify the point. Blistering is an important physical sign. A number of conditions such as pemphigus always blister, others occasionally do, like erythema multiforme. Pustules contain debris, leukocytes and micro-organisms as well as fluid but do not automatically indicate infection; the pustules of psoriasis for example are sterile. The exact location within the skin should be determined; are they perifollicular or subcorneal?

Where the epidermis is lost an erosion is formed and the consequent oozing of serous fluid which then dries produces crusts. Erosions will heal without damage to the skin but ulcers, produced by penetration into the dermis, will heal to give scarring. Erosions produced by different processes may be either above or just below the basement membrane of the epidermis. When they are below milia or tiny keratin cysts may form in the healing skin giving clues to the underlying pathological process.

Scaling is the accumulation of keratin, either normal or abnormal, on the skin surface. It may be the only visible change, as in some icthyoses or accompanied by inflammation as in psoriasis. Shedding of the horny layer is termed desquamation and can follow an inflammatory disorder such as an exanthem, drug reaction, or underlying cellulitis.

Outline

The margin of the individual lesions should be carefully examined. Some disorders give rise to lesions with a clearcut division between normal and abnormal skin whereas in others the abnormal blends into the normal. Generally a convex border indicates the direction of spread. Where multiple small lesions have coalesced to produce larger patches the margin will appear scalloped. Lichen planus (Fig. 16.4) is characteristically limited by the fine skin creases producing polygonal lesions. If the skin in the centre of a lesion returns to normal as it spreads an annular lesion is formed. Whilst typical of ringworm (Fig. 16.5) it is not pathognomonic. Linearity may imply either an underlying structural defect or a response to external factors applied to the skin in a linear fashion such as occurs in the Koebner phenomenon where non-specific injury results in productions of specific skin disease. This occurs most commonly in psoriasis.

Colour

The subtle differences in erythema between the lesions of different conditions can be very helpful in making the diagnosis but only practical experience will provide the necessary expertise. This also applies in interpreting colour changes in dark skins where redness may not be so obvious. As a general rule very bright red erythema indicates an active disorder and as activity begins to decline the lesions become paler, sometimes with the redness being replaced by post-inflammatory pigmentation, the staining from which can last for many months. Erythema can be distinguished from purpura by diascopy, that is pressing a glass slide against the skin; blanching will occur with erythema but not with purpura. Erythema which is occurring beneath an increased thickness of epidermis will tend to take on a slightly violaceous hue.

Texture

Is the surface of the lesion scaling or not? If it is difficult to determine the removal of surface grease using a little ether is helpful. If scaling is present and

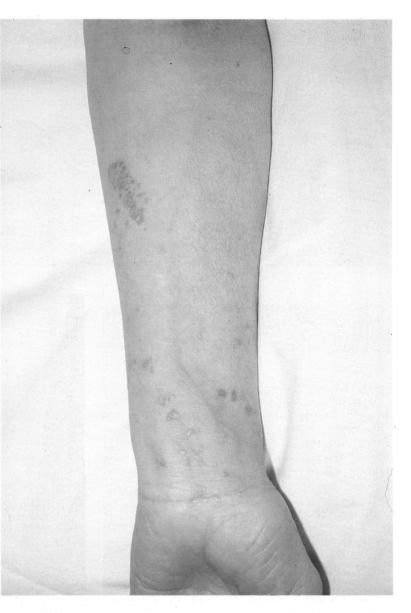

Fig. 16.4 Lichen planus. The itchy, shiny lesions of this rash vary but may be polygonal in shape and are commonly seen on the flexor surfaces of the wrist. It affects the young and middle-aged and is of unknown aetiology.

makes it difficult to see the base of the lesion a little oil can be applied to the surface. White scales are seen typically in the discoid lesions of psoriasis (Fig. 16.6).

Palpation

Palpation should never be omitted. As mentioned earlier it can be a great relief to a patient to know that you are not afraid to touch their skin. An extensive rash is an unpleasant to the patient as it would be to any of us: patients with skin disease are not a special subgroup of humanity. Their relatives and friends may keep a discrete distance and their sex lives may be non-existent so the last thing they want is a medical advisor who confirms their untouchability.

Palpation also conveys a lot of information. The skin may be thickened, in which case it should be

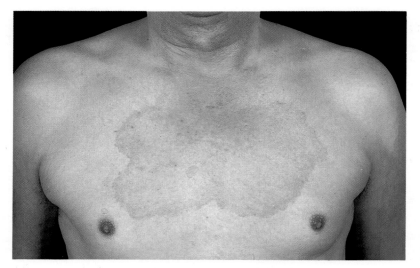

Fig. 16.5 Ringworm. The spreading edge is characteristic.

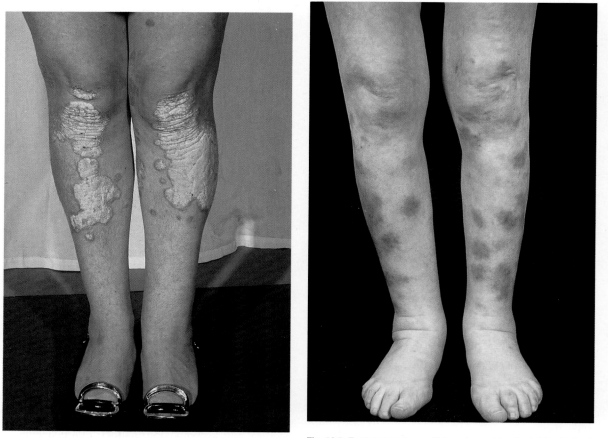

Fig. 16.6 Scaling lesions of discoid psoriasis. These occur at knees, elbows, scalp and sacral regions.

Fig. 16.7 Erythema nodosum. This rash consists of painful red raised nodules over the shins; these may become confluent with the reaction usually settling within a month.

possible to identify whether it is the epidermis which is thickened (lichenified) or the dermis. The lesion might spread much further than is evident visually, be calcified or cystic, cooler or warmer than the surrounding skin, as in erythema nodosum (Table 16.11 and Fig. 16.7) or atrophic with loss of dermal collagen.

Table 16.11. Causes of erythema nodosum

(a)	Infection	
	Streptococcus	Sometimes recurrent
	Primary tuberculosis	Early only, severe
	Deep mycoses	
	Cattle ringworm	
(b)	Sarcoidosis	
	Crohn's disease	
	Ulcerative colitis	
(d)	Sulphonamides	
(e)	Malignancies	After radiotherapy
(f)	Unknown	May be persistent

Crusts, when present, should be removed from a sample area so that the underlying surface can be inspected. As crusts are not firmly adherent to the surface the simplicity of removal will also help to distinguish them from keratin, which is an integral part of the lesion and can rarely be removed with ease. Any scale should also be tested for silveriness on scratching, a sign almost pathognomonic of psoriasis.

Other investigations

It is of course, not always possible to make a diagnosis on straightforward clinical grounds alone in which case further investigations may be indicated. The ability to isolate and identify an *Acarus* in scabies or fungal hyphae in suspected fungal infections should be regarded as extensions of the clinical examination as should the ability to use a Wood's light to detect fluorescence and varying degrees of pigmentation. A basic knowledge of entomology can also help in the identification of fleas, ticks, lice and bedbugs. Appropriate clinicopathological tests are often essential.

Biopsying the skin is a simple procedure which is likely to cause minimal upset to the patient and the specimen can be examined both under the light microscope and by immunofluorescent techniques, but it should be remembered that conditions which are atypical clinically are often atypical histologically as well!

References and further reading

Burton, JL. *Essentials of Dermatology*, 3rd edition. Edinburgh: Churchill Livingstone 1990.
Buxton PK. The skin and systemic disease. *British Medical Journal*. 1988; **296**: 916–17.
Champion RH, Burton JL, Ebling FJG (eds). *Textbook of Dermatology*, 5th edn. London: Blackwell, 1992.
Fitzpatrick, TB, Eisen AZ, Wolff K, Freedberg IM, Austen KF (eds). *Dermatology in general medicine*, 4th edn. New York: McGraw-Hill, 1993.
Fry L. *Dermatology. An illustrated guide*, 3rd edn. London: Butterworths, 1984.

17

The musculoskeletal system

N. J. Barton and P. J. Toghill

This chapter deals with muscles, joints and bones — tissues that are inextricably linked with support, protection and locomotion. First, we deal with the basic principles of examining joints and then, secondly, move on to the problems of some selected joints and the spine. These problems are, of course, expressed in the major rheumatic diseases and in a group of overlapping syndromes termed the connective tissue diseases. Finally we deal with acquired skeletal diseases.

The joints

Painful and stiff joints inflict much misery on patients, and may be caused by a wide range of disorders. To complicate matters further, arthritis may be a primary or secondary manifestation of disease.

Symptoms

Pain

Pain is the most common symptom, especially in the lower limbs and spine. The important questions are 'where' and 'when'?

Where? We need to ask the patient to point as accurately as he or she can to the place where the pain is worst.

When? Ask whether the pain is constant (in which case it is probably inflammatory) or intermittent (in which case it is probably mechanical). If the latter, what activity or positions make it worse; what gives relief? Many chronic joint disorders (and also healed fractures) are worse in cold or wet conditions, though the reason for this is not clear.

Stiffness

This may mean several different things. Usually it means a restriction in the range of movement of a joint. This may be due to an actual physical limitation of movement or because the movement is painful and therefore, in practice, is not made. Stiffness in the sense of an increased resistance to movement is probably rare in joint disease though, of course, it occurs in neurological disorders such as Parkinson's disease and multiple sclerosis.

Morning stiffness lasting up to 15 minutes is

common in many joint diseases, but if it lasts for an hour or more that suggests an inflammatory arthropathy. Intermittent restriction of movement which comes and goes suddenly indicates a mechanical disorder, usually in the joint but occasionally in a tendon which works the joint (e.g. trigger thumb); this is often described as locking. Stiffness after prolonged immobility is likely to be due to osteoarthritis.

Swelling

This symptom is common to many joint problems. If it follows an injury, the speed with which the swelling appears is important. Bleeding causes swelling within minutes, whereas a synovial effusion takes a few hours to develop. The site of the swelling obviously matters but so too may its shape. If it defines a synovial cavity, as in the knee, then the swelling is likely to be due to fluid within the joint.

Instability

This applies particularly to the weight-bearing joints of the lower limb. In the mechanical sense, an unstable situation is one from which, if the object is slightly displaced, it will collapse. Medically the term is not always used in this precise sense. It conveys a sense of insecurity: the patient feels that if he puts his weight on the leg something bad will happen, or finds from bitter experience that it does so! This may be due to weakness of the muscles which support the limb in the upright position (e.g. weakness of quadriceps allowing the knee to give way into flexion) or it may be that an abnormal movement takes place at a joint. Continuing with the knee as an example, it may angulate sideways. This in turn has two possible causes: (a) a torn or ineffective collateral ligament which no longer provides effective restraint; (b) altered shape of the bone (e.g. depressed tibial condyle) due to old fracture or to arthritis.

Locking

Loose bodies in joints (which include the loose portion of a torn meniscus in the knee) cause 'locking', i.e. a sudden block to part of the range of movement, usually extension, followed by sudden 'unlocking' when the loose body moves out of the way.

This is not a wholly logical usage, since a locked door cannot be moved either way. Patients may mean something different. Again, you must get them to explain what they do mean.

Clicking or clunking

Noises coming from joints are not necessarily pathological: some people produce harmless vacuum clicks and in others noises are produced by tendons slipping over bony prominences. However, some noises, particularly those accompanied by pain, are very significant.

Loss of function

In itself, this term is so vague as to be meaningless. You must find out what function is lost, and why. What exactly cannot the patient do that he wishes to do? What stops him from doing it: is it that the part simply won't move? If the latter, the examination will reveal whether the problem is paralysis or stiffness. These are the things which matter to the patient and also the things which matter if a decision is being made about treatment for a chronic condition.

Signs

For the examination of joints, the system based on that used by Apley is recommended (Table 17.1).

Table 17.1. System for the examination of joints	
When examining joints	LOOK FEEL MOVE ASSESS FUNCTION

If you vary the order you may miss out an important part of the examination by going straight to some obvious abnormality. In practice, however, the system is modified for individual joints; while you have the patient in a particular position, it may be sensible to carry out some part of the examination which would normally come later.

Look

The whole limb must be exposed and also the other arm or leg for comparison. Look for deformity (malalignment of the bones above and below the joint), swelling, wasting of muscles near the joint and scars.

Swelling which conforms to the outline of a synovial cavity should be distinguished from that which is either more localized or more diffuse. It is further elucidated by palpation.

Scars may be very important as indicating a previous infection or operation which the patient has forgotten to tell you about. Every scar around a painful joint must be explained.

Feel

While palpating the joint, watch the patient's face. Localization of tenderness is the single most important physical sign in joint disorders. Be gentle and feel systematically all around the joint, starting where it is least likely to be tender. Palpation will determine the limits of swelling more accurately.

Move

The joint must now be put through a full range of movement. The quickest way is to demonstrate the movement yourself and then to ask the patient to do the same, i.e. testing active movements. If the patient cannot do this, then take over and examine passive movements. Limitation of passive movement indicates something wrong in or around the joint. Full passive movements without pain means that the joint is all right but there is something wrong with the mechanism which moves it.

Movement should be measured in degrees with a goniometer (Fig. 17.1(a) and (b)), using the neutral zero method. In this, the anatomical position is zero and the degrees of flexion are measured from that point (Fig. 17.2). The measurements are not absolutely accurate, but they are considerably better than rough estimates such as 'good', 'bad' or 'indifferent' and are essential for following progress in individual patients. The measured range must then be written in the notes.

Whilst a joint is being moved, it is useful to keep one hand on it to feel crepitus or clicks.

It is also necessary to test abnormal movement, e.g. sideways movement at hinge joints. Laxity of collateral ligaments occurs in rheumatoid disease and after injury and seriously interferes with function.

Function

This is perhaps the most important part of the examination.

The legs are meant for standing and walking. It is not enough to examine them with the patient lying on a couch: you must get your patient to stand up and watch him walking, preferably unencumbered by much clothing. If the patient uses a stick, watch him walking both with and without the stick. This may tell you more than all the rest of the examination.

Similarly, if the complaint concerns the upper limb,

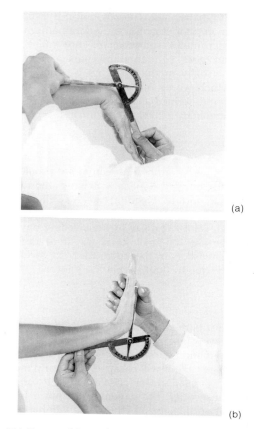

(a)

(b)

Fig. 17.1 The use of the goniometer to measure (a) flexion and (b) extension at the wrist.

get the patient to do or mime the thing which he finds difficult. You can always find a cup and fill it with water. You can usually find a kettle or a jug. Grasp of large objects can be tested on a bottle or box, and small ones by picking up a paper clip or pin from a flat surface. It is often helpful to watch the patient writing and to record this.

Now we must consider features of particular significance in important selected joints. The wrist and hand are of such crucial importance that they are dealt with separately in the following chapter.

The shoulder

The outstanding characteristic of the shoulder is that it is able to have a very large range of movements in all directions, by a ball and socket joint. To permit this, the socket is shallow and the joint is held

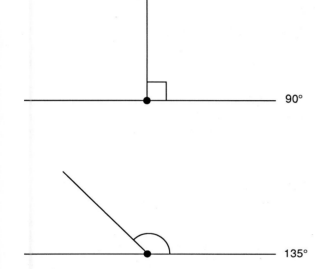

Fig. 17.2 The neutral zero method of measuring joint movement. This is internationally agreed and should always be used. Flexion is measured in degrees from the anatomical position, which is zero.

0°

45°

90°

135°

together by a musculotendinous cuff called the rotator cuff. Most patients with pain in the shoulder have pathology affecting the rotator cuff, not the articular surfaces. The two common examples are degenerative tears in the rotator cuff, causing a painful arc, and 'frozen shoulder' (a type of disorder apparently unique to this joint) in which all movements are restricted. A third possibility which must be borne in mind is referred pain from the neck, heart, diaphragm or an apical carcinoma of the lung (a Pancoast tumour).

It is very important to realize that only about two-thirds of the movement at the shoulder actually takes place at the glenohumeral joint: the other one-third is the result of movement of the scapula on the thoracic cage, where there is no synovial joint and which is controlled by different muscles. Contrary to what is often taught, it has been established beyond doubt that both movements occur throughout the whole range and that the deltoid and supraspinatus are both active in the whole process, not just in one part of it.

Symptoms

Pain Pain originating in the shoulder region is felt around the glenohumeral joint or the insertion of the deltoid. Pain felt across the top of the shoulder or around or between the scapulae is more likely to be referred from the cervical spine. Constant pain indicates an inflammatory arthritis or a frozen shoulder. In those conditions, attempted movement will make the pain worse, but in rotator-cuff tears and osteoarthritis (which is very rare in the shoulder) pain is only on movement, or if the patient lies on the shoulder at night.

Stiffness Here one must distinguish between a joint which won't move and a joint which is not moved because the movement causes pain.

Instability A patient who feels that his shoulder 'goes out of joint' may be describing recurrent dislocation, but it may be some lesser abnormal movement and careful examination and radiology are required.

Examination

Look for wasting of deltoid (Fig. 17.3), supraspinatus and infraspinatus. To see the last, examine the patient from behind. Most painful conditions cause only mild wasting; severe wasting occurs in damage to the axillary nerve and after neuralgic amyotrophy.

An altered shape of the front of the upper arm gives the clue to rupture of the tendon of the long head of biceps; this can be made obvious by asking the patient to flex the elbow against resistance.

Feel carefully to localize tenderness. This may enable you to distinguish between glenohumeral disorders, acromioclavicular problems, or more specific bony tenderness.

Move A simple scheme, which can be carried out very quickly, will show you if your patient has full active shoulder movements. Ask the patient to:

- 'lift your arms right up like this' while you demonstrate full active abduction (Fig. 17.4(a))
- hold it up for 10 s or so

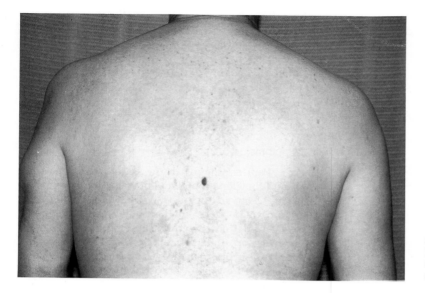

Fig. 17.3 Wasting of the left deltoid muscle. Note the concavity of the outline of the muscle from the back as compared with the normal convexity.

- 'now let your arm down slowly' and watch the face while she does so: a painful arc is often more evident on the downstroke than on the upstroke
- 'put your hands behind your head like this'. (This tests external rotation (Fig. 17.4(b)))
- 'put your hands behind your waist like this' to test internal rotation (Fig. 17.4(c))

If the patient cannot do these movements, you must help him, i.e. the test becomes one of passive movements. Proceeding slowly and gently, you may be able to ease the arm through a painful mid-arc of elevation and up into a painless position of full or nearly full elevation (Fig. 17.5). This indicates pathology in the rotator cuff and usually in the supraspinatus part of the cuff. A painful arc in the top part of the range points to a disorder of the acromioclavicular joint. If movements of the shoulder in all directions are limited, you are dealing with either a frozen shoulder or intra-articular pathology. In the former the x-ray is normal, but in the latter abnormal.

At this stage, you should distinguish between glenohumeral and scapulothoracic movements. It is usually recommended that the examiner uses one hand to fix the lower pole of the scapula and then asks the patient to lift the arm up: when the scapula begins to move the glenohumeral component of abduction has been completed. It is actually much easier to stabilize the scapula from above by putting a hand firmly on the top of the shoulder.

Function Although it is convenient to examine abduction in the coronal plane, the movements which are of more importance in daily life are flexion (to reach a shelf or hook in front), internal rotation (to wipe one's bottom and do up clothes which fasten behind) and external rotation (to do your hair).

The hip

The hip resembles the shoulder in that it is a ball-and-socket joint allowing movement in all directions. In the hip the socket is deeper, allowing a smaller range of movement but providing greater inherent stability. Whereas shoulder pain usually arises in the periarticular structures, hip pain usually arises in the joint itself. In both, the movement of the limb is mostly at the ball-and-socket joint but partly more proximally: in the case of the hip, movements of the lumbar spine allow a fair range of movement of the leg even if the hip joint has been fused. Examination must distinguish between movement at these two sites.

Symptoms

Pain arising in the hip joint is usually felt in or around the groin, though it may go down the thigh. Pain felt mainly in the buttock is more likely to be a limited form of sciatica, referred from the lumbar spine. Pain arising from the hip is usually worst when it is bearing the greatest load, i.e. when the

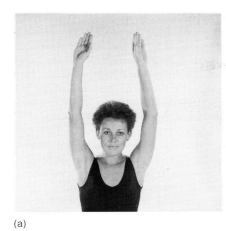

(a)

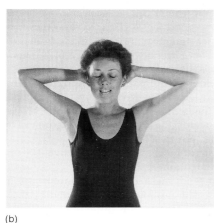

(b)

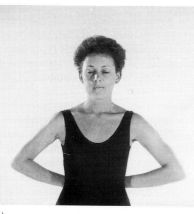

(c)

Fig. 17.4 Assessment of shoulder movements: (a) full active abduction; (b) external rotation; (c) internal rotation.

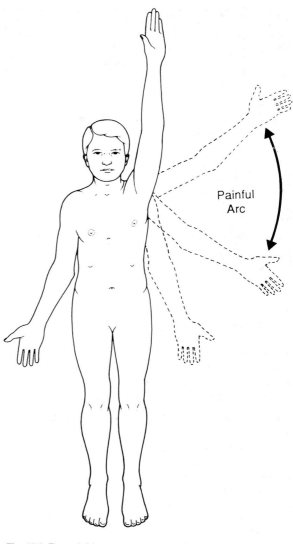

Fig. 17.5 The painful arc.

patient is standing or walking, though it may also disturb sleep when the patient turns over.

Referred pain is one of the most common pitfalls in connection with the hip. Pathology in the hip may present with a complaint of pain in the knee and vice versa. The importance of this cannot be over-emphasized. Examination of the hip must always include also examination of the knee.

Limp The commonest cause of a limp is pain, causing the patient to move his weight quickly off that leg onto the other one. This is called an antalgic gait and produces an altered rhythm of gait: a type of limp which can be heard as well as seen.

Mechanical causes of limp are:

1. A short leg. The pelvis on that side is lower during the stance phase of gait (when the leg is on the ground).
2. Inefficient abduction of the hip. This is important, but slightly complicated. Walking involves standing on each leg alternately, during which the hip abductors must contract to keep the pelvis level or in fact slightly raised on the other side so that the other leg can swing through. The effect of this is to create a load across the hip joint of 2.5 times the body weight; artificial hips as well as normal ones have to be designed to withstand this. If the abductor muscles cannot work properly, the pelvis drops on the other side, i.e. during the swing phase of gait. This is called a Trendelenburg limp and may be due to paralysis of the abductors or loss of their fulcrum due to dislocation of the hip or fracture of the femoral neck.
3. Other mechanical causes of limp, which may be in hip, knee or ankle, include stiffness, weakness, instability of joints, an artificial leg or a fracture.

Stiffness   Loss of movement at the hip can to some extent be overcome, as has been said, by movements of the lumbar spine so that the whole pelvis tilts in the required direction and carries the leg with it. The most common deformity to cause symptoms is an adduction contracture, which makes access to the perineum difficult and may interfere with sexual intercourse: severe contractures may make one leg cross over the other.

Clicking   As a symptom, this is usually due to the tensor fascia lata slipping over the greater trochanter which, though it may be uncomfortable, is of no great importance.

Examination

Look   This starts as the patient enters the room and sits down (if the hip is very stiff, he may prefer to stand). With the patient lying down, look for abnormal posture of the legs, muscle wasting, scars around the hips and shortening. Shortening may be apparent or real. Unfortunately there is no uniformity of terminology so it is essential that you know what you mean and can convey it clearly to someone else. A leg may look short because it really is short (true shortening). If you straighten your left knee and bend your right knee to about 45°, the right leg now looks short (apparent shortening) though it is not really. You have probably flexed your hip too and a flexion contracture of the hip will also cause apparent shortening. So, also, will an adduction contracture of the hip; with the erect patient, to get the legs parallel, the pelvis has to be lifted on that side which makes that leg appear short. In this definition, which we prefer, apparent shortening means the amount by which the leg appears short but is not really, i.e. the effect of contractures.

However, some doctors use 'apparent shortening' to mean the amount by which the leg appears short, i.e. the sum of true shortening and the effect of contractures. This is measured with a tape-measure from the umbilicus to the medial malleolus on both sides.

To eliminate the effect of contractures (i.e. the amount by which the leg appears, but is not really, short) the good leg is put into the same position as the bad leg and measurements made from the anterior superior iliac spine to the medial malleolus on each side. This gives the true shortening.

Now look at the patient standing up and ask him to lift one leg off the ground. Normally the pelvis will rise on that side, to move the centre of gravity of the body towards the other side. If the pelvis drops on that side (positive Trendelenburg test) it means that the abductor mechanism is ineffective, for one of the reasons mentioned above.

Feel   for tenderness (especially important in infections). As the hip joint is surrounded by the thickest muscles in the body, it is difficult to feel details other than the greater trochanter and the front of the neck of the femur.

Move   It is difficult to explain all the different hip movements to a patient, so in this joint it is usual to measure passive movements. It is also difficult to use a goniometer and for the hip an estimate of the range of movement in degrees is acceptable.

1. Extension: the patient may have 30° loss of extension but be able to put the thigh flat on the table by extending the spine. To eliminate this, put one hand behind the lumbar spine and with the other hand flex the patient's opposite hip fully to flatten out the lumbar spine. Now any loss of extension (fixed flexion) on the side you are examining will be revealed (Fig. 17.6(a)).
   During the rest of the examination, keep one hand on the pelvis as, when it starts to move, the limit of the hip movement has been reached.
2. Flexion.
3. Abduction (Fig. 17.6(b)).
4. Adduction: you also have to flex the hip slightly

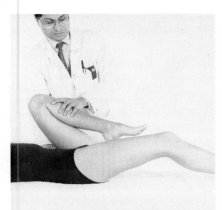
(a)

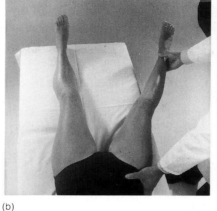
(b)

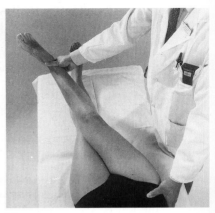
(c)

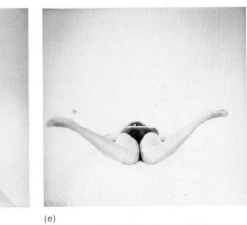
(d)

(e)

Fig. 17.6 Clinical examination of the hip. (a) the concealed fixed flexion of this patient's right hip is revealed by fully flexing the opposite hip to flatten out the lumbar spine (see text). (b) Abduction of the hip. Note that the position of the pelvis has been fixed by the examiner's left hand. (c) Adduction of the hip. (d) With the patient prone this is a useful way of checking external rotation. (e) Internal rotation of the hip with the patient prone.

so that the leg can adduct in front of the other (Fig. 17.6(c)).
5. External rotation (Fig. 17.6(d)).
6. Internal rotation, loss of which is often the earliest sign of osteoarthritis of the hip and is also an important sign in slipped upper femoral epiphysis (Fig. 17.6(e)).

Again do not forget that pain felt at the hip may be referred from the knee which must also be examined.

The elbow

The elbow is a hinge joint which on its posterolateral and posteromedial aspects is quite close to the surface of the skin. Here again, however, one is dealing with two adjoining joints, the other being the superior radioulnar joint. Rheumatoid arthritis may affect one

or both and it is important to try and find out which predominates in causing the symptoms.

Symptoms

The commonest cause of elbow pain is not in the joint but in the common origin of the extensors of the wrist and fingers: tennis elbow. It is important therefore to find out precisely where the pain is felt. Slight loss of extension is common after injuries and in early rheumatoid arthritis or osteoarthritis but causes little functional problem; lack of flexion is what interferes with the patient's life. Long-standing elbow disorders may cause a tardy ulnar palsy and thus present as weakness or loss of feeling in the hand.

Examination

Look for swelling on either side of the olecranon. This may be due to fluid in the joint.

Feel for it too. In tennis elbow, the tenderness is on the lateral side of the elbow, though it may be above, at, or below the level of the joint. Golfer's elbow is the corresponding condition on the medial side, at the origin of the flexors of the wrist and digits.

Move Measure the range of active flexion and extension with a goniometer held over the lateral side of the arm. In severe rheumatoid involvement, the movement is so painful that it may be made very slowly and in a jerky manner. Assess and record the range of pronation and supination. This is the only exception to the 'neutral zero' method, the neutral position for this purpose being in mid-rotation with the thumb and radius anterior (or rather superior, as the test is best carried out with the elbow flexed to 90°), from which there should be 90° of supination and 90° of pronation. Try to find out from the patient whether the range of movement of the elbow or the rotation of the forearm is the most painful movement and feel for crepitus while these movements are being made.

Function Flexion of the elbow is needed to bring the hand to the mouth or face; thus limitation of flexion is an enormous disability.

The knee

The knee is also essentially a hinge, but biomechanically a very complicated one, with a moving axis and allowing some rotation around a longitudinal axis when flexed. There are actually three joints: one between each femoral and tibial condyle and one patello-femoral. In addition, the presence of menisci introduces a whole new range of pathology. Injuries to the knee are common and it is particularly important to ask about any possible trauma. Remember also that the symptoms may be referred from the hip.

Symptoms

Pain

Distinguish between constant pain (as in synovitis) and pain on bearing weight (as in damage to the joint surface). Localization of pain is important: patello-femoral arthritis needs quite different treatment to that arising from the femoro-tibial joints. Injuries to structures with a blood supply cause a haemarthrosis which appears within minutes; this includes ligamentous tears and fractures. Injuries to the avascular menisci produce a synovial effusion which takes an hour or two to develop. Bruising

similarly indicates damage to a vascular structure but may be simply due to contusion of the skin and subcutaneous tissues.

Stiffness

Limitation of both flexion and extension are common in the arthritic knee. Loose bodies and torn menisci cause 'locking' — a sudden block to full extension followed by sudden unlocking, usually after some manipulation or twisting movement by the patient.

Instability

The knee joint has no inherent stability. The two surfaces are only held in their normal relationship by the cruciate and collateral ligaments, injuries to which cause various complex types of instability.

Giving way

Even if the ligaments are intact, the quadriceps must contract powerfully to keep the knee straight during the stance phase of gait. This muscle wastes within a few weeks of the onset of knee problems so that the knee may give way, i.e. flex when it should not have flexed. This may cause the patient to fall down suddenly. Patients with long-standing paralysis of the quadriceps due to poliomyelitis develop hyper-extension of the knee and are able to stabilize it in that position, the strain being taken by the posterior capsule.

Examination

Look With the patient supine look for swelling. Does it follow the outline of the synovial cavity with its suprapatellar pouch (haemarthrosis or synovitis) (Fig. 17.7) or is it localized to one side of the joint (contusion or cystic meniscus)? Look also for wasting of the quadriceps which is most obvious in the distal part of vastus medialis. It is best to measure the circumference of both thighs (say at 14 cm above the superior pole of the patella) to detect less obvious wasting. An unusual but interesting sign is an area of callosity on the thigh which develops in a patient with paralysed quadriceps who, whenever he takes a step, has to push his thigh backwards to hold the knee in extension.

Look also for sideways angulation (knock-knee or bow-leg) though this will be more obvious when the patient stands. Sometimes the angulation of the knees is the same on both sides, the so-called wind-swept

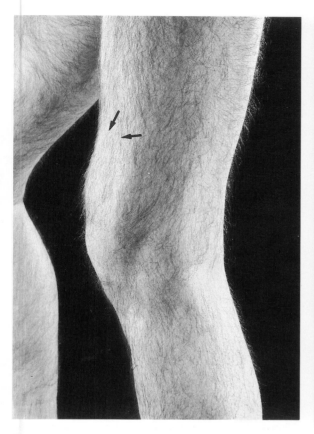

Fig. 17.7 Swelling of the knee due to synovial fluid. Note the bulge of the suprapatellar pouch (arrowed) which extends to 5 cm above the upper border of the patella. The quadriceps muscle in this patient is markedly wasted.

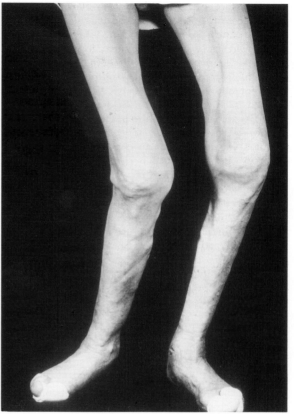

Fig. 17.8 Wind-swept knees in rheumatoid arthritis.

knees (Fig. 17.8). It is also worth getting the patient to flex the knee to 90° (if he can) and looking at the knee from the side: if the posterior cruciate ligament is ineffective, the tibia will sag backwards. This angle of inspection will also reveal the swelling of the tibial tuberosity seen in Osgood–Schlatter's osteochondritis.

Feel Palpation is necessary to detect a small effusion. The 'patellar tap' test only works if there is exactly the right amount of fluid in the knee and is therefore of limited use. A better method involves a combination of feeling and looking. Normally there is a hollow on the anteromedial aspect of the knee, behind the patella and in front of the femoral condyle. An effusion will fill up this hollow, but slight filling is not obvious just by looking at the knee. However, if this area is massaged gently, the fluid can be displaced into the rest of the synovial cavity. Tapping

on the other (lateral) side of the knee smartly with the flat of the fingers will cause visible sudden filling of the medial hollow as the fluid is pushed back to that side of the joint. This sounds complicated but is easy to do and is a valuable sign.

Localization of tenderness is one of the most important signs in the knee, especially following injuries, as the collateral ligaments usually tear at their ends (i.e. over the femoral or tibial condyle) whereas meniscal injuries cause tenderness over the joint line. It is only possible to feel the bony landmarks properly with the knee flexed to about 90°, though sometimes pain makes this impossible.

Move Measuring active flexion and extension of the knee is straightforward. A large goniometer should be used. While the movement is being made, feel for crepitus or clunking; try to decide whether it is arising from the patello-femoral or tibio-femoral joints.

Normally the extended knee allows no lateral movement. If the collateral ligament is torn but the cruciates remain intact, there is still no sideways laxity so it is best to test for this with the knee slightly flexed, say to 20°. Watch the patient's face when looking for either pain (as occurs with a partly torn or 'sprained' collateral ligament) or abnormal movement (if the ligament is completely torn). Injury to the cruciate ligament allows the tibia to be drawn forwards or pushed back in relation to the femur — the drawer sign. Do not forget to ask the patient to turn over and lie face-down. Swelling in the popliteal fossa may be an aneurysm, a cyst, or an expression of a synovial effusion ('Baker's cyst'). In rheumatoid disease, the latter may extend down into the calf; this can then rupture causing pain and tenderness which mimics a deep-vein thrombosis. Before the patient gets off the couch, examine the hip, in case the 'knee' pain is referred from above.

Function   Watch the bare-legged patient walking to and fro. This is very informative, particularly in revealing the outward thrust of the knee seen in osteoarthritic bow-legs, which sometimes reaches extraordinary proportions.

The spine

This is a chain of joints or rather of joint-complexes because each vertebra is joined to the next one by an intervertebral disc (a syndesmosis which, as everyone knows, is very prone to mechanical disorders) and by two posterior facet joints (which, like any synovial joints, are subject to osteoarthritis). Degenerative changes in the discs are known as spondylosis. This must be distinguished from the two mechanical abnormalities: spondylolysis, a defect in the pars interarticularis, and spondylolisthesis in which one vertebra slips forwards on the one below. Spondylitis implies inflammation and in practice is only used for ankylosing spondylitis, one of the inflammatory arthropathies.

Symptoms

Pain

This is much the commonest symptom. Disc disorders are commonest in the lower cervical and lower lumbar regions and cause pain there, but if a nerve root is compressed, there may be referred pain down the arm or down the leg (the latter being called sciatica). The pain from lumbosacral disc lesions is often felt at the sacroiliac joint. Sometimes the symptoms are

virtually confined to the limb and the patient does not complain of neck or back pain at all.

Disc lesions can occur in the thoracic spine but are uncommon, because the ribs splint that part of the spine and limit its movement. Pain around or between the shoulder blades may be due to pathology in the thoracic vertebral bodies, but is more often referred from a cervical disc lesion.

Back pain may also arise from the facet joints or even from the muscles, but it usually arises from disc strain or, in more severe cases, disc prolapse or vertebral collapse.

Weakness and sensory changes

Collapse or disease of vertebrae or associated structures may cause cord damage either by direct compression or ischaemia (Fig. 17.9). Weakness or actual paralysis and/or sensory impairment in association with spinal disease demand very urgent investigation and treatment. Of critical importance is involvement of the sacral nerve roots causing difficulty in micturition and loss of sensation to pin-prick in the perineum: if the compression is not relieved by surgery within hours there may be permanent incontinence.

Deformity

The different types of deformity are considered below, but may in themselves be the presenting complaint, especially in an adolescent girl developing scoliosis. Deformity of the feet may be an expression of muscle imbalance caused by a spinal abnormality such as diastomatomyelia.

Severe scoliosis interferes with the function of the lungs and heart and, in untreated cases, this usually causes premature death.

Stiffness

This can be due to many spinal diseases, but if it is the dominant complaint the diagnosis of ankylosing spondylitis must be considered. For instance, a lorry driver may be unable to turn his head to reverse his lorry because of fixity of the whole spine.

Examination

Look at the undressed patient from the side and from behind:

• a pure lateral deformity is called a tilt. This may be due to a short leg or a fixed adduction contracture

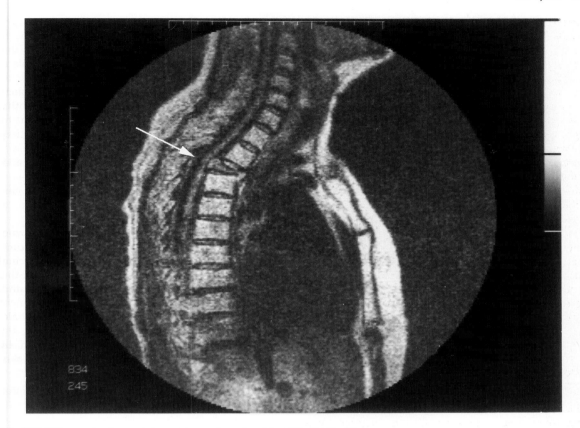

Fig. 17.9 MRI scan showing cord damage by a collapsed vertebra following trauma.

of the hip (causing apparent shortening of the leg) or to a spinal lesion, usually an acute intervertebral disc prolapse

- an abnormally flexed position of the spine, usually in the thoracic region, is called a kyphosis if it is a smooth curve over many vertebrae (as in tuberculosis or ankylosing spondylitis) (Figs 17.10 and 17.22) or a kyphos if there is a sharp angle at one point (due to destruction of a vertebral body by metastasis) (Fig. 17.11). Severe osteoporosis produces what is clinically a kyphosis but is actually due to compression fractures of several vertebral bodies (see Fig. 4.7)
- an abnormally extended position of the spine is called lordosis. This uncommon deformity is seen in its most extreme form in severe spina bifida. The cervical and lumbar spines are normally in a position of slight lordosis: loss of this (i.e. that part of the spine becomes straight) is common in disc disorders
- The most severe spinal deformities take the

form of scoliosis. This is a combined lateral and rotational deformity (Fig. 4.6). Clinically it may look like a kyphosis but this is an illusion due to the twisting: actually the anterior longitudinal ligament is longer than the posterior longitudinal ligament, i.e. there is a lordosis. The term kyphoscoliosis should, therefore, not be used. Scoliosis may be due to poliomyelitis or to a congenital abnormality in the spine, but in Britain is usually idiopathic. The type which occurs in infant boys is usually convex to the left and often resolves spontaneously. The commonest type is in adolescent girls, is usually convex to the right, and can produce appalling deformity which turns a normal 12-year-old girl into a 14-year-old hunchback. The reason for these differences is not understood. Some people appear to have a scoliosis when standing up but when they bend forwards the lateral deformity in the spine disappears. If it persists in flexion, the scoliosis is structural and needs to be assessed by an orthopaedic surgeon.

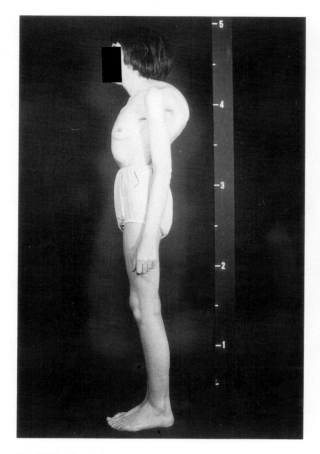

Fig. 17.10 A kyphosis due to collapse of several adjacent vertebrae.

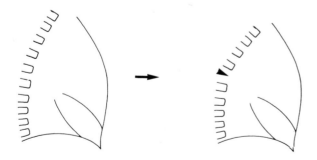

Fig. 17.11 The production of a kyphos with a sharp angle at one point.

Move   While the patient is standing up, assess the flexion, extension, lateral flexion and rotation each way. It is hard to measure these accurately and for most purposes it is probably enough to estimate it as

a quarter, half, three-quarters or full. Don't forget that a patient with a stiff spine may be able to touch his toes by flexing the hips: you must look at the lumbar spine to be sure that flexion is taking place there. For greater accuracy, use a tape-measure to find the distance between two fixed points, such as the spinous processes of T12 and L5, with the patient standing up straight; then ask the patient to bend forwards and see how much this distance has increased.

If the back is very painful, it is unreasonable and unkind to ask the patient to touch his toes, but you can ask him to bend forwards as much as he can comfortably manage. With a lumbar disc lesion, it may be straightening up again which is difficult.

Even if your patient cannot move his back you must get him to move his legs to carry out a neurological examination of the lower limbs. In a recent injury which may have caused a spinal fracture, the patient should be moved as little as possible and rolled over in one piece like a log.

Feel   Ask the patient to lie face-down on the couch. Localization of tenderness is valuable.

Neurological examination   Three special points need to be made about neurological examination in this context:

- straight leg raising is a very important sign. First flex the hip and knee simultaneously to make sure the hip will flex. Then, with the patient lying face up, lift the leg slowly with the knee straight while watching the patient's face so that you stop when it hurts. If straight leg raising is limited to 20° or 30°, there is probably a prolapsed intervertebral disc. Ask the patient where it hurts: pain in the back suggests a more central disc prolapse, whereas pain in the leg points to a lateral prolapse compressing the nerve root. Pain in the other leg (the one you are not lifting up) is rare but strongly suggests disc prolapse

- consider root levels (see Tables 8.5 and 8.7). Much the commonest cause of backache is a lumbar disc lesion. The purpose of neurological examination is to try to localize this. When testing the ankle-jerk, what you really want to know is whether the S1 nerve root is working normally. Similarly, the patient is asked to extend the big toe against resistance because extensor hallucis longus is principally supplied from the L5 nerve root and you want to test that. These are the two roots most often affected by disc lesions.

You should also know the sensory dermatomes in the arm and leg (Fig. 17.12) so you can 'think root' when testing sensation

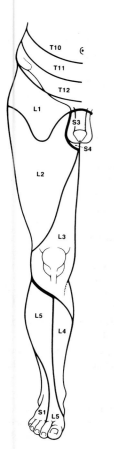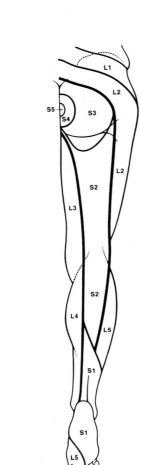

Fig. 17.12 The sensory dermatomes of the leg.

- difficulty in micturition associated with backache is a surgical emergency. In all patients with acute back pain, you should test sensation to pin-prick on both sides of the anus, unpleasant though this is, because perianal analgesia indicates involvement of the sacral roots which also supply the bladder

Some causes of various abnormalities of spine structure and function are listed in Table 17.2.

Diagnosis of joint problems

Joint problems may arise as part of a primary arthritic syndrome or secondary to other diseases. In view of this we have to take account of the differential diagnosis of the arthritides in conjunction with the exam-

ination of individual joints. Often the essential distinction is whether there has been an injury or not. This may not be as straightforward as you would think. Some patients give a history of injury, recalled retrospectively, which they feel must be responsible for their symptoms though in fact it is irrelevant. The time-scale is usually the best clue: if the symptoms developed within a day or two of a definite injury they are probably due to it, whereas, if they developed weeks or months later, they are probably due to some other cause. On the other hand, the symptoms may be due to injury but the history of trauma is not forthcoming, either because the patient cannot give a history because he is too young, too drunk, or too comatose or because the injury was sustained in a discreditable manner and is therefore concealed. The most important and extreme example of the last is the battered baby, who may present with a painful swollen joint but a history of injury is denied.

The treatment of injuries is generally a surgical matter and in the limbs comes within the sphere of the orthopaedic surgeon. For this reason, the symptoms and signs of joint injury will not be discussed in detail in this chapter, but the physician must always keep this possibility in mind.

What are the other causes of a painful and/or swollen joint? These may be classified as being of synovial or cartilaginous origin but in practical terms the causes may be considered as follows:

- infection
- non-infective inflammatory conditions (rheumatoid arthritis and the seronegative arthritides)
- gout
- osteoarthritis
- osteochondritis
- connective tissue diseases

Infection

Infection is an eminently treatable condition and failure to diagnose it and therefore to treat it correctly is a calamity. Acute septic arthritis is an urgent matter: pus dissolves articular cartilage rapidly. It is no longer very common in the Western world but doctors in any speciality, and of course in general practice, may encounter it and must be able to recognize it. It should be obvious when a joint is very painful, hot and swollen and when the patient is febrile and toxic, but milder forms are becoming increasingly common. Unfortunately they can damage the joint just as badly and early diagnosis remains essential. Septic arthritis often originates as

Table 17.2. Abnormalities of spine structure and function

Physical abnormality of spine	Young	Middle-aged or elderly
Scoliosis	Congenital Idiopathic acquired Neurological (e.g. poliomyelitis)	As a result of disorders in youth
Kyphosis or kyphos	Congenital Ankylosing spondylitis Spinal tuberculosis Scheuermann's disease	Osteoporosis Secondary carcinoma Myelomatosis Tuberculosis Ankylosing spondylitis
Stiffness and pain	Ankylosing spondylitis Disc lesions Injuries	As in the young Spondylosis Myelomatosis Lymphoma Secondary carcinoma Chronic infections
Loss of height	Injuries	Osteoporosis Myelomatosis Secondary carcinoma Crush injuries Paget's disease

osteomyelitis in the adjoining bone, especially at the hip joint. The distinction between these two may therefore not be absolute. Bony tenderness suggests bony infection. Failure to improve greatly in 24 hours requires an orthopaedic opinion urgently (i.e. that day) as immediate surgical exploration is usually needed.

Of chronic infections, tuberculosis remains the most common and even in Britain is still seen from time to time. In some undeveloped countries it remains a common problem. It is important to realize that rheumatoid joints are subject to infection as it is easy to miss this and regard it just as a 'flare-up'. When in doubt, aspirate the synovial fluid and send it for culture.

Rheumatoid arthritis

Unquestionably rheumatoid arthritis (RA) is the most common inflammatory arthropathy in Britain but a precise diagnosis may be difficult in the early stages of the disease. The disease is most usually seen in young or middle-aged women commencing as a symmetrical, small-joint arthropathy affecting hands and feet. Pain, swelling and morning stiffness are characteristic features with wrists, metocarpo-

phalangeal (MCP) and proximal interphalangeal (PIP) joints being affected at an early stage (see Chapter 18). Later, other joints may be involved such as ankles, knees and hips, together with elbows and shoulders. Rheumatoid nodules at the elbows provide good confirmatory evidence of the disease (Fig. 17.13). These subcutaneous nodules are seen in about 20 per cent of patients with RA and usually indicate activity and seropositivity (i.e. rheumatoid factor is found in the blood). Similar lesions may be seen sometimes over other surfaces subjected to pressure, such as the thumb or sacrum.

It is important to remember that whilst in its typical form RA is a polyarthritis, it may start as a monoarthritis, the diagnosis of which may prove elusive in the early stages.

A small group of patients with RA progress to crippling disease with extensive joint destruction and deformity. In most, the course of the disease is characterized by relapses and remissions.

It is essential to remember that RA is a multisystem disease affecting heart, lungs, blood vessels and eyes and in any inflammatory arthropathy the history and physical examination must include a search for possible complications (Fig. 17.14). Felty's syndrome is a rare variant of rheumatoid arthritis character-

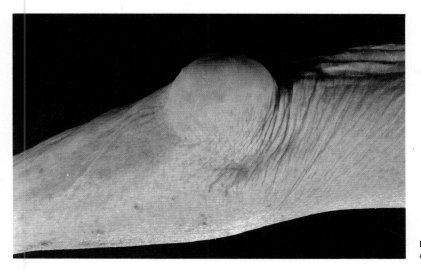

Fig. 17.13 A rheumatoid nodule at the elbow. Sometimes these lesions ulcerate.

ized by associated splenomegaly, leucopenia and lymphadenopathy.

Other inflammatory arthropathies

A wide range of joint disorders is included in this category. One of the closest to rheumatoid arthritis in its clinical pattern is psoriatic arthropathy. In true psoriatic arthritis (see Chapter 18) distal interphalangeal (DIP) joint involvement occurs, distinguishing it from rheumatoid arthritis (Fig. 17.15). However, another characteristic feature of psoriatic arthritis is the 'sausage' digit where simultaneous involvement of distal and proximal IP joints and the MCP or metatarsophalangeal (MTP) joints occurs. In a rare form of psoriatic arthropathy, arthritis mutilans, absorption of periarticular bone takes place with consequent gross shortening and deformity of the hands or feet (see Fig. 18.21). Spondylitis with sacroiliitis, sometimes unilateral, is found in about 5 per cent of patients.

Acute rheumatic fever is now rare in the developed world but is still common in the tropics. A flitting, large-joint arthropathy following a streptococcal infection should bring to mind this possibility, confirmed by the associated carditis.

Polyarthritis may complicate infections elsewhere, the term 'reactive arthropathy' being used to describe this type of association. The best known of these is Reiter's syndrome which is mainly a 'below-the-belt' arthritis associated with conjunctivitis and urethritis (see Chapter 21). A similar reactive arthropathy may be seen with gut infections by organisms such as *Shigella* or *Yersinia*.

Ankylosing spondylitis is a relatively rare form of arthritis affecting 0.05 per cent of the population in the United Kingdom with a strongly male predominance. The hallmark of ankylosing spondylitis is a sacroiliitis, but with advancing disease the vertebral and costovertebral joints are involved. Fifteen per cent of sufferers have peripheral joint involvement which sometimes precedes the spinal symptoms. Most patients develop symptoms in their 20s or 30s with aching, low backache and increasing stiffness. Over subsequent years, as the spinous ligaments ossify, the spine becomes more stiff but sometimes less painful. Eventually the patient acquires a completely rigid back and his incapacity may be increased by worsening arthritis of the hips which are often involved later. Systemic associations of ankylosing spondylitis include upper-lobe pulmonary fibrosis, aortic incompetence and iritis.

Patients with ankylosing spondylitis, Reiter's syndrome and psoriasis with arthritis have a close association with the histocompatibility antigen HLA B27, suggesting a genetic susceptibility and predisposition.

Gout

Gout is the most commonly seen form of crystal synovitis. Acute attacks usually occur first in the first MTP joints and are exquisitely painful. Chronic gout produces knobbly asymmetrical swellings of the

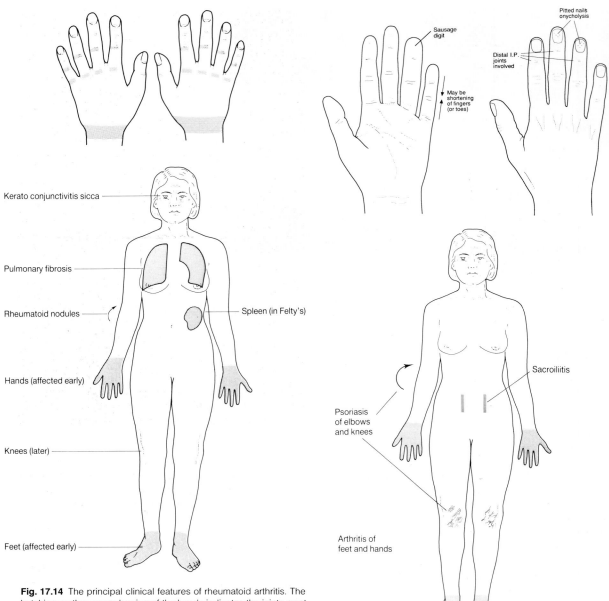

Fig. 17.14 The principal clinical features of rheumatoid arthritis. The hatching on the upper drawing of the hands indicates the joints most likely to be affected, but not necessarily simultaneously.

Fig. 17.15 The principal clinical features of psoriatic arthropathy.

fingers and feet (Fig. 17.16(a)), which may ulcerate and discharge a white, chalk-like debris of urates. A hallmark of gout is the tophus which may be seen on the hands, feet or ears (Fig. 17.16(b)). Sometimes the disease may be complicated by a uric-acid nephropathy.

Osteoarthritis (or osteoarthrosis)

Neither term is entirely satisfactory. There is no acute inflammation, which distinguishes the condition from the inflammatory arthropathies described

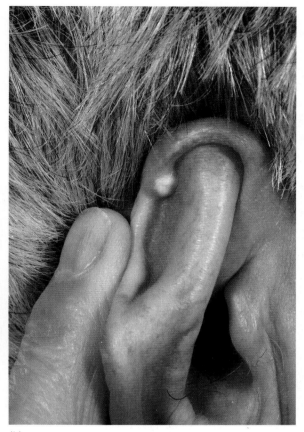

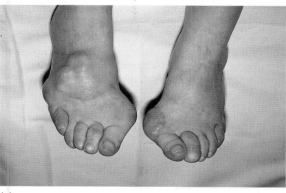

(a)

Fig. 17.16 (a) Chronic gouty swellings of the feet. The first metatarsophalangeal joint is characteristically the initial site of attacks of acute gout. (b) A gouty tophus of the ear (now an infrequently seen physical sign).

(b)

earlier. In basic terms, osteoarthritis is a 'wear-and-tear' phenomenon. In the primary form no obvious predisposing cause is apparent though some familial patterns emerge. In secondary osteoarthritis a predisposing condition is obvious such as an old injury which has caused irregularity of the joint surface, altered mechanics, or defective nerve supply. With this last defect, a painless and grossly disorganized joint may result (Charcot's joint).

In osteoarthritis, joints are not usually painful at rest; it is movement or load-bearing which brings on the pain. The physical signs are due to the changes in cartilage and bone; these cause grating on movement, loss of movement, osteophytes, and angular deformity. Osteoarthritis is predominantly a disease of the weight-bearing joints — the spine, hips and knees (Fig. 17.17). Nodules on the dorsal or lateral aspect of the distal interphalangeal joints of the middle-aged or elderly, are called Heberden's nodes (see Fig. 18.23); these are really just osteophytes and

though often classified as osteoarthritic they are not necessarily associated with osteoarthritis elsewhere. These nodes are ugly but usually painless.

Osteochondritis

This is another unsatisfactory term embracing three different types of disorder, based on the x-ray appearance:

- 'crushing' osteochondritis, of which the most important is Perthes' disease of the epiphysis of the head of the femur. Here osteonecrosis of one or both femoral heads occurs in children aged 4−10 years
- 'pulling' osteochondritis such as Osgood−Schlatter's disease of the tibial tuberosity, due to traction by the patellar tendon
- 'splitting' osteochondritis or osteochondritis dissecans. This occurs on the convex surface of joints,

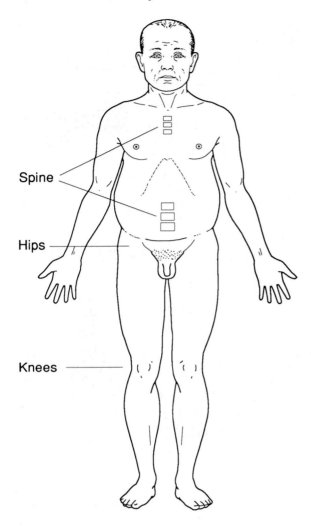

Spine

Hips

Knees

Fig. 17.17 Joints most often affected by osteoarthritis.

especially the knee. The cause is probably trauma in most cases, for example the impact of the patella on the femoral condyle. Later the affected area may split off altogether and fall into the joint where it forms a loose body

The connective tissue diseases

Though not strictly primary disorders of the musculoskeletal system, the connective tissue diseases can be conveniently considered at this stage. They have been grouped together under this title because a common feature in their pathology is fibrinoid change in the connective tissue. The diseases included in this category are:

- rheumatoid arthritis
- systemic lupus erythematosus
- systemic sclerosis (scleroderma)
- dermatomyositis
- polyarteritis nodosa
- Sjögren's syndrome

They predominantly affect women and although they do not share the same aetiology they have many common features. These include systemic disease, overlapping pathological and clinical features and significant immunological abnormalities. Although fairly rare these diseases are described individually because many have physical features that are striking and often diagnostic. However, not all the syndromes are distinct and patients are seen with overlap syndromes which do not fit happily into any particular diagnostic category.

Systemic lupus erythematosus (SLE)

This relatively uncommon disease affects young women during the reproductive period of life. Some ethnic groups such as Negroes in the USA and the Chinese seem particularly vulnerable. The commonest problem is non-erosive, symmetrical small-joint disease, similar in distribution to that of rheumatoid arthritis. Associated with the arthritis in the majority of cases are skin lesions including butterfly erythema of the face, photosensitivity, cutaneous vasculitis and alopecia. Systemic involvement occurs in about 50 per cent of patients with renal disease, neuropsychiatric problems and pleurisy. Constitutional symptoms are common and these include fatigue, weight loss and fever. Some of the clinical features are summarized in Fig. 17.18.

Systemic sclerosis (scleroderma)

The hallmark of this disease is thickening and tethering of the skin by dense fibrosis. Similar diffuse fibrosis affects internal organs such as the gut, heart and lungs. Characteristically this is a disorder of middle-aged women and it is recognized by puckering of the skin round the mouth and tightening of the skin of the face particularly the forehead (see Fig. 2.3). The patients have stiff, tight hands which are the site of Raynaud's phenomenon. Over the years, areas of ischaemic necrosis may scar the finger ends. In some patients there is loss of the pulp of the fingertips with digital gangrene (Fig. 18.6). A true

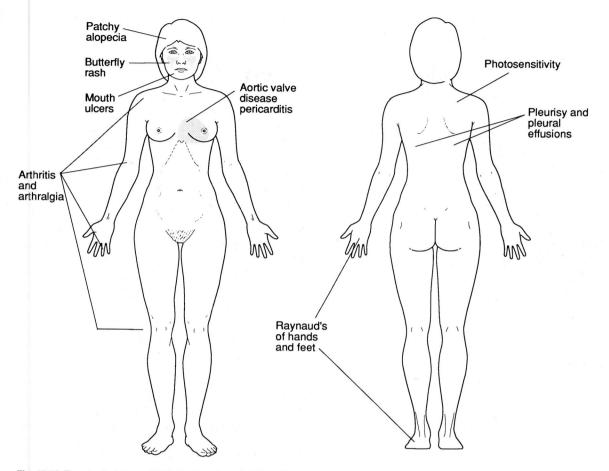

Fig. 17.18 The physical signs of SLE showing the main joints affected.

small-joint arthropathy is a feature of the disease in 25 per cent of patients (Fig. 17.19).

Dermatomyositis

This rare syndrome of middle-aged women is dominated by two clinical features, a rash and muscle weakness. The rash is situated round the eyes and on the cheeks; the eyelids have an unusual, reddish-purple (heliotrope) coloration. There may also be some facial oedema. The muscle weakness due to proximal myositis, may cause difficulties in climbing stairs or lifting the arms above the head. Hyperaemia of the nail-folds is a frequent finding as are elevated plaques over the knuckles (Gottron's papules). Underlying malignancy, mainly carcinoma of the ovary, lungs or breast, occurs in 10 per cent of patients with dermatomyositis.

Polyarteritis nodosa (Fig. 17.20)

This is the only member of the group of connective tissue diseases which is commoner in men. The basic lesion is a necrotizing arteritis affecting small and medium arteries and, as a result, the clinical manifestations are protean. A symmetrical polyarthritis is an early feature of polyarteritis but progressive deformity is unusual. The majority of patients (70 per cent) suffer renal involvement with haematuria and albuminuria and may develop hypertension and renal failure. Skin lesions include livedo reticularis, ulcers and areas of infarction. Involvement of the peripheral nerves is common to give either a mononeuritis or polyneuritis.

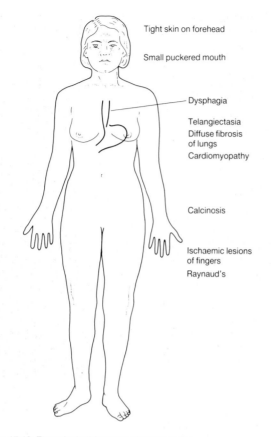

Fig. 17.19 The principal features of scleroderma.

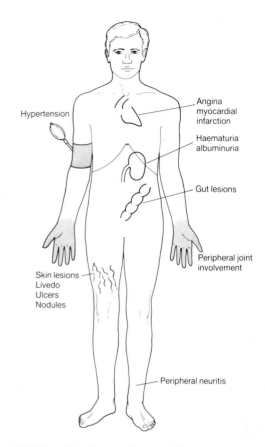

Fig. 17.20 The clinical features of polyarteritis nodosa.

Acquired disease of the skeleton

During adult life the shape of the skeleton changes with progressive ageing. In the 20s and 30s, an almost imperceptible loss of height begins which continues through middle age. In old age obvious loss of height occurs. This is mainly due to trunk shortening with thinning of the intervertebral discs and loss of height of the vertebral bodies. The loss of height may be accentuated by vertebral collapse. Old men and women often stand with knees and hips slightly flexed and this, with increasing dorsal kyphosis, further emphasizes the loss of height.

In addition to these age changes four diseases may alter the shape of the skeleton:

- Paget's disease (osteitis deformans)
- osteoporosis
- malignant disease of bone (mainly metastatic cancer and myelomatosis)
- osteomalacia, rickets

Paget's disease (Fig. 17.21(a) and (b))

This is a disorder of unknown aetiology seen mainly in men of European stock and occurring predominantly in the second half of life. Although evidence of Paget's disease is revealed in 3 per cent of autopsies in the United Kingdom it is only the more severe forms which rise to clinical disease. Pathologically it is due initially to increased osteoclastic activity causing softening followed by osteoblastic activity with bone resorption and deposition. These changes result in thick but soft bones, and loss of differentiation between cortex and medulla.

Clinically the skull increases in size and the cranial nerve foraminae may be occluded to give deafness,

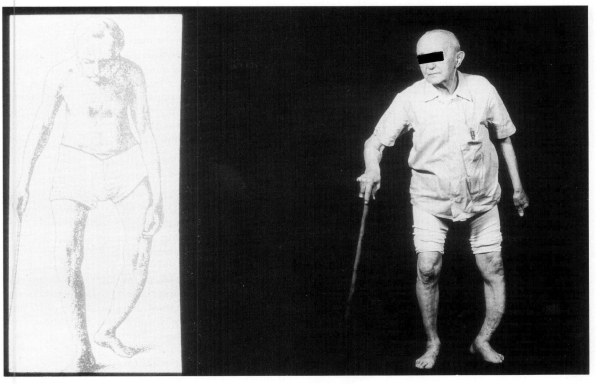

(a)

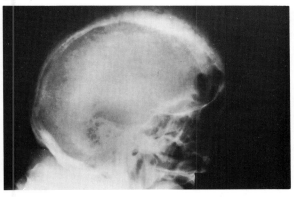

(b)

Fig. 17.21 (a) An elderly patient with Paget's disease matched with a drawing of one of Paget's original cases. Note the large skull, deaf-aid and bowed left tibia. (b) Radiographic appearances of the skull in Paget's disease.

blindness and facial weakness. One or both tibiae may enlarge and bow; because of the increased blood supply affected tibiae usually feel warm. Kyphosis is common. Paget's disease itself seldom causes

pain, which suggests a complication such as fracture, sarcoma or osteoarthritis.

Osteoporosis

This term refers to a group of diseases characterized by a reduction of bone mass secondary to loss of bone matrix. To a certain extent the process is physiological, occurring in postmenopausal women and in old age. However, many other causes may be responsible (Table 17.3).

Table 17.3. Some causes of osteoporosis

Physiological	Post-menopausal, ageing
Mechanical	Immobility
Idiopathic	Juvenile or adult
Endocrine	Thyrotoxicosis
	Cushing's syndrome
	Hypogonadism
Metabolic	Chronic liver disease
	Malabsorption
Drugs	Steroids
Toxins	Chronic alcoholism

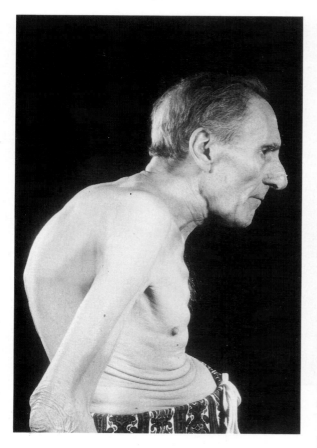

Fig. 17.22 A rapidly acquired kyphotic spine with collapse of multiple vertebral bodies due to myelomatosis.

Clinically the main features are shortening of the trunk due to compression or collapse of the vertebral bodies. This produces an exaggeration of the normal dorsal kyphosis. In advanced cases the ribs may ride on the iliac crests and the short trunk produces transverse abdominal creases (see Fig. 6.2(a) and (b)). Bones fracture easily, particularly the neck of the femur and the wrist.

Malignant disease of the skeleton

Whilst many primary carcinomas, such as breast, prostate, kidney, bronchus and thyroid, metastasize to bone, they usually present with pain and pathological fractures rather than with skeletal deformity. Trunk shortening, kyphosis (Fig. 17.22), rib and limb fractures are commonly seen in myelomatosis, one of the few diseases which results in fracture and deformity of the sternum.

Osteomalacia

The failure of calcification of newly formed osteoid caused by vitamin D deficiency causes rickets in the child and osteomalacia in the adult. Simple dietary deficiency causing rickets or osteomalacia is uncommon in the United Kingdom but deficiency may result from malabsorption or chronic renal disease. In childhood rickets the clinical features are those of tender swellings at the growing ends of the bones, stunting of stature, bossing of the skull and bowing, usually laterally, of the legs. In adults osteomalacia is characterized by bone pains (pseudofractures) and proximal muscle weakness. Strictly speaking, osteomalacia in the adult rarely causes acquired skeletal defects though, of course, it may be grafted onto childhood rickets.

References and further reading

Apley AG, Solomon L. *Apley's system of orthopaedics and fractures*, 6th edn. London: Butterworth, 1982.
Dickson RA, Wright V. *Musculo-skeletal disease*. London: Heinemann, 1984.
Freeman MAR. Reconstructive surgery in arthritis. In Hadfield J, Hobsley M (eds). *Current surgical practice*, vol. 3, pp. 211–29. London: Edward Arnold, 1981.
McRea R. *Clinical orthopaedic examination*, 2nd edn. Edinburgh: Churchill Livingstone, 1983.

18

The hand

N. J. Barton and P. J. Toghill

Symptoms
Examination
The wrist
References and further reading

Man's dominant position is due to the development of his brain, but the way in which his brain implements the required action involves the hand, which has been called the 'cutting edge of the mind'. The importance of the hand is shown by its very large representation in the cerebral cortex, where the thumb alone has more grey matter controlling it than all the thoracic and abdominal viscera.

The most obvious function of the hand is its motor activity which ranges from the power grip of the labourer to the delicate manipulations of the musician, but the hand is also a sensory organ used to explore the surfaces of objects. Moreover a hand with motor power but without sensation does not work properly because the patient does not know how hard he is gripping or how hard he should grip. The hand is also used as a means of physical contact with other people, loss of which is considered by patients to be one of their greatest deprivations.

Symptoms

Pain

Constant pain occurs in inflammatory conditions: acute infection or the synovitis of inflammatory arthropathies. Intermittent pain occurs with constriction of tendons or nerves or with arthritis of joint surfaces. Symptomatic osteoarthritis is uncommon in the hand except in the carpometacarpal joint of the thumb. Patients with end-stage rheumatoid deformities of the hands usually no longer have severe pain, but those with active disease suffer aching pain worse with movement and associated with early morning stiffness. The wrist is often more painful than the hand itself.

Sensory disturbances

Sensory symptoms (Fig. 18.1) may be a local manifestation of a generalized neurological disorder (see Chapter 9) but certain syndromes are of particular importance in the hand.

The carpal tunnel syndrome causes painful pins-and-needles which wake the patient at night and are relieved by movement or a change in position. The paraesthesiae are mainly in the median nerve distribution though it is hard to localize paraesthesiae exactly, especially in retrospect. The patient usually feels the symptoms more on the palmar surface of the hand. There may be retrograde radiation to the elbow, but not above.

Cervical spondylosis causes pain or deadness in the appropriate root distribution in the arm and/or the hand. The patient usually points to the back of the hand but may have little or no pain in the neck.

Ulnar nerve lesions also cause deadness or loss of feeling, but not the same kind of symptoms as carpal tunnel syndrome.

Deformity

In temperate climes in cool weather, the face and hands may be the only parts of the body that are visible. The hand is thrust forwards in greeting, in

SENSORY DISTURBANCES IN THE HAND

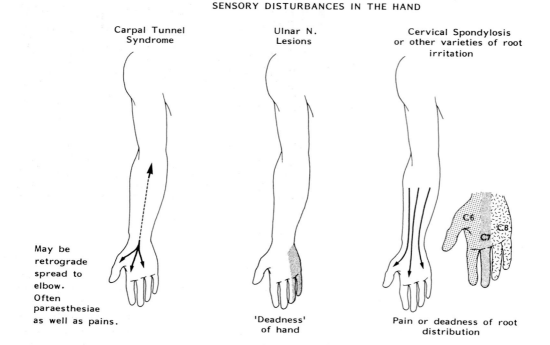

Fig. 18.1 Common sensory disturbances in the hand.

giving and taking, and quickly draws attention to itself; patients are much more concerned about the cosmetic appearance of their hands than is generally realized.

Clumsiness

This is a difficult symptom to define. 'Dropping things' is usually a sensory symptom. However, deformities and stiffness also contribute to clumsiness. Few things are more awkward than a single bent finger which will not straighten or a single straight finger which will not bend. For instance, patients with Dupuytren's contracture often complain that, when they wash their faces, the bent fingers get in the way.

Stiffness

Intermittent obstruction to movement occurs in trigger finger or thumb. Permanent restriction of extension develops in Dupuytren's and other contractures (see Fig. 18.11) after injuries to the interphalangeal joints or flexor tendons, and in many rheumatoid patients due to joint disease or rupture

of extensor tendons. In rheumatoid arthritis (RA), the severe stiffness on waking eases after an hour or so. Restriction of active flexion occurs in RA and after injuries to the flexor or extensor tendons. Loss of abduction of the thumb occurs in RA or osteoarthritis and in Dupuytren's disease involving the thumb web.

'Disability'

This is in inverted commas because it is an inadequate description and really it is not much better than asking a patient if he is ill. It is essential to find out which function is lost. 'Give me an example of something you can't do with your hand, or which you find difficult.' This symptom embraces a huge range of problems such as being unable to unscrew bottle-tops because of rheumatoid arthritis, having difficulty in winding a watch because of peripheral neuropathy or being incapable of buttoning a coat because of Parkinson's disease. For the patient this loss of function is the over-riding consideration. This is what he would like us to improve and that is why we must define it precisely.

Examination

All patients have, to a certain extent, a selective examination of the parts suggested by the history; not infrequently something turns up during the examination that sends one back to the history to ask further questions which may in turn lead to further examination. However, there is no excuse for failing to examine the hand; the patient does not even have to undress. Even the psychiatrist may find it rewarding; a tremor and sweaty palms may be the only objective signs of alcoholism.

The examination of the hand should be in three stages (Fig. 18.2).

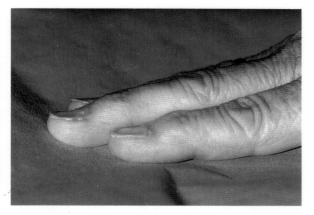

Fig. 18.3 Koilonychia. This patient had chronic iron-deficiency anaemia due to menorrhagia.

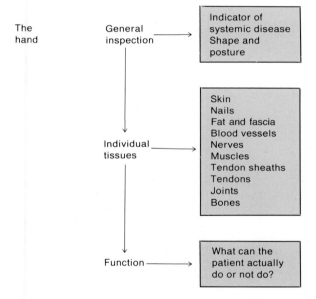

Fig. 18.2 A scheme for examining the hand.

Inspection

The hand as an indicator of systemic disease

The hand may signal disease elsewhere in the body. Start with the nails; they may show clubbing (see Fig. 4.1 and Tables 4.7 and 4.8), koilonychia or splinter haemorrhages. Whilst the last may be an important sign of subacute bacterial endocarditis, their significance has been exaggerated and they are usually the result of trauma. Spoon-shaped nails (koilonychia) are seen with chronic iron-deficiency anaemia (Fig. 18.3).

During periods of poor health, the nails grow slowly and defectively; because of this, serious ill-nesses, treatment with chemotherapy and episodes of malnutrition may be marked by white bands and abnormal zones of nail growth (Fig. 18.4). White flecks on the nails are of no particular significance in relation to health; they are due to trauma. A fascinating account of the growth of his own nail has been painstakingly recorded by William Bean.

The texture of both skin and tissues requires attention. With advancing years, particularly in women, the skin of the hands thins and is easily injured. The back of the hand is a common site for senile purpura (see Fig. 9.4), which may arise without obvious injury. These changes are all aggravated by steroid therapy giving rise to 'tissue-paper skin' (Fig. 18.5). The skin changes in scleroderma may be preceded by Raynaud's phenomenon for several years. As the disease progresses the skin becomes shiny, tight and immobile and the patient may have increasing stiffness of the fingers. In advanced cases there is ischaemic necrosis at the tips of the fingers (Fig. 18.6). In the CREST syndrome (*C*alcinosis, *R*aynauds, *O*esophageal hypomotility, *S*cleroderma, *T*elangiectasia) calcified nodules may ulcerate through the skin (Fig. 18.7). Similar though less severe changes without calcinosis may be found in mixed connective tissue disease. Telangiectasia of the nail-beds may be seen as a feature of both systemic lupus erythematosus and dermatomyositis.

In patients suspected of having familial hypercholesterolaemia, a careful search should be made for xanthomata around the Achilles tendon, knee and dorsum of hand (Fig. 18.8). These may be associated with xanthelasma and arcus juvenilis or senilis. Whilst tendon xanthomata are virtually diagnostic of

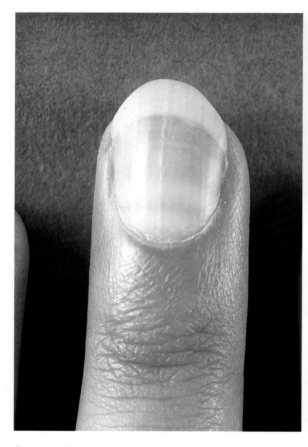

Fig. 18.4 White bands on the nails following chemotherapy for acute lymphoblastic leukaemia. Beau's lines are transverse depressions on the nails, also associated with defective nail-growth.

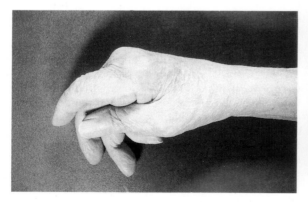

Fig. 18.5 Tissue-paper skin in a lady with rheumatoid arthritis who had been on steroid therapy for several years.

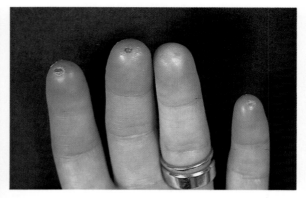

Fig. 18.6 Ischaemic necrosis of the fingertips in a patient with scleroderma.

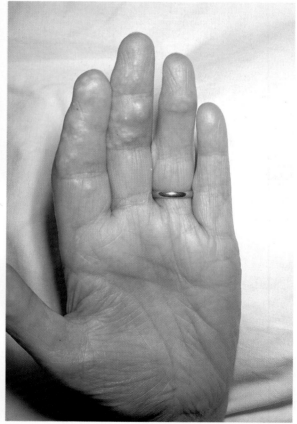

Fig. 18.7 Calcified nodules in a patient with the CREST syndrome.

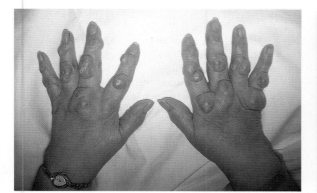

Fig. 18.8 Tendon xanthomata in a patient with familial hypercholesterolaemia.

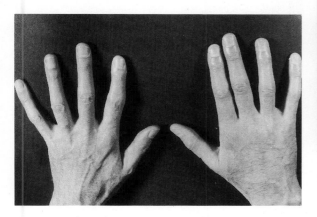

Fig. 18.9 Long, spidery fingers (arachnodactyly) in Marfan's syndrome.

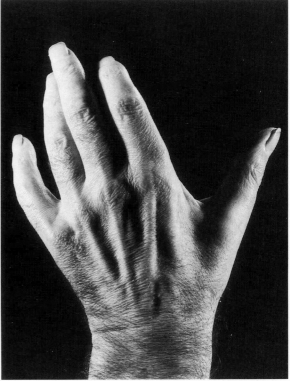

Fig. 18.10 Wasting of the small muscles of the hand. Here wasting of the dorsal interossei followed a gunshot injury to the brachial plexus.

familial hypercholesterolaemia, the other two features are less specific.

Unusually big hands are a characteristic feature of acromegaly (see Fig. 12.12) but those working manually such as carpenters and stonemasons may also develop thick, heavy hands. This is in contrast with the long, thin, spidery fingers of the arachnodactyly (Fig. 18.9) in Marfan's syndrome. Broad hands with stubby fingers, including curved little fingers, and a single transverse crease characterize Down's syndrome.

Shape and posture of the hand

Swelling due to infection or injury is most marked on the back of the hand where the skin is looser. Wasting of the small muscles may also be obvious (Fig. 18.10) and may be due to any nerve lesion from anterior horn cells to the ulnar or median nerves, a generalized neurological disorder, or simply disuse atrophy as in old age.

Of the abnormal postures, it is the 'claw hand' which is the most characteristic. This is a hand with hyperextension of the MCP joints and lack of extension of the interphalangeal (IP) joints due to weakness or paralysis of the interossei. Damage to the medial cord of the brachial plexus at birth or by subsequent trauma may result in clawing, as may ulnar and median nerve injuries. Isolated ulnar nerve lesions only cause clawing of the ring and little fingers. Wasting of the small muscles with extreme old age or peripheral neuropathy may also be responsible for unusual postures. In rheumatoid arthritis, the arthropathy combined with the small-muscle wasting may result in the hand and fingers adopting characteristic appearances.

A flexed finger (which may first be noticed while shaking hands with the patient) may be caused by Dupuytren's contracture, old injury, or a severe trigger finger.

Individual tissues

Skin

Look very carefully for scars. They can be hard to see in the hand, where most people have a few scars anyway, but may be the clue to the whole problem; for example an old, forgotten, or concealed cut or a penetrating injury may result in the later development of an inclusion dermoid cyst or a discharging abscess or sinus. Excessive sweating is usually due to anxiety but may be due to thyrotoxicosis or alcoholism. Some people have embarrassingly profuse sweating of the hands (hyperhidrosis). Lack of sweating follows division of peripheral nerves.

Finger-nails

The most common cause of an abnormal nail is an old injury which has damaged the nail-bed. Several dermatological conditions affect the nails (see Chapter 16). Of these, one of the most important is psoriasis which may cause pitting of the nails and arthropathy of the distal interphalangeal (DIP) joint. Separation of the distal part of the nail from the nail-bed (onycholysis) may also be seen in psoriasis.

Subcutaneous fat and palmar fascia

The most frequent and important condition affecting this layer is Dupuytren's disease which is much more common than is generally appreciated (Fig. 18.11). In older patients, especially men, Dupuytren's contracture is very common, with a prevalence over 65 years of more than 20 per cent.

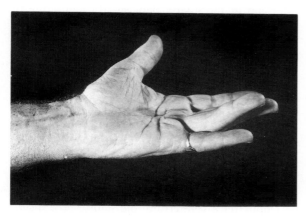

Fig. 18.11 Dupuytren's contracture.

Blood vessels

The hand receives most of its blood supply through the ulnar artery which can be palpated more easily if the radial artery is occluded. If the palm is exsanguinated by making a fist and both arteries then occluded by the examiner squeezing them over the wrist, the patency of each can be determined by extending the fingers again and releasing the arteries one at a time (Allen's test).

Haemorrhages in the nail-folds suggest vasculitis which may be a feature of RA, scleroderma or dermatomyositis. Vasculitic lesions of the fingers, particularly of the tips, are a common feature of RA (Fig. 18.12).

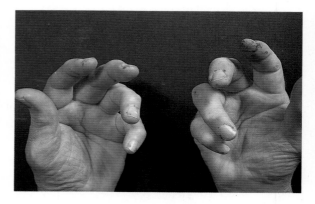

Fig. 18.12 Vasculitic lesions in rheumatoid arthritis. These lesions are usually seen in long-standing seropositive disease but with relatively inactive synovitis.

A common vascular disorder of the hand is Raynaud's phenomenon. On exposure to cold, the fingers turn first white, numb and cold, then blue, and eventually red, hot and painful. If the attacks are prolonged and troublesome it is called Raynaud's disease. Often Raynaud's phenomenon affects young women and is without obvious cause. In this group the symptoms are mild and tend to regress with increasing age.

Raynaud's phenomenon starting later in life is usually secondary to some structural abnormality or underlying disease such as cervical ribs, scleroderma or mixed connective tissue disease. It may also be due to prolonged use of vibrating tools such as pneumatic drills. Here recurrent episodes of digital ischaemia lead to pulp atrophy, ischaemic lesions of the skin and recurrent infections. Trivial injuries are slow to heal. Eventually episodes of gangrene of the finger-tips lead to shortening and stiffening of the fingers. Severe rest-pain due to ischaemia may necessitate surgical amputation. Some of the causes of Raynaud's phenomenon are shown in Table 18.1.

Table 18.1. Some causes of Raynaud's phenomenon

Common	Primary Raynaud's disease Scleroderma Mixed connective tissue disease β-blocker therapy
Less common	Platelet emboli from subclavian artery stenosis or aneurysm Myxoedema
Rare	Cryoglobulinaemia Cold agglutinins Vibrating tools Exposure to vinyl chloride

Nerves

Any approach to nerves depends upon the circumstances. With a cut on the arm or hand, a very careful examination must be made of motor and sensory function in the territory of any nerve which could conceivably have been injured, bearing in mind that a long, thin blade or sliver of glass entering obliquely can divide a nerve remote from the cut in the skin.

Since nerve damage often involves both sensory and motor defects it is more convenient to examine both nerve and muscle function together. The essential features of the typical sensory and motor innervation are summarized in Fig. 18.13. It is important to remember that 20 per cent of patients have arrangements of the nerves in the hands which are not those described in the anatomical textbooks.

Do not forget that nerve root lesions are very commonly due to cervical disc damage and may mimic a more peripheral nerve lesion. Always 'think root'; ask about neck symptoms and examine the neck.

Ulnar nerve A lesion of the ulnar nerve will cause sensory loss over the ulnar aspect of the ring finger and both sides of the little finger as in the diagram. On the motor side there is paralysis of the interossei (causing true clawing) and the third and fourth lumbricals, the hypothenar muscles and adductor pollicis. However, as the lumbricals cannot be tested they can ignored from the clinical point of view. The

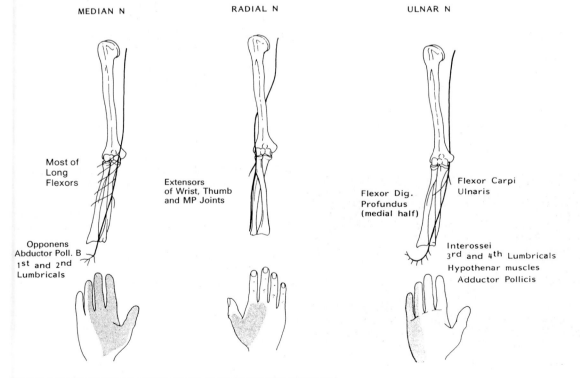

Fig. 18.13 The motor (above) and the sensory (below) innervation of the hand.

easiest muscles to test are abductor digiti minimi, the first dorsal interosseous and adductor pollicis. Weakness of the first dorsal interosseous muscle can be tested by asking the patient to abduct the index finger against resistance (Fig. 18.14(a)). Weakness of adductor pollicis can be tested by asking the patient to grip a newspaper between the extended thumb and the radial side of the clenched fingers. When the adductor is not working, the thumb flexes at the IP joint because the head of the thumb metacarpal cannot be pulled down on to the index finger (Fig. 18.14(b)).

In a patient who presents with sensory symptoms of ulnar distribution but no injury, the first requirement is to identify the level of the lesion. This requires a knowledge of the branching pattern of the nerve and how to test the different muscles it supplies. For example ulnar neuritis arising at the elbow will affect all parts of the ulnar nerve distal to the elbow, including the dorsal cutaneous branch which arises about 5 cm above the wrist and supplies the skin over the back of the little and ring fingers and their metacarpals. Compression of the ulnar nerve at the wrist will not affect the dorsal cutaneous branch which arises more proximally, but will cause weakness of the small muscles. A lesion a little further distal, beyond the nerve which supplies abductor digiti minimi, will spare that muscle but affect the others, so the little finger will tend to stick out sideways. It is thus often possible to localize the level of the lesion without electrical tests; once you know the level you can make a good guess at the pathology.

Median nerve   The median nerve supplies, in the majority of patients, the palm of the hand (Fig. 18.13) and the palmar surfaces of the thumb, index and middle fingers and the radial side of the ring finger.

It also supplies the backs of the fingers to the PIP joints where the radial nerve takes over. However, there is much variation between individuals.

On the motor side, abductor pollicis brevis is almost always supplied wholly by the median nerve. Opponens is usually median but ulnar in 20 per cent of patients. Abductor pollicis brevis should be tested by placing the patient's hand palm upwards on the table with the thumb-nail vertical. The patient then tries to lift the thumb vertically upwards against resistance with the thumb-nail remaining at right-angles to the palm (Fig. 18.15). A long-standing median nerve palsy causes wasting of the thenar eminence.

Radial nerve   A radial nerve lesion causes sensory loss over the back of the hand, mainly over the web of the thumb, and weakness of extension of the wrist (Fig. 18.16), thumb and the MCP joints of the fingers but not the IP joints which are extended by the ulnar-innervated intrinsic muscles.

Autonomic nervous supply   If you stay in a hot bath too long, your fingertips wrinkle up. The mechanism of this is not known but it may be mediated by the sympathetic nervous system. After complete division of a nerve it does not happen. In children and malingerers it is therefore useful to soak the hand in water as hot as the patient can tolerate for 20 or 30 min and then inspect the fingertips immediately after removal from the hot water.

Tendon sheaths

Thickening of the fibrous sheath of the tendons of abductor pollicis longus and extensor pollicis brevis causes a visible and palpable lump over the radial styloid (de Quervain's stenosing tenovaginitis). In

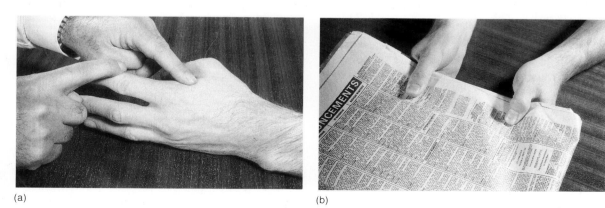

(a)   (b)

Fig. 18.14 (a) Testing the first dorsal interosseous muscle (ulnar nerve). With the fingers and palm flat on the table, the patient attempts to abduct the index finger against resistance. The belly of the muscle should be felt with the fingertip. (b) Testing the normal (patient's right) and paralysed (left) adductor pollicis muscle (ulnar nerve). This is Froment's sign.

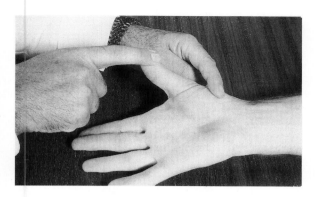

Fig. 18.15 Testing the abductor pollicis brevis (median nerve).

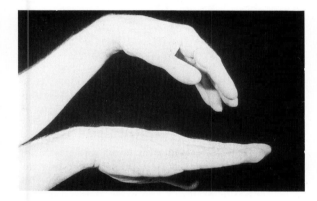

Fig. 18.16 Wrist-drop due to a radial nerve lesion.

trigger finger this is harder to feel, but you can feel the click at the base of the fibrous sheath as the finger snaps back into extension: a phenomenon almost impossible to describe in words but unmistakable once seen.

In rheumatoid disease, thickening of the synovial sheaths of the tendons causes swelling on the back of the wrist and front of the fingers and wrist. It is important to realize that the synovium of tendons is just as likely to be affected as the synovium of joints.

A diagnosis of 'tenosynovitis' should not be made unless there is actual thickening of tenosynovium; to most patients 'tenosynovitis' means that their symptoms have been caused by their work and a law-suit will ensue. If you don't know the cause, it is better to avoid the 'tenosynovitis' label.

Tendons

Any cut on the wrist or hand may divide tendons; if the wound is caused by a long, thin object entering

obliquely, the injury to the tendon may be removed from the cut in the skin. There are 24 tendons crossing the wrist and it may be necessary to test all of them.

Flexor digitorum profundus (FDP), which flexes the DIP joint, crosses the PIP joint and therefore contributes to flexion of that too. To test this tendon, the examiner must hold the PIP joint in extension and ask the patient to flex the DIP joint.

Removing the action of FDP in order to test the flexor digitorum superficialis (FDS) which flexes the PIP joint is more difficult but is possible because, whereas FDS can be regarded as four separate muscles each with its tendon, FDP has a common muscle belly with four tendons and therefore a mass action. If three fingers are held by the examiner in full extension, the profundus muscle cannot contract and any flexion in the free finger is limited to FDS and the PIP joint. This may not work in the little finger where FDS is often congenitally underdeveloped.

If the tendons are in continuity but not working fully, the limitation can be recorded quite simply (though not very accurately) by measuring the distance by which the tip of the actively flexed finger falls short of the transverse palmar creases.

Joints

Each of the relevant joints of the hand must be examined according to the principles outlined in the previous chapter.

Rheumatoid arthritis In this very common disease, the changes in the hands may progressively deteriorate from mild spindling of the PIP joints (Fig. 18.17) to gross, floppy disorganization of the hand with subluxation of the joints and wasting of the small muscles (Fig. 18.18). The disease may be arrested at any stage and does not necessarily deteriorate inexorably. The initial stages of the disease are characterized by pain and stiffness in the MCP and PIP joints. Though the hands are affected early, the DIP joints are seldom involved in RA.

As the disease advances the articular cartilage is destroyed, the bony attachments of the joint capsules become eroded and periarticular tissues become inflamed. In the late stages, inflammation is less marked and the hands may even be painless. Softening and laxity of the joint capsules with uneven pull of the tendons leads to subluxation and deformities, particularly ulnar drift of the fingers.

The fingers in RA may take up a variety of Z-shaped postures, such as 'swan-neck' deformity, i.e. hyperextension of the PIP joint and flexion of the DIP joint (Fig. 18.19(a)). If the central portion of the extensor expansion weakens and ruptures the

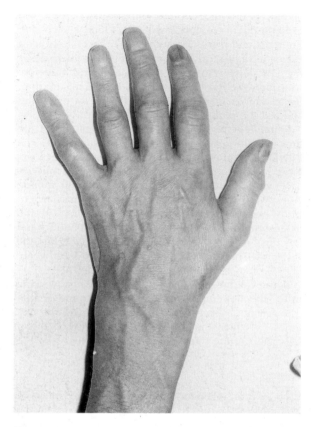

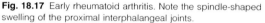

Fig. 18.17 Early rheumatoid arthritis. Note the spindle-shaped swelling of the proximal interphalangeal joints.

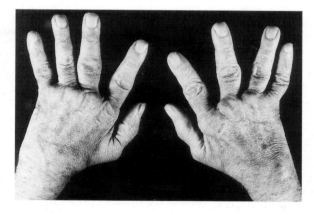

Fig. 18.18 Advanced rheumatoid arthritis. There is subluxation and ulnar deviation of the fingers at the metacarpophalangeal joints.

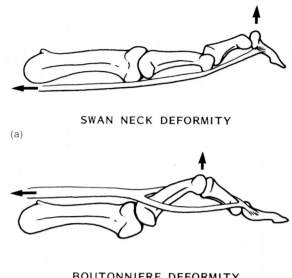

Fig. 18.19 (a) Swan-neck deformity; (b) boutonnière deformity in rheumatoid arthritis.

proximal interphalangeal joint flexes and protrudes through the 'pathological buttonhole' to produce the so-called boutonnière deformity (Fig. 18.19(b)). This is the opposite of the 'swan-neck' deformity. The fingers may deviate towards the ulnar side of the hand (ulnar drift) and the thumb may take up a Z shape (Fig. 18.20).

Psoriatic arthropathy   About 5 per cent of the psoriatic population have arthritis. Of these, the majority have just one or a few scattered joints involved which are in general less severely affected than in RA. This asymmetrical oligoarticular type of arthritis is found in 70 per cent of patients. The DIP joints are sometimes affected in one specific type of psoriatic arthropathy, when adjacent nails may be pitted. In one form of psoriatic arthropathy, arthritis mutilans, there is much bone destruction around joints, which results in shortening of the digits (Fig. 18.21).

Chronic tophaceous gout   Because of energetic treatment with uricosuric agents, tophaceous gout is now rarely seen. However, in untreated patients, deposits of monosodium urate appear around joints, over pressure points, over the elbow (where they may be confused with large rheumatoid nodules) and in the helix of the ear. Gout most commonly attacks the MTP joint of the great toe and with advanced gout, tophi may be seen in the hands (Fig. 18.22).

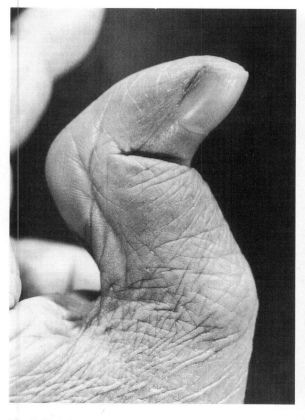

Fig. 18.20 A Z thumb in rheumatoid arthritis.

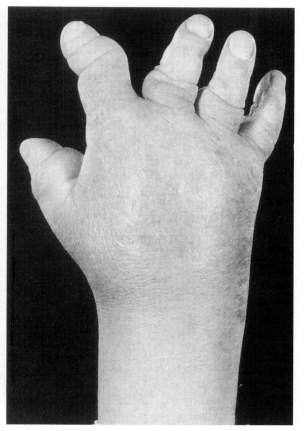

Fig. 18.21 Psoriatic arthropathy (arthritis mutilans).

Heberden's nodes   These commonly cause swellings of the fingers particularly in middle-aged and elderly women. They are really just osteophytes at the DIP joint (Fig. 18.23) and are not usually painful.

Bones

Fractures, bony prominences and congenital abnormalities can be detected clinically but x-rays yield more information about bony lesions.

Function

This is more important in the hand than anywhere else and is often the most instructive part of the examination.

The history may have established, for example, that the patient finds it difficult to pick up a cup. The next question is 'Why is it difficult?' and the easiest way to find out is to get the patient to try to do it in

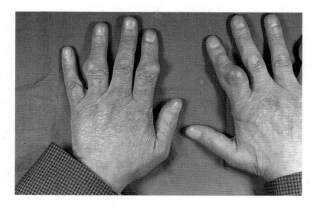

Fig. 18.22 Gouty arthritis of the hands.

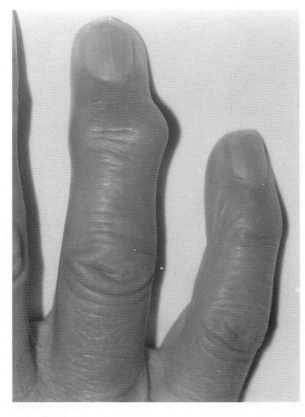

Fig. 18.23 A Heberden's node.

front of you so that you can see exactly what happens. In this example, it may be that there is laxity of the ulnar collateral ligament of the metacarpophalangeal joint of the thumb so that the thumb retreats before the pressure of the index finger instead of pressing against it. (The patient may be able to manage an empty cup: it should have some water in it to simulate normal use.)

It is easy to get a patient to do up buttons and undo them, to write, to pick up coins, paper-clips or pins from a flat surface and to lift some heavy object. All these are readily available in any clinic: in our hand clinic we keep a variety of other objects which have been mentioned by patients, including a kettle, a brick, some knitting and a steering wheel.

The wrist

Between the radius and ulna and the five metacarpals are eight carpal bones: any of these 15 bones may be fractured, most commonly the distal radius and the scaphoid. Between these bones are many small joints, any of which may be affected by arthritis or injury, though certain patterns predominate. Crossing the wrist are 11 flexor tendons (+ palmaris longus) and 12 extensor tendons, any of which may be injured or damaged by rheumatoid disease. Also crossing the wrist are the median nerve (within the carpal tunnel) and the ulnar nerve (outside the carpal tunnel) which may be compressed or cut, plus the terminal sensory branch of the radial nerve.

Thus there is a lot of machinery in a small space and careful clinical examination is necessary to find out exactly where the pathology lies. Increasing understanding of the biomechanics of the wrist is revealing what a complicated area this is and there are now books and courses on the wrist alone.

Symptoms

Pain

Pain is much the commonest complaint. The most important part of the history is to get the patient to localize the pain as precisely as possible. Ask him or her to point with one finger of the other hand to where the pain is felt or, if that is difficult, to where the pain is worst.

If the pain can be well localized, there is a good chance of finding an organic cause which can be cured. If it is diffuse, you are going to have problems.

Swelling

The nature of this will emerge on examination. A complaint of swelling when none can be found poses problems; however, ganglia do come and go.

Stiffness

This is usually due to arthritis or injury, but is surprisingly seldom the thing of which the patient complains. Only about half the full range of wrist movement is used in ordinary life; patients can in fact manage with only a third of the normal range, by adjusting the way they do things. Indeed arthrodesis (complete stiffening) of the painful wrist is an excellent operation with which the patient is usually very pleased.

Clicking

This may be of little significance or great importance — see below.

'Weakness'

This is put in inverted commas because usually the patient means that pain on trying to lift something prevents him from doing so. This may also be described as 'giving way'.

Examination

Look

The deformity of an old malunited Colles' fracture is said to resemble a dinner-fork. Cerebral palsy or a stroke often leads to the wrist being held in flexion, usually with pronation of the forearm.

A round lump is likely to be a ganglion, either on the back of the wrist or on the front under the radial artery. Small dorsal ganglia can only be seen when the wrist is flexed: these do not need treatment. Large ganglia are transilluminant.

A more diffuse swelling on the back of the wrist is usually due to rheumatoid arthritis causing tenosynovitis around the extensor tendons, though indistinguishable appearances may occur in tuberculosis. Tenosynovitis does not occur in the absence of specific diseases such as these; unfortunately this diagnosis is commonly made without a shred of evidence, by doctors too lazy to make a proper diagnosis and apparently too ignorant to know the medicolegal implications.

Medical certificates by doctors alleging 'tenosynovitis' are the source of official statistics according to which 30 per cent of office workers suffer from tenosynovitis. The public believes this impressive-sounding statistic and concludes that tenosynovitis is common and that it is probably the cause of their pain; thus the problem is compounded. If you do not know the cause of the pain, write on the certificate 'pain in arm' or 'pain in wrist', even if the patient believes the trouble to be caused by his work.

True rheumatoid or tuberculous tenosynovitis may also affect the flexor tendons. Here the strong flexor retinaculum prevents the swollen tissues from bulging out visibly in that area, so one sees swelling above the wrist and in the palm (compound palmar ganglion). The swelling within the carpal tunnel, because it cannot expand outwards, increases the pressure to compress the median nerve. Thus true tenosynovitis can cause carpal tunnel syndrome, but in the huge majority of patients with this very common condition the synovium is normal.

Feel

Nowhere is it more important to localize tenderness precisely than in the wrist, for the reasons given above. Feel with one finger, gently but firmly, starting where you don't think it will be tender and working in towards the most painful area.

Every carpal bone except the trapezoid is palpable and so are the joints between them. Most can be felt best from the dorsal side, but the pisiform and the hook of the hamate must be examined from the front. Different parts of the scaphoid can be felt from the back, the front and the radial side (in the 'anatomical snuffbox'), but everybody is tender in the snuffbox if you press hard enough because you are pressing on the terminal sensory branches of the radial nerve. This examination must, therefore, always be done in comparison with the other wrist.

Palpation will also help you to define the extent and margin of lumps.

Move

It is usually adequate to measure extension and flexion (= 'dorsiflexion' and 'palmarflexion') but in some cases one must also assess abduction and adduction (= radial and ulnar deviation). As in other joints, the neutral zero method should be used (Fig. 18.24). In the absence of injury, significant stiffness is usually due to arthritis: rheumatoid arthritis is the most common, but osteoarthritis can affect the wrist after injury and is very common on both sides of the trapezium in women over the age of 50.

Do not forget to put the forearm through a full range of pronation and supination, holding the mid-forearm to ensure you are only moving the radioulnar joints and not the wrist as well.

Carpal instability is a complicated problem, not fully understood; but it is clear that abnormal movements between the carpal bones can occur, especially after ligamentous injuries and can cause symptoms. These may be detected by various provocative tests in which a shearing stress is applied to a particular joint; details of these will be found in books on the wrist.

Listen

Four different sounds have been described as emanating from the wrist:

- a 'catch-up clunk', when ligamentous damage or laxity allows one carpal bone to linger behind its

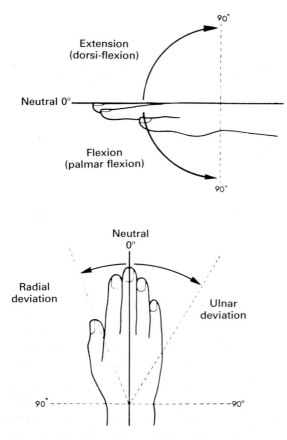

Fig. 18.24 Movements of the wrist. This provides an excellent example of the use of the 'neutral zero' method of recording movements at joints. (Reproduced by permission of the International Federation of Societies for Surgery of the Hand.)

Broadly speaking, the louder and more consistent the sound, the more significant it is, especially if it is painful. Ask the patient to make the movement which causes the sound: that is more likely to be productive than passive movements carried out by the examiner.

Function

If the patient complain˜ of difficulty in a particular activity, ask him to do it in front of you; this may help to reveal the cause of the difficulty. In some cases, it is worth sending the patient away to use the wrist intensively for an hour and then examining him again immediately afterwards. This may produce signs which could not be detected before.

References and further reading

Aids to the examination of the peripheral nervous system. London: Ballière Tindall, 1986.

Barton NJ. Surgery of the arthritic hand. In: Hadfield J, Hobsley M (eds) *Current surgical practice*, Vol 3. London: Edward Arnold, 1981.

Bean WB. Nail growth. *Archives of Internal Medicine.* 1968; **122**: 359−61.

Brown DE, Lichtman DM. Physical examination of the wrist. In: Lichtman DM (ed.) *The wrist and its disorders.* Philadelphia: Saunders, 1988.

Lister G. *The hand: diagnosis and indications*, 2nd edn. Edinburgh: Churchill Livingstone, 1984.

moving neighbours so that it suddenly has to move fast to catch up. This can make a loud noise which may be accompanied by pain and is an important physical sign
- a repeatable snap may be caused by a loose flap of cartilage
- a vacuum click: this low-pitched sound is of no importance and cannot be repeated for 20 minutes
- tendons slipping over a bony prominence may cause a high-pitched click

19

Dealing with diseases related to tropical exposure

G. C. Cook

The clinical history
Physical examination
References and further reading

During the last two decades international travel has increased at a colossal rate. Tourism to countries in the tropics and subtropics is now a frequent and commonplace pursuit for very many thousands of people living in temperate climates, many of whom had not previously left the land of their birth. Businessmen, air crews, diplomats, civil servants, academics, teachers, workers in voluntary service organizations, sportsmen and women, children on school holidays, students on 'electives', missionaries and seamen constitute other groups who are at potential risk regarding diseases which are especially common in tropical countries. Another major category consists of immigrants who are members of ethnic groups in the United Kingdom — mostly from the Indian subcontinent, Africa and the Caribbean — who, as well as frequently being infected with one or more 'tropical' disease when they arrive here, are also in a position to contract an infection (e.g. malaria or schistosomiasis) when returning to the country of their birth for holidays and/or to visit relations. African students who have spent a year or two in the United Kingdom and then return to their country of origin can be at a serious potential risk for malaria because their level of immunity may have declined during their sojourn here.

Modern travel is so rapid that almost any disease known to man can be conveyed from a tropical to a temperate environment in a matter of hours. Therefore, some knowledge of the world distribution of disease (geographical medicine) is essential in the practice of medicine in the United Kingdom in the latter years of the twentieth century. While most communicable and 'tropical' diseases are widely distributed, some (e.g. schistosomiasis, leishmaniasis, filariasis, yellow fever and various rickettsial infections) have their own limited and characteristic geographical areas.

In the United Kingdom undergraduate teaching is usually oriented towards making a single diagnosis; in tropical and subtropical countries many individuals harbour more than one infective agent — viral, bacterial, rickettsial, mycotic, protozoan and/or helminthic — and unless this is appreciated important diagnoses will not be made. In medical practice in a tropical country, the use of an interpreter is often necessary, there being so many foreign languages and local dialects. Local customs must be clearly understood; traditional medicine and its proponents frequently dominate the diagnostic and therapeutic scene.

The clinical history

The precise ethnic origin of the individual under consideration must be ascertained if possible; certain diseases, e.g. haemoglobinopathies, adult hypolactasia, familial Mediterranean fever, etc., have a genetic basis. The sickle cell gene in its heterozygous form is partly protective against *Plasmodium falciparum* malaria. Detailed information regarding geographical factors and countries visited (with precise dates) must be recorded; this applies equally to British travellers, members of the minor ethnic groups in the United Kingdom and indigenous people in or from a tropical or subtropical country. It is also important to establish whether residence has occurred in urban or rural settings; the disease patterns may well be very different.

As much information as possible about previous vaccinations and inoculations should be obtained; Table 19.1 summarizes some of the possibilities. A special effort should be made to acquire accurate information on the precise type and duration of malaria prophylaxis. Table 19.2 summarizes some of the possible chemoprophylactic agents in current use; others possessing foreign trade names, which are not included in this list must be recorded carefully. As with any other clinical history, accurate dates are important (calendar dates should be recorded, and not *x* or *y* days after this or that has happened!). It is important to know about any previous treatment; an antimalarial agent, other antiprotozoan drug or antibiotic might, for example, have altered the classical presentation of malaria, amoebiasis, or typhoid fever.

A good dietary history is essential: fasting by the Muslim pilgrim to Mecca (hypoglycaemia), indulgence in pig feasts in the Papua New Guinea Highlands ('pig bel' disease), or ingestion of raw fish or seafood in Southeast Asia (anisakiasis or gnathostomiasis) might produce crucial 'diagnostic' information.

The presenting features should be recorded as related by the patient (frequently via an interpreter). 'Fever' (and rigors) often dominate the history; Table 19.3 lists some important causes of a febrile illness. Generalized malaise/tiredness is commonly present in schistosomiasis (bilharzia). However, the majority of symptoms are system-related; Table 19.4

Table 19.1. Vaccinations and inoculations which the traveller might (or might not) have received

Vaccine	Recommended frequency of 'booster' (years)
Yellow fever*	10
Cholera	0.5
Typhoid fever	3
Poliomyelitis	10
Tetanus	10
Hepatitis A (HAV)†	0.5
Hepatitis B (HBV)	5
BCG	—
Rabies	1–2
Diphtheria	10
Plague	0.5
Tick-borne encephalitis	1
Japanese B encephalitis	‡
Meningococcal (A and C)	3

* Compulsory for most of 'tropical' Africa and South America.
† Human normal immunoglobulin (HNIG) offers short-term protection (<3 months) against hepatitis A. 'Havrix' has a ten year duration.
‡ Prior to re-exposure, when relevant.

Table 19.2. Some malarial chemoprophylactics which might (or might not) have been taken before, during, or after a journey abroad

Chemoprophylactic agent	Adult dose
Proguanil ('Paludrine')	100–200 mg daily
Chloroquine	300 mg weekly
'Maloprim' (pyrimethamine + dapsone)	1 tab weekly
Proguanil + chloroquine	200 mg daily + 300 mg weekly
'Maloprim' + chloroquine	1 tab weekly + 300 mg weekly
Mefloquine 250 mg weekly	

Table 19.3. Some common causes of 'fever' in a tropical and subtropical context

Viral
  Influenza
  EBV (Epstein–Barr virus)
  CMV (cytomegalovirus)
  Lassa fever and other viral haemorrhagic fevers
  Dengue
  HAV (hepatitis A) infection
  HIV-related disease
Bacterial
  Tuberculosis (pulmonary or extrapulmonary)
  Pneumococcal pneumonia
  Typhoid fever
  Brucellosis
  Leptospirosis
  Legionnaires' disease
  Relapsing fevers
  Plague
  (Pyogenic infections)
Rickettsial
  Coxiella (Q fever)
  Typhus
Protozoan
  Malaria
  Entamoeba histolytica (invasive hepatic disease)
  Kala-azar (visceral leishmaniasis)
  African trypanosomiasis

Table 19.4. Some important communicable and 'tropical' diseases listed under the likely presenting symptom(s)*

Diarrhoea
  Travellers' diarrhoea
  Salmonellosis
  Shigellosis
  Campylobacter jejuni
  Typhoid/paratyphoid
  Yersinia enterocolitica
  Giardiasis
  Cholera
  Entamoeba histolytica
  Schistosomiasis (*S. mansoni* and
    japonicum)
  Postinfective malabsorption (tropical
    sprue)
  Inflammatory bowel disease (usually
    ulcerative colitis)
Diarrhoea and vomiting
  'Food poisoning'
Rash
  Mycotic (fungal) infections
  Typhus (tick)
  Cutaneous leishmaniasis
  African trypanosomiasis
Respiratory
  Pneumococcal pneumonia
  Tuberculosis
  Legionnaires' disease
Headache
  Dengue
  Meningococcal meningitis
  Malaria
  Typhoid
  Tuberculous meningitis
  Trypanosomiasis
Jaundice
  Viral hepatitis
  Epstein–Barr virus (EBV)
  CMV
Sore throat
  EBV
  Diphtheria
  Lassa fever
Haematuria
  Schistosoma haematobium
Pruritus ani
  Threadworm
Tiredness/malaise
  Schistosomiasis
Worm phobias
  Tapeworm
  Ascaris lumbricoides

* For those associated with 'fever', also see Table 19.3.

summarizes some relatively common communicable and 'tropical' diseases arranged under the major presenting symptom. A detailed history should be sought regarding a snakebite, or exposure to a mammal likely to be infected with rabies; identification of the animal is important.

The gastrointestinal tract is often involved in 'tropical' disease; therefore, much can be gained from a detailed history (for this system does not readily yield its secrets simply on clinical examination). Nausea and vomiting might merely result from 'food poisoning', or if accompanied by 'cramps' could possibly suggest sodium deficiency resulting from heat exhaustion. Haematemesis (or melaena) could complicate peptic ulceration, but yellow fever or another haemorrhagic fever, or hepatosplenic schistosomiasis (with portal hypertension), should be included in the list of differential diagnoses. Abdominal pain must be carefully assessed; while a sickle-cell (SS) crisis might be responsible, amoebic liver 'abscess' (sometimes associated with right shoulder-tip pain), or splenic enlargement (or infarct) in *P. falciparum* infection or SS disease should also be considered. Diarrhoea is an important presenting feature; Table 19.5 summarizes some characteristic features of different types of diarrhoea. The location of the infection within the gastrointestinal tract can often be delineated reasonably accurately from a careful history. A clinical diagnosis of liver disease may be difficult because cutaneous signs are often impossible to detect in a black or brown skin (see below); however, a history of 'yellow eyes' might suggest this.

In pulmonary tuberculosis, a history of respiratory symptoms associated with night sweats and weight loss may be present (Chapter 4). Legionnaires' disease should perhaps be suspected if the patient has recently stayed at an hotel with a cooling system, suspect or otherwise.

Acute rheumatic fever may present commonly in a tropical country with classical symptoms, including a 'flitting' arthropathy (Chapter 17); a high index of suspicion for bacterial endocarditis is also required and the cause might be an unusual organism, e.g. *Coxiella*.

Meningitis and meningoencephalitis are common in tropical countries; in the latter case a careful history from a friend or relation might be crucial in arriving at a correct diagnosis.

Bloody urine (especially at the end of micturition) often suggests a *Schistosoma haematobium* infection; 'blackwater fever' or acute haemolysis from another cause can often be diagnosed from the history.

Suspicion of a sexually transmitted disorder might

Table 19.5. Characteristic features of small intestinal and colo-rectal diarrhoea

Stool appearance	Faecal microscopy	Causes
High, volume, watery (secretory) (small intestinal)	(*Vibrio cholerae*)	*Vibrio cholerae* *Campylobacter jejuni* Salmonellae *E. coli* (enterotoxigenic) *Clostridium perfringens* *Staphylococcus aureus* (*Plasmodium falciparum*) Hypolactasia
Large, bulky, fatty (malabsorption) (small intestinal)	Fat globules	Tropical sprue *Giardia lamblia* *Strongyloides stercoralis* Other non-infective causes
Small, bloody, with mucus and pus (invasive) (colo-recta)	Pus cells, red blood cells	Shigellae *Yersinia enterocolitica* *Clostridium difficile* *Campylobacter jejuni* Enteroinvasive *E. coli* *Entamoeba histolytica* Inflammatory bowel disease

also originate from the history; HIV (1 and 2) infection and the acquired immune deficiency syndrome (AIDS) has reached epidemic proportions in Africa and Asia, the importance of careful questioning of members of both indigenous and expatriate populations about sexual practices, and past and recent activity must be re-emphasized (see Chapter 21).

Psychiatric histories are nearly always difficult to obtain in developing tropical countries. Generalized 'weakness', unusual feelings of 'hotness' and 'coldness', and parasthesiae (which may take various forms) are common presenting symptoms. Sexual incapacity, including impotence, is also a common symptom and an organic cause is usually absent. The psychiatric manifestations of AIDS are becoming increasingly important in Africa and Asia. Worm phobias — of parasites emerging from any orifice and/or through the skin — are common in expatriate travellers, especially women, to the tropics; extensive investigation is usually necessary, but ultimately yields negative results in most cases.

Physical examination

General physical condition

In the general examination of a patient in the tropics

certain features require more concentrated attention than is usual in a temperate country. Overall nutritional status should be assessed; the end result is often similar whether the cause is primary, secondary (to various infections, including tuberculosis (Fig. 2.8)), or a consequence of malabsorption. Associated vitamin deficiencies should also be sought. Anaemia, frequently of a hypochromic, iron-deficiency type is common, particularly with hookworm disease. Jaundice is an important sign, which only manifests itself in the conjunctivae of individuals with black or brown skins; it may be haemolytic (in, for example, a *P. falciparum* infection), hepatocellular (in various forms of hepatitis, cirrhosis and hepatoma), or of mixed type (in, for example, the jaundice associated with systemic bacterial infection). Painless enlargement of the parotid glands is often present in severe malnutrition (kwashiorkor) and the chronic calcific pancreatitis syndrome — a frequent cause of malabsorption in Africa and other tropical areas.

Fever

The temperature chart warrants especially careful attention. Some causes of 'fever' are listed in Table 19.3; in some (e.g. tuberculosis, typhoid and malaria) the chart may give a valuable clue to the aetiological factor(s) involved (Fig. 19.1). In malaria, especially

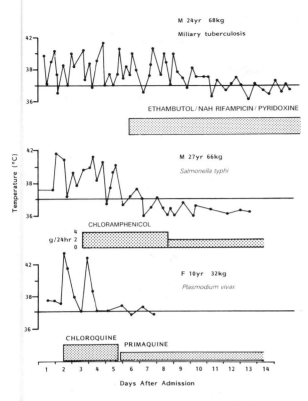

M 24yr 68kg

Miliary tuberculosis

ETHAMBUTOL / NAH RIFAMPICIN / PYRIDOXINE

M 27yr 66kg

Salmonella typhi

CHLORAMPHENICOL

F 10yr 32kg

Plasmodium vivax

CHLOROQUINE

PRIMAQUINE

Days After Admission

Fig. 19.1 Temperature charts in patients suffering from (a) pulmonary tuberculosis; (b) Typhoid (*Salmonella typhi*) fever; (c) *Plasmodium vivax* malaria.

that caused by *P. falciparum*, a 'classical' chart with sharp peaks every 48 h is unusual; it is therefore important not to regard a 'tertiary' or 'quartan' peak as a consistent finding, otherwise the correct diagnosis may not be made.

The skin

Many cutaneous lesions, e.g. erythematous and macular rashes (e.g. in measles), cutaneous stigmata of hepatocellular dysfunction (including 'spider naevi') and 'rose spots' (in typhoid fever), are difficult or impossible to visualize in people with black or brown skins. Furthermore, excessive humidity and underhydration can make diagnosis difficult. Pruritus, followed by intense scratching and secondary infection, can also mask an underlying lesion, e.g. scabies (*Sarcoptes scabei* var. *hominis*).

Table 19.6 lists some communicable and 'tropical' diseases arranged under common dermatological

manifestations. Several helminthic infections can produce characteristic dermatological signs.

Larva migrans (Fig. 19.3), larva currens, dracontiasis, and loaiasis (raised erythematous lesions sometimes outlining subcutaneous worms) are some examples. Transient oedematous swellings (loaiasis, gnathostomiasis and trichiniasis), and chronic lymphoedema (*Wuchereria bancrofti* and *Brugia malayi* (Fig. 19.8)) are other manifestations. Tumbu fly (*Cordylobia anthropophagus*) infection is often followed by secondary furunculosis.

Drug-induced reactions, e.g. those associated with antituberculous and antileprosy chemotherapy, are common. 'Temperate' dermatological conditions, e.g. pityriasis, erythema nodosum and erythema multiforme also occur in tropical countries.

Gastrointestinal tract

Special attention should be given to examination of the mouth which is one of the two accessible segments of the gastrointestinal tract. Dry lips may result from climatic factors or from dehydration. Fissures at the stomal angles often result from vitamin B deficiency. A 'magenta' tongue may be a feature of pellagra; in severe tropical sprue (postinfective malabsorption) the tongue is often smooth (with loss of papillae) and aphthous ulcers may be present. Koplik's spots are diagnostic of measles, a very common viral infection in many parts of the tropics, notably west Africa, especially in childhood.

Abdominal palpation is frequently far easier in tropical compared with temperate countries, because a high percentage of individuals are under-, rather

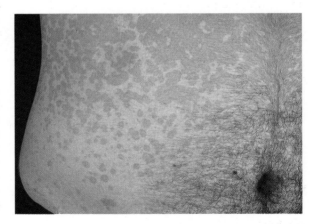

Fig. 19.2 Tinea versicolor — this is a common skin eruption seen in Europeans working in the tropics.

Table 19.6. Dermatological manifestations of some communicable and 'tropical' diseases

Macular
Rickettsial infections
Leprosy
Pinta
Tinea versicolor (Fig. 19.2)
Onchocerciasis (river blindness)

Papular
Secondary syphilis
Leprosy
Larva migrans (Fig. 19.3)
Larva currens
Onchocerciasis
Scabies
Flea bites
Tungiasis
Myiasis
Kaposi's sarcoma (AIDS) (see Fig. 21.3(a) and (b))

Maculopapular
Measles
Rickettsial infections

Vesicular
Chickenpox
Monkeypox
Herpes simplex and zoster

Pustules
Herpes simplex and zoster
Pyoderma
Paracoccidioidomycosis

Crust (scab)
Impetigo
Anthrax
Tick typhus ('eschar') (Fig. 19.4)
African trypanosomiasis (chancre)

Circinate erythema
Erythema multiforme
African trypanosomiasis

Ulcers
Tropical ulcer
Cancrum oris
Primary syphilis
Leprosy
Buruli ulcer
Sporotrichosis
Cutaneous leishmaniasis (oriental sore) (Fig. 19.5)

Urticaria/wheal
Acute schistosomiasis (Katayama fever)
'Allergies'

Petechiae/ecchymosis
Viral haemorrhagic fevers
Meningococcal bacteraemia

Scaly dermatitis
Pellagra (exposed surfaces) (Fig. 19.6)
Onchocerciasis

Depigmented patches
Leprosy (Fig. 19.7)
Yaws
Post-Kala-azar dermal leishmaniasis

Nodules
Yaws
Leprosy
Chromomycosis
Sporotrichosis
Maduromycosis
Onchocerciasis
Paracoccidioidomycosis
Myiasis
Kaposi's sarcoma (AIDS) (see Fig. 21.3(a) and (b))

than overweight. Colonic carcinoma is very unusual in most developing countries and a palpable colon or colonic 'mass' is far more likely to result from amoebic (amoeboma) or schistosomal colitis (sometimes complicated by polyposis, most commonly in Egypt and Sudan). An ileocaecal mass and/or enlarged mesenteric lymph glands often result from tuberculosis, an underdiagnosed cause of gastrointestinal disease in most tropical countries. Ascites is frequently secondary to intra-abdominal tuberculosis; however, it might also accompany portal hypertension com-

plicating macronodular cirrhosis, hepatoma or hepatosplenic schistosomiasis (Fig. 19.9).

Hepatomegaly (with or without splenomegaly) is found in a high proportion of communicable and 'tropical' diseases. Table 19.7 summarizes some diseases associated with hepatomegaly. Splenomegaly may be present either alone or in combination with hepatomegaly; Table 19.8 summarizes some of the aetiological agents involved.

A renal mass is most likely to result from a hydronephrosis complicating a *S. haematobium* infection,

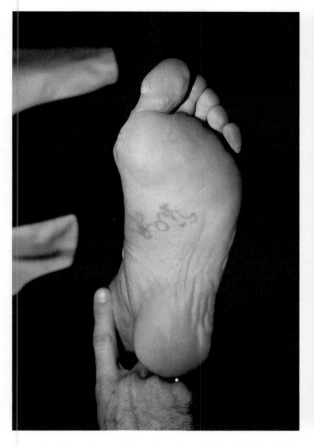

Fig. 19.3 Larva migrans of the sole — the result of walking barefoot on the beach during a Caribbean holiday.

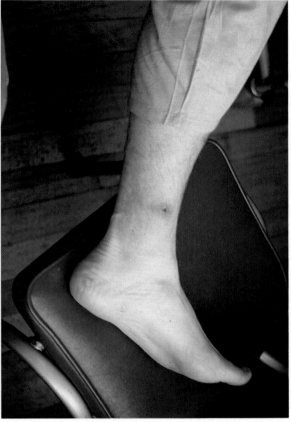

Fig. 19.4 Characteristic 'eschar' occurring at the site of a tick bite in a young man suffering from tick-typhus contracted in an East African game park.

hydatid involvement of the kidney, or tuberculosis. A nephrotic syndrome associated with *P. malariae* infection (Fig. 19.14) is a further possibility.

Rectal prolapse is occasionally caused by *Trichuris trichiura*, especially in children. Proctoscopic and sigmoidoscopic examinations are important clinical investigations in shigellosis, amoebic colitis, schistosomal colitis, pseudomembranous colitis, and inflammatory bowel disease.

Cardiovascular disease

The examination of this system has been described in Chapter 3. Although chronic rheumatic cardiac disease is now relatively unusual in the United Kingdom it is commonly seen in the developing countries of the 'Third World' following acute rheumatic fever. The signs of mitral and aortic valve damage, as a feature of chronic rheumatic heart disease, are therefore frequently encountered.

A disproportionately rapid tachycardia in relation to body temperature may result from African trypanosomiasis and Chagas' disease (South American trypanosomiasis) when myocarditis is present. A disproportionate bradycardia in a febrile patient suggests yellow fever or typhoid (enteric) fever. Other causes of myocarditis are leptospirosis, trichinosis (trichiniasis) and toxoplasmosis. In addition to rheumatic fever, pericarditis may be present in yellow fever, typhus, amoebiasis (where it is associated with an especially poor prognosis), and African trypanosomiasis.

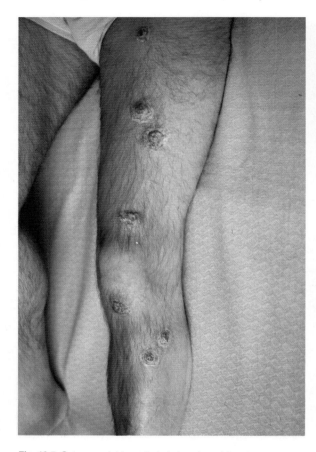

Fig. 19.5 Cutaneous leishmaniasis (oriental sore) in a young man who had contracted the disease in Saudi Arabia.

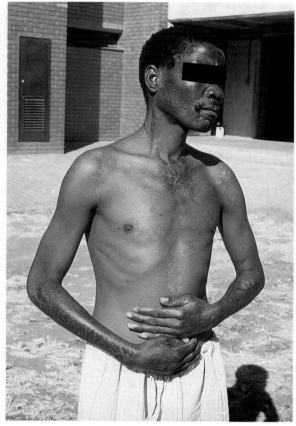

Fig. 19.6 Casal's necklace; scaly rash on the exposed parts in a Zambian man suffering from pellagra (tryptophan—niacin deficiency).

Cardiac failure is a common sequel to chronic rheumatic cardiac disease, cardiomyopathies of varying aetiologies and endomyocardial fibrosis (EMF) (especially in Africa). The severe anaemia of hookworm disease is a further common cause. Schistosomiasis (usually caused by *S. mansoni* and complicated by cor pulmonale), Chagas' disease, hydatidosis and nutritional deficiencies (including kwashiorkor and beriberi) are other causes which are encountered in tropical countries.

Respiratory system

The detailed examination of this system is covered in Chapter 4 but certain features are of especial importance in the tropics. Finger and toe clubbing are relatively common physical signs often resulting from long-standing bronchiectasis (Fig. 19.12).

Although now less common in temperate countries, classical lobar pneumonia (usually resulting from a *Streptococcus pneumoniae* infection) remains a major cause of morbidity and mortality in developing countries; bronchiectasis is usually a sequel to inadequately treated disease. Pulmonary tuberculosis, which is also now an unusual infection in temperate countries, still causes much morbidity and mortality in subtropical and tropical areas; florid physical signs are frequently present.

During migration through the lungs, several nematodes, including *Ascaris lumbricoides*, *Strongyloides stercoralis*, and *Toxocara canis*, can cause bronchospasm and patchy radiological changes in

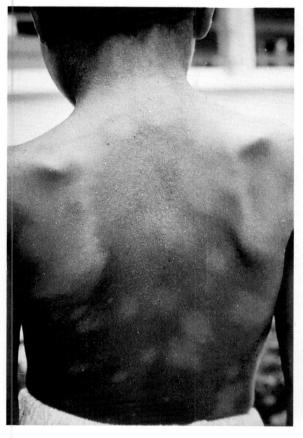

Fig. 19.7 Depigmented anaesthetic patches in tuberculoid leprosy. The patient was from Papua New Guinea.

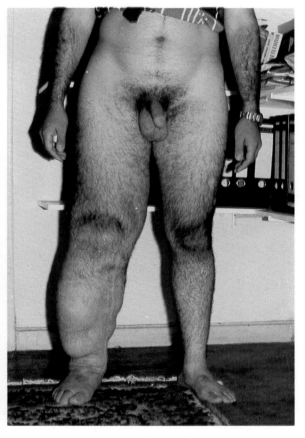

Fig. 19.8 Unilateral elephantiasis (lymphoedema) in an Egyptian man with 'burnt-out' lymphatic filariasis.

the pulmonary parenchyma (Löffler's syndrome). In acute schistosomiasis (Katayama fever), similar pulmonary involvement, which is most common with *Schistosoma japonicum* and *S. mansoni* infection, occurs some 4–6 weeks after the initial infection. In southern India and Sri Lanka, tropical pulmonary eosinophilia (TPE) occasionally results from a filarial infection. Although a high peripheral eosinophilia is usually present, filariae are frequently absent in peripheral blood films.

Acute pulmonary oedema may be a consequence of a *P. falciparum* infection; frequently (but not always) this is a corollary to overhydration by the intravenous route.

Several other parasitic diseases can also present with chronic pulmonary disease. In hepatic amoe-

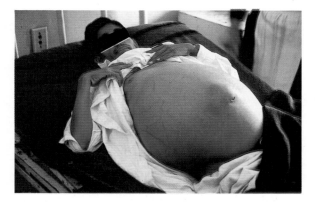

Fig. 19.9 Gross ascites in a young Egyptian man suffering from hepatosplenic schistosomiasis with portal hypertension.

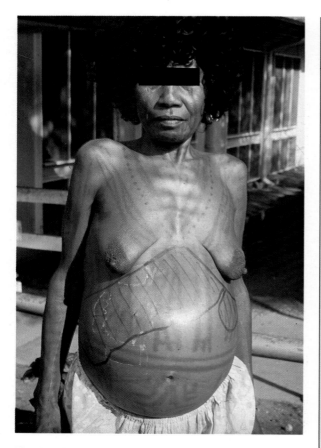

Fig. 19.10 Papua New Guinean woman with gross hepatosplenomegaly and ascites caused by hepatocellular carcinoma associated with chronic HBV infection.

Table 19.7. Some causes of hepatomegaly (with or without splenomegaly) in communicable and 'tropical' disease

Tender
'Hepatitis' (viral, EBV, CMV, etc.)
Jaundice associated with systemic bacterial infection
Malaria
Amoebic liver 'abscess' (invasive amoebiasis)
Brucellosis
Leptospirosis
Relapsing fever
Migratory helminthiases (e.g. ascariasis and *Toxocara canis* infection)
Yellow fever
South American trypanosomiasis (Chagas' disease)
Veno-occlusive disease (VOD)
Sickle-cell disease and thalassaemia
Beriberi

Non-tender
Cirrhosis
Hepatocellular carcinoma (hepatoma) (Fig. 19.10)
Schistosomiasis
Haemosiderosis (Bantu siderosis)
Bartonellosis
Plague
African trypanosomiasis
Kala-azar
Hydatid disease
Clonorchiasis/opisthorchiasis
Fascioliasis
Malnutrition (kwashiorkor)

Table 19.8. Some causes of splenomegaly (with or without hepatomegaly) in communicable and 'tropical' disease

Tender
Malaria (acute)
Typhoid
Brucellosis
Relapsing fever
Bartonellosis
Typhus
Trypanosomiasis (African and South American)

Non-tender
Malaria (chronic, endemic)
Tropical splenomegaly syndrome (Fig. 19.11(a))
Schistosomiasis with portal hypertension
Leptospirosis
Kala-azar (visceral leishmaniasis (Fig. 19.11(b))
Hydatidosis
Sickle-cell disease and thalassaemia

biasis, signs in the right lower chest are often present; an age-old clinical axiom states that pathology in the right lower lung in an individual who has experienced tropical exposure should always be considered to result from invasive hepatic amoebiasis until that diagnosis is positively disproved. Pulmonary paragonimiasis can present with apical cavitation, chronic cough and haemoptysis which can easily be confused with pulmonary tuberculosis. Multiple hydatid cysts can also give rise to significant pulmonary symptoms and signs.

Central nervous system

Signs and symptoms resulting from meningitis and

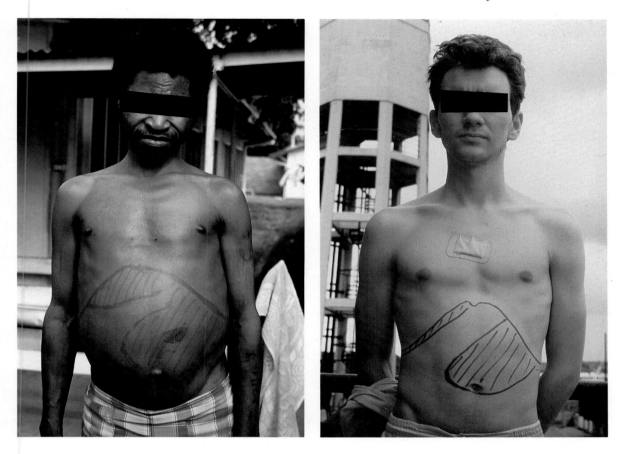

Fig. 19.11 Gross splenomegaly in (a) a young Papua New Guinean man suffering from the tropical splenomegaly syndrome (TSS); (b) an Englishman with visceral leishmaniasis (kala-azar) acquired in Malta.

encephalitis are important in the practice of clinical medicine in developing countries; Table 19.9 summarizes some relevant aetiological agents. Bacterial meningitis is common and the causes similar to those in the Western world. With many of the other forms of meningitis and encephalitis a knowledge of the local epidemiology is crucial. The high prevalence of HIV infection in Central Africa and Asia influences the pattern of disease seen there.

Fits, delirium, and coma are important neurological events in developing countries; Table 19.10 summarizes some of the infective causes. Differentiation of space-occupying lesions is frequently difficult because computerized tomography (CT) scanning is a rare luxury in undeveloped countries; a trial of antituberculous chemotherapy is often justified if a tuberculoma is suspected. Do not forget that patients in tropical and subtropical regions may

also have non-infective causes for fits and coma (see Table 8.10).

Cord lesions and transverse myelitis are relatively common. Many viruses, including HTLV-I, can be involved in spastic paresis and *S. mansoni* can produce a transverse myelitis. Pott's disease of the vertebral column is usually suspected from the corresponding skeletal deformity (kyphosis).

Peripheral nerve lesions are common. 'Burning feet' may result from pellagra. Thiamine deficiency can, in addition to wrist and foot drop, give rise to wasting of the lower extremities. In leprosy (Hansen's disease), there may be thickening of subcutaneous nerves, especially the ulnar, posterior tibial, external popliteal and greater auricular. Anaesthesia, paralysis, trophic changes and neuropathic skin, bones and joints are also long-term complications of this disease.

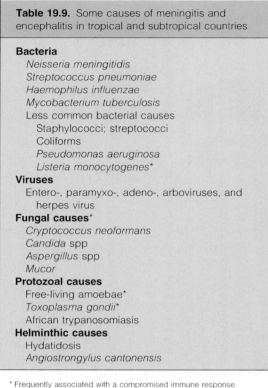

Table 19.9. Some causes of meningitis and encephalitis in tropical and subtropical countries

Bacteria
  Neisseria meningitidis
  Streptococcus pneumoniae
  Haemophilus influenzae
  Mycobacterium tuberculosis
  Less common bacterial causes
    Staphylococci; streptococci
    Coliforms
    Pseudomonas aeruginosa
    *Listeria monocytogenes**
Viruses
  Entero-, paramyxo-, adeno-, arboviruses, and
    herpes virus
Fungal causes*
  Cryptococcus neoformans
  Candida spp
  Aspergillus spp
  Mucor
Protozoal causes
  Free-living amoebae*
  *Toxoplasma gondii**
  African trypanosomiasis
Helminthic causes
  Hydatidosis
  Angiostrongylus cantonensis

* Frequently associated with a compromised immune response.

Table 19.10. Some infective causes of fits, delirium and coma in tropical and subtropical countries

Plasmodium falciparum
  Cerebral malaria
Other parasitic causes
  Cysticercosis (*Taenia solium*)
  Hydatidosis
  African trypanosomiasis
  Toxoplasma gondii (especially in AIDS)
  Schistosoma japonicum
Bacterial causes
  Tuberculoma (see also Table 19.9)
Viral causes
  Japanese B encephalitis
  Other viral encephalitides
  (Kuru)

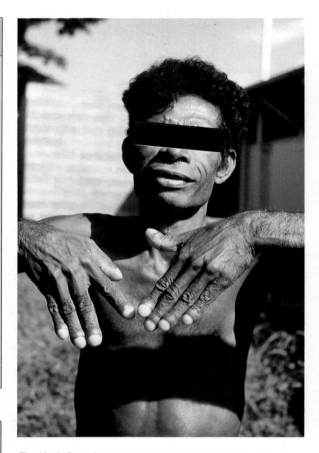

Fig. 19.12 Gross finger clubbing in a young Papua New Guinean man suffering from bilateral bronchiectasis which had complicated a severe chest infection in childhood.

Ophthalmic examination

Ophthalmic problems are common in tropical countries; careful examination of the eyes is therefore imperative. Vitamin A deficiency may be accompanied by xerophthalmia, keratomalacia, corneal perforation and subsequent blindness. Photophobia associated with vascularization of the sclera can follow riboflavin deficiency. Trachoma, caused by *Chlamydia trachomatis*, often presents with small, pale follicles in the palpebral conjunctivae of the upper lids and is a major cause of blindness throughout the tropics. Subconjunctival haemorrhages can occur in leptospirosis and the viral haemorrhagic fevers. In leprosy, the eyebrows and eyelashes may be scanty or absent, but more importantly in acute exacerbations of lepromatous disease there is hypersensitivity within the uveal tract, inability to close the eyes, and subsequent corneal ulceration and blindness.

Several parasitic infections also produce eye signs: African trypanosomiasis and Chagas' disease can produce unilateral palpebral and facial oedema and

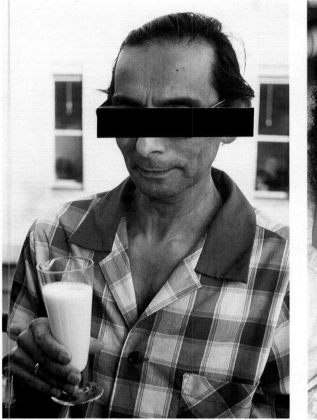

Fig. 19.13 Chyluria in a Sri Lankan man with 'burnt-out' lymphatic filariasis.

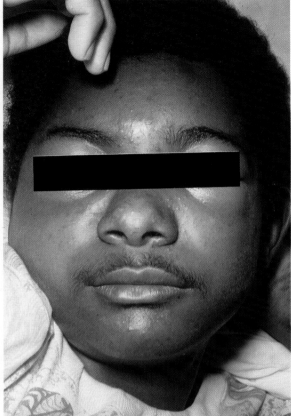

Fig. 19.14 Severe nephrotic syndrome in a Ugandan boy; the disease was caused by a chronic *Plasmodium malariae* infection.

in loaiasis conjunctival irritation occurs when the adult worm crosses the conjunctiva. Onchocerciasis (river blindness) causes 'snow-flake' opacities, sclerosing keratitis and blindness. Toxocariasis rarely causes choroidoretinitis, with subsequent blindness, usually in children; retinoblastoma is an important differential diagnosis.

Genitourinary examination

Frank haematuria (classically towards the end of micturition) is a sign of *S. haematobium* infection; this may be associated with dysuria, cystitis (with bladder changes) and subsequently hydroureter and hydronephrosis. In severe haemolysis during a heavy *P. falciparum* infection, haemoglobinuria may be of such a degree that very dark or even black urine is produced ('blackwater fever'). In lymphatic filariasis, chyluria (Fig. 19.13) occasionally results from involvement of the bladder and ureteric lymphatic vessels; the milky urine, especially that produced after a fatty meal, contains a high density of chylomicrons.

Renal failure has multiple causes. Poststreptococcal glomerulonephritis is common throughout the developing countries especially in children. Oliguria, anuria and tubular necrosis can all result from *P. falciparum* malaria. *P. malariae* infection can give rise to a nephrotic syndrome, especially in African children (Fig. 19.14).

Table 19.11. Some sexually transmitted diseases occurring predominantly in tropical and subtropical areas

Disease	Major abnormalities, including those involving the external genitalia	Region
HIV	Acquired immune deficiency syndrome (AIDS); Kaposi's sarcoma; opportunistic infections	Central Africa and Asia; rapidly spreading to other areas
Chancroid (*Haemophilus ducreyi*)	Anogenital ulceration Painful inguinal glands	SE Asia Africa Central America
Lymphogranuloma venereum (*Chlamydia trachomatis*)	Endocervicitis, destructive genital lesions, painful inguinal glands	Asia Africa S America
Granuloma inguinale (*Calymmatobacterium granulomatis*)	Destructive genital lesions; carcinoma	Papua New Guinea India

Renal and ureteric stones are occasionally encountered in medical practice in tropical countries, especially in expatriates whose fluid intake is frequently suboptimal.

Thorough examination of the external genitalia is essential. Sexually transmitted diseases in tropical and subtropical countries are common, as indeed they are in the Western world (see Chapter 20). Those that are seen predominantly, though not exclusively, in tropical and subtropical areas are listed in Table 19.11.

References and further reading

Cook GC. *Tropical gastroenterology*. Oxford: Oxford University Press, 1980.

Cook GC. *Communicable and tropical diseases*. London: Heinemann, 1988.

Cook GC. Parasitic disease in clinical practice. Berlin, London: Springer-Verlag, 1990.

Dawood R. (ed.) *Travellers' health*, 3rd edn. Oxford: Oxford University Press, 1992.

Harries JR, Harries AD, Cook GC. *100 Clinical problems in tropical medicine*. London: Baillière Tindall, 1987.

Walker E, Williams G, Raeside F. *ABC of healthy travel*, 4th edn. London: British Medical Association, 1993.

20

The symptoms and signs of genitourinary disease

C. Bignell

> Symptoms
> Examination
> Disseminated manifestations of sexually transmitted infection
> References and further reading

Sexually acquired infections are common and are not confined to the promiscuous or to sexually active young adults, but may occur at any age and be acquired by 'the respectable'. Neonates may contract infections intrapartum from their mothers and sexually transmitted infection in a child may be the consequence of sex abuse.

Symptoms

Patients with sexually acquired infections commonly present with genital symptoms to their general practitioners or directly to a genitourinary department. The most frequent symptoms are urethral discharge and/or dysuria in men, vaginal discharge and/or vulval irritation in women, or a genital rash. The manifestations of sexually transmitted infections are not confined to the genital tract and the initial presentation of an infection may, for example, be a painful arthropathy of sudden onset, a generalized rash, or a neurological deficit. Asymptomatic infection is not uncommon, particularly in women, and there is a need to dispel the commonly held myth that 'feeling-well' equates with absence of infection. Many asymptomatic patients attend genitourinary departments because a sexual partner has been found to have an infection, or for screening for infection when uncertain about the well-being of a recent partner. The management of such patients centres on examination, microbiological testing and the nature of the partner's infection.

It is not uncommon for more than one genital infection to be present concurrently and it is essential to perform a full examination and comprehensive range of genital tests on all patients, even though one infection might be apparent and responsible for the symptoms. Approximately 50 per cent of women with cervical gonorrhoea have concurrent cervical infection with *Chlamydia trachomatis*, and routine antimicrobial therapy for gonorrhoea is usually inadequate to treat this second infection.

More than 25 per cent of patients with genital warts have other sexually acquired infections, notably gonorrhoea, infection with *C. trachomatis*, nongonococcal urethritis or trichomoniasis; it is clearly inappropriate management just to inspect and treat the warts without full screening for other infections.

Sexually acquired infections must have been acquired from someone and may have been passed on to another. An essential aspect of the management of sexually acquired infections is the eliciting of a history of recent sexual relationships and initiating contact-tracing measures where appropriate and feasible. It is futile to treat, for example, a man with gonorrhoea and for him to then sleep with an untreated partner who may have been the source or recipient of his infection. Serious complications of infection, such as infertility, may be prevented by prompt contact-tracing.

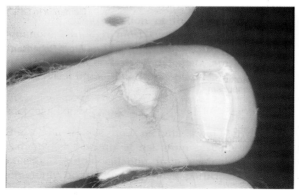

Fig. 20.7 A typical pustular lesion on the toe of a young woman with disseminated gonorrhoea.

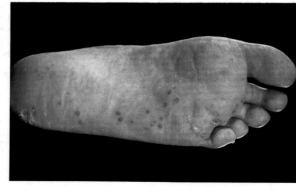

Fig. 20.9 The sole in keratodermia blenorrhagica. The appearances may be confused with psoriasis.

affects the feet and hands and resembles psoriasis (Fig. 20.9). The arthropathy invariably persists for more than a month and distal joints are most commonly affected, notably the knees, ankles and feet. Iritis and cardiac involvement, causing pericarditis, conduction defects and aortic incompetence, occur very rarely.

References and further reading

Adler MW. *ABC of sexually transmitted diseases*, 2nd edn. London: British Medical Association, 1990.

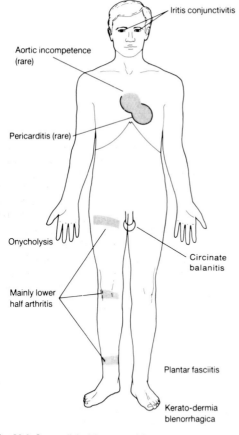

Iritis conjunctivitis

Aortic incompetence (rare)

Pericarditis (rare)

Onycholysis

Circinate balanitis

Mainly lower half arthritis

Plantar fasciitis

Kerato-dermia blenorrhagica

Fig. 20.8 Some clinical features of Reiter's syndrome.

21

Human immunodeficiency virus (HIV) infection and AIDS

C. Bignell

Introduction
Clinical history
Natural history of HIV infection
Definition of AIDS
Diagnosis
HIV counselling
Prognosis
Further reading

Introduction

HIV infection and AIDS have been surrounded with mystique since their clinical recognition as a new disease in 1981. They have challenged health-care workers to re-examine many working practices, particularly highlighting the importance of communication with patients and having regard for the social, psychological and legal consequences of diagnosing a chronic, incurable disease. Sadly the challenge and new demands made by HIV disease have deterred some doctors from discussing this infection with patients or becoming involved in the care of infected individuals. HIV-related disease encompasses a wide spectrum of clinical presentations, may involve multiple body systems and invariably presents the clinician with a challenge in clinical management. Much general medicine can be learnt by becoming involved with HIV-infected individuals, who are usually young, articulate and well-informed about the disease.

HIV infection has attained pandemic proportions, with more than ten million individuals estimated to be infected worldwide. It has become a significant cause of morbidity and mortality in young adults, particularly men, and infection in children is increasing. It is predominantly acquired through penetrative sexual intercourse. Parenteral transmission (notably injecting drugs and transfusion of blood products) and vertical transmission from mother to child account for the remaining infections. In the United Kingdom, 9290 cases of AIDS have been reported from 1982 to May 1994 and there have been 21 718 reports of HIV infection from 1984 to March 1994. Of the reported AIDS cases, 6283 (68 per cent) are known to have died. Reported figures underestimate the true prevalence of HIV infection, which is not increasing in Northern Europe as fast as was once feared. Most young people and adults are aware of HIV and well-informed about how it is acquired.

Clinical history

Although many individuals with HIV infection are asymptomatic, a significant proportion of those presenting for health care with AIDS or symptomatic disease have had no prior test for HIV infection and are unaware they are infected. In the United Kingdom, HIV infection is closely linked to risky sexual behaviour such as male homosexual penetrative sexual intercourse, heterosexual intercourse with an overseas partner or partner with other known risk-factors for HIV, injecting drug use and treatment with infected blood products. These categories are not exclusive and the epidemiology of HIV infection has seen dramatic changes outside Northern Europe, with an increasing proportion of cases acquired heterosexually.

The sensitive eliciting of a patient's sexual and illicit drug-taking history should be part of routine clinical history-taking, especially in younger adult patients. It should be approached in a way that does not make the patient feel uncomfortable or oneself feel embarrassed and at a level relevant to the clinical problem at hand. Privacy and confidentiality are of crucial importance when asking questions about personal sexuality and curtains around a bed in an open ward rarely afford a satisfactory environment. Use of treatment rooms or side-rooms is to be encouraged. Additionally, it is inappropriate either to make detailed notes of a sexual history in front of the patient or to enter a detailed account of the history in the hospital case-notes unless of direct relevance to the diagnosis and management of the presenting clinical problem.

Recent sexual lifestyle surveys show that most sexually active adults in the United Kingdom are in monogomous relationships and have not had very many previous sexual partners, if any. Direct questions 'out of the blue' about personal sexuality are likely to be greeted with the response: 'Is that relevant, doctor?'. The topic needs introducing. If the patient has a clinical presentation where HIV infection is a realistic differential diagnosis, it may be appropriate to approach the topic directly: 'Your present illness could be the result of infection. One possible infection is HIV. Do you think you have ever put yourself at risk of getting this infection?'. In other situations, sexual history-taking requires a more general introduction, perhaps along the lines: 'This may not be directly relevant to your present problem, but some illnesses relate to infection picked up through sexual intercourse. May I ask if you have a partner/boyfriend/girlfriend? . . . and do you have sex?'. Questioning can usually be quickly but gently steered to elicit the duration of the relationship, whether contraception is used, past sexually acquired infection and whether any partner has been from abroad. If the patient is married, the sentence introducing the topic of sexual activity can be followed with something like: 'I notice you are married. How long have you been together with your wife/husband? . . . One question we routinely ask, and I hope you won't be offended by my asking it, is

whether you have had sex with anyone else during that time?'. If the marriage relationship is of short duration, it would be appropriate to ask about sexual relationships before marriage.

Sexual orientation is often apparent or sensed as the conversation progresses. If one feels in any doubt or one senses homosexual contacts may have occurred but not been explicitly mentioned, it is in order to ask a direct question, such as: 'May I ask if you have ever had sex with another man?'. If the man is homosexual or bisexual, it does not necessarily mean that he has been at risk for HIV infection. A follow-up question to the acknowledgement of gay sex might be: 'Have you ever had risky sex and put yourself at risk of HIV infection?'. If the response is 'No', it is sometimes appropriate to clarify the issue by asking: 'Have you ever had penetrative sex with another man?'. Any identified risk can be assessed by a few further questions, including an enquiry as to whether the patient has ever had an HIV antibody test.

Natural history of HIV infection

Infection with HIV is a necessary precondition for someone to develop AIDS. Acquisition of HIV is followed by a period of unchecked viral replication before a vigorous immune response is mounted. An acute illness may occur at the time of seroconversion, usually within six weeks of infection. The symptoms of the seroconversion illness often take the form of a glandular fever-like illness, with fever, malaise, lethargy, myalgia, arthralgia, lymphadenopathy and sore throat. A self-limiting aseptic meningoencephalitic-like illness has also been described. The non-specific nature of the seroconversion illness related to HIV infection results in many such episodes passing unrecognized. Seroconversion is followed by a dramatic reduction in viraemia and an asymptomatic phase of long duration. Viral replication has been shown to continue in lymphoid tissue during this phase, which may be accompanied by generalized lymphadenopathy. Immune dysfunction is demonstrable but absolute immunodeficiency has yet to develop. Dermatological problems may occur (Table 21.1) or be exacerbated during this phase and thrombocytopenia can develop.

Those infected with HIV show progressive immune impairment centred on the destruction of CD4+T lymphocytes over a period of years. The clinical illnesses of HIV infection reflect the loss of the immune-modulating role of CD4+T lymphocytes with the host becoming increasingly vulnerable to opportun-

Table 21.1. Common skin problems in HIV disease

Seborrhoeic eczema
Tinea — cruris and pedis
Candidiasis — perianal and vaginal
Herpes simplex virus infection — genital, perianal, oral
Herpes varicella zoster
Bacterial folliculitis

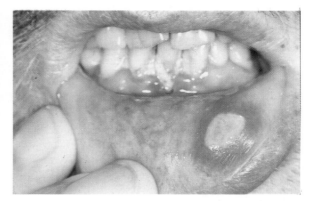

Fig. 21.1 Oral ulcer and gum disease in HIV infection.

istic pathogens and reactivation of dormant infection acquired earlier in life. Quantification of CD4+T lymphocytes in the peripheral blood is used as an imperfect monitor of disease progression, offering a useful guide to when life-threatening infection may occur. HIV-infected individuals are usually very aware of the implications of CD4+T lymphocyte counts and are keen to know their own results. Significant opportunistic infection is related to CD4+T lymphocyte counts (Table 21.2).

Table 21.2. Common opportunistic infections in relation to CD4+T lymphocyte count

CD4+T lymphocyte count ($\times 10^6$/l)	Opportunistic infection
200–500	Candidiasis *Mycobacterium tuberculosis*
<200	*Pneumocystis carinii* pneumonia Cerebral toxoplasmosis Cryptococcal meningitis Cryptosporidial enteritis
<100	*Mycobacterium avium* complex Cytomegalovirus infection

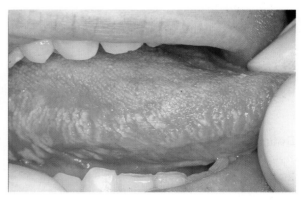

Fig. 21.2 Oral hairy leukoplakia.

As immune deficiency develops, infected individuals commonly develop mucous membrane problems in the mouth (Fig. 21.1), skin problems (Table 21.1), constitutional symptoms (lethargy, weight loss, fever and night sweats) and non-infective diarrhoea. Some clinical signs at this stage of disease are diagnostic or strongly suggestive of HIV infection, notably oral hairy leukoplakia (Fig. 21.2). Progressive immune deficiency results in the increasing likelihood of clinical disease and AIDS developing. Serious disease is usually manifest in the lung, central nervous system, gut or constitutionally. Disease is generally attributable to opportunistic infection, malignancy (Kaposi's sarcoma and lymphomas) and the direct effects of HIV. The more common disease presentations are shown in Table 21.3. The relative frequency of the different clinical presentations of AIDS is changing with the introduction of widespread use of prophylaxis against certain opportunistic infections, notably *Pneumocystis carinii* pneumonia.

Kaposi's sarcoma is a malignant tumour that appears to arise from vascular endothelium. Lesions are usually multiple, often appear before the development of serious opportunistic infection and can involve both cutaneous and internal sites (Fig. 21.3(a) and (b)). On the skin, the appearance is of red or purplish-blue areas of discoloration which progress into raised nodules and plaques. Kaposi's sarcoma is seen in approximately 20 per cent of homosexual men with AIDS and is exceedingly rare in other patients with HIV infection. The incidence of Kaposi's sarcoma appears to be declining.

Table 21.3. Major clinical presentations in late-stage HIV infection

System	Clinical features	Common pathogens/cause
Pulmonary	Increasing dyspnoea Dry cough Fever	*Pneumocystis carinii* pneumonia Mycobacterial pneumonia *Strep. pneumoniae* *Haem. influenzae*
GI tract	Painful swallowing High-volume diarrhoea Abdominal pain/bloody diarrhoea	Candidal oesophagitis Cryptosporidial enteritis Microsporidial enteritis Cytomegalovirus colitis
Central nervous system	Dementia Meningitis Focal signs Fits	HIV encephalitis — direct effect *Cryptococcus neoformans* *Toxoplasma gondii* — intracerebral abscesses Primary cerebral lymphoma
Constitutional	Persistent fever Weight loss Debilitating fatigue Anorexia Anaemia	Disseminated infection, particularly *Mycobacterium avium* Lymphoma HIV wasting Drug toxicity

Definition of AIDS

In the United Kingdom, an individual with HIV infection is defined as having AIDS when he or she develops one of the 24 or so internationally agreed indicator diseases associated with profound cellular immune deficiency. The definition of AIDS has undergone a number of revisions since 1982 to reflect an increasing appreciation of the diversity of HIV disease. In the United States, an expanded definition of AIDS was introduced in 1993 and now includes all individuals seropositive for HIV and who have a CD4+T lymphocyte count below 200/µl. By this definition, an infected individual could have AIDS and still be asymptomatic. This revised definition has not been adopted in Europe, where AIDS remains defined by clinical indicator diseases.

Diagnosis

Diagnosis of HIV infection is based on HIV antibody tests. Antibodies usually develop within two months of infection, although longer intervals to seroconversion have occasionally been reported, and they persist for life. Screening tests are based on enzyme-linked immunosorbant assay (ELISA) technology and most modern tests detect both subtypes of HIV. Positive results generally undergo confirmatory testing by alternative methodology. These tests will not detect very early infection and exclusion of infection requires consideration of recent risk exposures in addition to serological tests.

Testing for HIV should only be performed with the explicit informed consent of the patient. A structured discussion, termed pre-test counselling, is undertaken to ensure the patient is aware of the meaning and implications of a positive test result and to enable them to make an informed decision whether to be tested or not. Pre-test counselling also provides an opportunity for a patient to consider what support might be required in the event of a positive result, to review the ways they may have put themselves at risk of infection and to consider strategies to protect their health and that of others in the future.

HIV counselling

Counselling is an important aspect of comprehensive patient management, whatever condition afflicts a patient. It has become well developed in the management of those infected with HIV and for uninfected

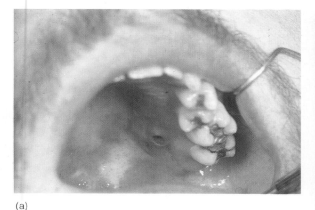

(a)

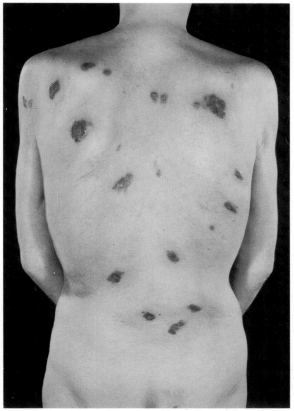

(b)

Fig. 21.3 (a) Oral Kaposi's sarcoma; (b) cutaneous Kaposi's in a homosexual man.

individuals with concerns about this infection. HIV counselling involves much more than giving information and advice and is exercised at a number of levels of complexity. It is a skilled process which provides emotional and psychological support, encouraging patients to live more fully and satisfyingly in the face of an incurable condition, uncertainty, reduced life-expectancy and possible rejection. Vulnerability to rejection is perhaps the major difference faced by patients with HIV infection compared with other fatal illnesses.

Prognosis

The outcome of HIV infection is usually defined in terms of the development of significant clinical disease, the development of an AIDS-defining condition and death. Less than 5 per cent of adults infected with HIV-1 develop AIDS within three years of infection. However, 10–11 years after infection approxi-

mately 50 per cent of adults will have progressed to AIDS and a further 25–30 per cent will have symptomatic disease. Median survival after the onset of AIDS is currently about two years, with survival depending on the indicator condition occurring. Some predictions suggest that all infected with HIV will eventually develop symptomatic disease, but this has yet to be observed in practice. Figure 21.4 shows the time-course of HIV infection.

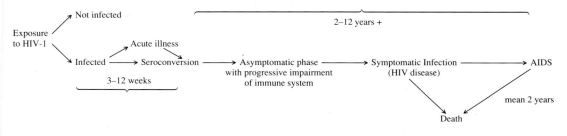

Fig. 21.4 Schematic representation of the time-course of HIV-1 infection.

Further reading

Adler MW (ed.) *ABC of AIDS*, 2nd edn. London: British Medical Association, 1991.

Bor R, Miller R, Johnson M. A testing time for doctors: counselling patients before an HIV test. *British Medical Journal*. 1991; **303**: 905–7.

Mindel A. (ed.) *AIDS: a pocket book of diagnosis and management*. London: Edward Arnold, 1990.

22

The eye as a diagnostic indicator of systemic disease

N. R. Galloway

Eye signs without instruments

Eye signs with basic instruments

Ophthalmoscopic signs of systemic disease

Generalized infections manifesting themselves
  ophthalmoscopically

Drugs affecting the eyesight

References and further reading

Apart from being the sensory organ of vision, the eye is an important site for early signs of disease elsewhere in the body. This is because one can make a direct examination of nerve tissue and blood vessels in and around the eye. A knowledge of the appearance of the normal eye and its variations is needed if diagnostic errors are to be avoided. Before making a diagnosis of systemic disease from eye signs it is often important to exclude disease limited to the eye itself. For example, before considering the intracranial causes of optic atrophy one must exclude chronic glaucoma or before embarking on invasive investigations of an unusual defect in the visual field, one must exclude the possibility of a retinal detachment.

Many sophisticated and ingenious instruments are now part of the ophthalmologist's armamentarium but it is still possible for the non-specialist to make useful observations without instruments apart from the ophthalmoscope. In this chapter the types of systemic diseases that manifest themselves in the eye are considered from the point of view of the non-specialist.

Eye signs without instruments

Changes in the eyelids

Swelling of the eyelids may simply be the result of oedema occurring overnight in a middle-aged person without obvious systemic upset but it can accompany both hypo- and hyperthyroidism (see Fig. 12.6(a)) as well as being a feature of renal disease, heart failure or superior vena caval obstruction. Acute swelling of the eyelids can result from a systemic hypersensitivity reaction, for example after an injection of penicillin, or from a local reaction after handling certain plants and rubbing the skin of the eyelids. Firm, chronic swelling of the eyelids is a rare complication of sarcoidosis or lymphoma. Xanthelasma (see Fig. 6.21) is a common, yellowish deposit seen in the elderly usually affecting the skin of the medial part of the eyelids. In some patients it may be a manifestation of hypercholesterolaemia. A peculiar kind of lid swelling resembling the appearance after over-exposure to the sun, is sometimes seen in patients with dermatomyositis; it is known as 'heliotrope eyelids'. Atopic eczema and psoriasis of the eyelids are not uncommon but need no further mention being part of the more evident generalized disease.

The commonest infection to cause acute lid swelling

is staphylococcal infection of a lash follicle (a stye) or a meibomian gland. Herpes zoster should always be kept in mind, especially if there has been a preceding headache, but the development of the rash usually accompanies or precedes the swelling. Although herpes zoster is a unilateral condition, bilateral lid swelling may occur and cause considerable anxiety if both eyes become closed (see Fig. 2.2). A rare but potentially serious cause of bilateral lid swelling, with inflammation, is erysipelas.

A capillary haemangioma of the eyelids and side of the face known as the 'port-wine stain' may be part of the Sturge–Weber syndrome. Such individuals should have their intraocular pressure checked to detect glaucoma as well as investigations for meningeal involvement (see Fig. 8.20).

Inspection of the eyelids may show proptosis or forward protusion of the globe. There are many causes of proptosis (Table 22.1), hyperthyroidism being a common one, but symptomless proptosis should alert one for the possibility of an orbital neoplasm. Sometimes one eye is larger than the other giving the false impression of proptosis. The larger eye is myopic and thus the diagnosis of an abnormally large eye can be made by refraction (measurement for spectacles). Exophthalmos also means forward protusion of the eyes but the term is usually restricted to the appearance seen in ophthalmic Graves' disease (Fig. 22.1(a) and (b)).

The simplest way to assess proptosis is to stand behind the seated patient and to look down to compare the position of the globes from above.

Table 22.1. Causes of proptosis

Basic disorder	Features
Muscle palsy	About 1 or 2 mm of proptosis accompanies palsies of the extraocular muscles
Thyrotoxicosis	This is the commonest cause of unilateral or bilateral proptosis; the other eye signs should be noted
Infection	Orbital cellulitis usually from neighbouring sinuses requires urgent otorhinological investigation
Trauma	Proptosis can occur as a result of retro-orbital haemorrhage
Tumour	Haemangioma is the commonest primary neoplasm of the orbit but other tumours such as meningiomas may occur (Fig. 22.1(b))
Pseudotumour	A localized, chronic, inflammatory swelling of unknown cause which responds to systemic steroids but tends to recur
Mucocele of sinuses	Diagnosed by x-ray
Lymphomatous tumour	
Pseudoproptosis	An apparent forward displacement due to enlargement of the globe or sometimes posterior displacement or shrinkage of the other eye

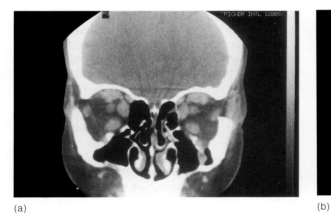

(a)

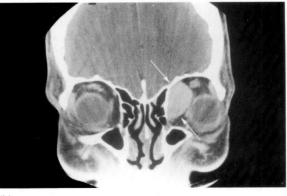

(b)

Fig. 22.1 (a) CT scan of the orbit showing enlargement of the extraocular muscles in ophthalmic Graves' disease. (b) Protrusion of the globe by an orbital neurofibroma (arrowed).

This simple method avoids errors due to abnormal widening of the palpebral aperture. One must remember that not only does the palpebral aperture become narrower with age but the position of the lids becomes lower in relation to the globe. More accurate measurements of protrusion of the globe can be recorded using appropriate instruments (Fig. 22.2).

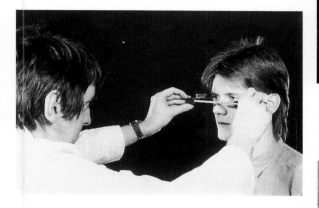

Fig. 22.2 The use of exophthalmometry to assess patients with ophthalmic Graves' disease.

Swellings of the lachrymal glands and lachrymal sac (Table 22.2)

Unilateral swelling of a lachrymal gland may rarely be seen with tumours such as carcinomas or lymphomas. Bilateral swelling is not uncommon as with Sjögren's syndrome, lymphoma, chronic lymphatic leukaemia or sarcoidosis (Fig. 22.3). Dacrocystitis or inflammation of the lachrymal sac causes a red tender swelling below the inner canthus (Fig. 22.4).

Table 22.2.	Swellings of lachrymal glands
Unilateral	Tumours such as carcinomas or lymphomas
Bilateral	Sarcoidosis
	Sjögren's syndrome
	Lymphoma ⎫
	Chronic lymphatic leukaemia ⎭ rare

Changes in the conjunctiva and sclera

The 'white' of the eye undergoes interesting microscopic changes in disease but for the physician colour change can be of vital importance. It must be

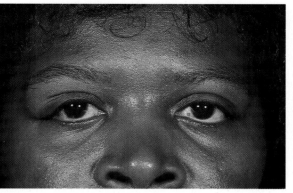

Fig. 22.3 Enlargement of the lachrymal glands in sarcoidosis. This disease often runs a more aggressive course in Afro-Caribbean patients.

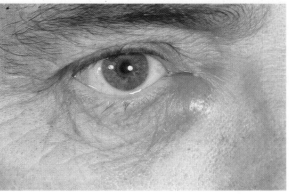

Fig. 22.4 Dacrocystitis. Inflammation of the lachrymal sac is not unusual in chronic lymphatic leukaemia as was the case with this patient.

remembered that the appearance of the 'white' of the eye is not only dependent on the colour of the sclera but also on changes in the overlying bulbar conjunctiva (that is the conjunctiva over the globe of the eye as opposed to the palpebral conjunctiva which lines the eyelids).

The conjunctiva

Examination of the palpebral conjunctiva of the lower lid by pulling the lid gently down with the finger can give some indication of anaemia. Jaundice, even when slight, may be evident as yellowing of the bulbar conjunctiva and of the sclera. When the conjunctiva is oedematous, the thickened, glistening membrane can bulge slightly at the lid margin giving the impression that the eyes are brimming with tears (chemosis). This 'tear that never drops' is seen in thyrotoxicosis and in other oedematous states such as congestive heart failure. There are also a number of local causes, for example, it may be seen after glaucoma surgery.

The red eye in systemic diseases

Subconjunctival haemorrhage   Apparent spontaneous leakage of blood subconjunctivally is a common cause of a sudden 'red eye'; usually the individual is otherwise healthy. Recurrent subconjunctival haemorrhages may make one suspect diabetes mellitus or blood dyscrasia. Vomiting, strangulation, or extreme respiratory effort may cause subconjunctival haemorrhages (Fig. 22.5).

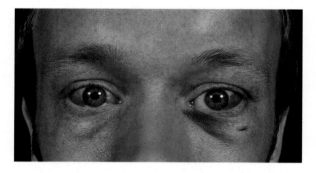

Fig. 22.5 Bilateral subconjunctival haemorrhages in a patient who had had an episode of cardiorespiratory arrest.

Episcleritis   This term refers to an inflammation of the connective tissue underlying the conjunctiva. It tends to be more painful than conjunctivitis and there is no purulent discharge. Episcleritis may be an important sign of rheumatoid arthritis. It is seen in certain other acquired diseases of joints and connective tissue, in particular Reiter's syndrome. Less commonly the sclera may be involved in a similar inflammatory process known as scleritis. This tends to be more painful and in severe cases may lead to necrosis of the sclera. After healing the thin areas of sclera appear bluish-black.

Associated with skin disease   Atopic eczema may be associated with disease of the skin of the eyelids and occasional involvement of the eye itself. The patient may present with a red eye when allergic conjunctivitis is a main feature. The eyelids become thickened and the lashes disappear after years of recurrent irritation and scaling of the skin. Atopic individuals show an increased tendency to develop cataracts and also a less common condition affecting

the cornea known as keratoconus or conical cornea.

Acne rosacea of the eyelids and cornea is nearly always associated with the typical changes on the cheeks. The main features are erythema, pustule formation, telangiectasia and rhinophyma. Recurrent blepharitis and meibomian cysts are found and tongues of vascularized scarring encroach on the cornea.

Stevens—Johnson syndrome is a rare severe form of erythema multiforme (see Fig. 5.12). The eruption on the skin is accompanied by conjunctivitis which may lead to the formation of adhesions between lids and globe. The cornea becomes opaque, dried and keratinized.

Keratoconjunctivitis   Patients with chronic rheumatoid arthritis may complain of recurrent soreness and redness of the eyes due to keratoconjunctivitis sicca. The secretion of tears is reduced and slit-lamp microscopy is needed to confirm the diagnosis. Schirmer's test of tear flow may also be helpful. When the eyelids fail to close properly during blinking or sleep the conjunctiva and cornea may be inflamed often with chronic discharge (exposure keratoconjunctivitis). This is typically seen in patients with thyrotoxic eye disease or with seventh cranial nerve palsies.

Telangiectasia   More permanent redness of the conjunctiva is seen in some rare conditions associated with telangiectasia. Examples are hereditary haemorrhagic telangiectasia (Osler—Weber—Rendu syndrome) (see Fig. 5.4), where there are similar lesions in the skin and mucous membrane, and ataxia telangiectasia. The latter is an autosomal recessive disorder involving the central nervous system, skin and lymphoreticular system as well as the eye. Cerebellar ataxia and deficiency of IgA are important features.

Other associations   Patients with polycythaemia occasionally present with red eyes. Chronic alcoholics have red eyes due to dilatation of the conjunctival vessels and similar changes are seen in patients with renal failure. Some patients with migraine, particularly migrainous neuralgia, develop a red eye on the affected side at the time of the attack.

The red eye may therefore be a useful indicator of systemic disease but never forget the possibility of intraocular causes of red eyes, for example glaucoma and iridocyclitis. These may lead to blindness unless treated promptly.

Blue sclera

The normal white of the eye takes on a bluish hue if the sclera is thin allowing the underlying dark pigment to show through. This appearance is seen under the upper lid more than in the exposed areas in patients with rheumatoid arthritis who have suffered recurrent scleritis. It is seen sometimes in the Ehlers–Danlos syndrome, a generalized inherited disorder of connective tissue showing hyperelasticity of the skin and hypermobility of the joints. Blueness of the sclera is also a feature of fragilitas ossium or brittle-bone disease, the rare condition which may lead to the mistaken impression of non-accidental injury to children.

Brown sclera and conjunctiva

Diffuse, flat, brown pigmentation may be due to precancerous melanosis of the conjunctiva. In fact this type of pigmentation may be observed for many years without evidence of malignancy. Ochronosis is an exceptionally rare disorder of the metabolism of homogentisic acid. A brown-black pigment derived from homogentisic acid is deposited in the tissues including the cornea and sclera.

Extraocular muscle weakness

Eye movements can simply be tested by asking the patient to follow a light or the tip of a pencil into the cardinal positions of gaze. One eye may appear to be off-line and the eyes may fail to be directed together to the point of regard (i.e. a squint) but this does not necessarily indicate any muscle weakness. In fact most cases of childhood squint show a full range of eye movements and are due to a failure of co-ordination between convergence and accommodation.

When a patient presents with a squint due to defective eye movements then a more serious under-

lying cause must be suspected. Sometimes the eye movements may be restricted by a congenital musculofascial anomaly and this may give the erroneous impression of a cranial nerve palsy. More detailed ophthalmological examination can distinguish the true nerve palsy. Squint occurring suddenly in adult life may occasionally be due to the breakdown of a long-standing muscle-balance problem but it is more likely to be due to a cranial nerve palsy and demands urgent investigation. Such squints of sudden onset are accompanied by diplopia. If the diplopia becomes worse during the day or when tired then myasthenia gravis may be the underlying cause especially if accompanied by ptosis (see Fig. 8.10). Systemic causes of acquired weakness of eye muscles are shown in Table 22.3. The distinction between the various causes usually depends upon more extensive ophthalmological and neurological investigation (see Chapter 8) but a carefully taken history can go far towards realizing the true situation.

Nystagmus (see also Chapters 8 and 23)

Simple testing of the eye movements will reveal the presence of nystagmus if this was not evident on first seeing the patient. As a rule of thumb, nystagmus of an irregular roving type, rotary or horizontal, present in all positions of gaze, without the subjective sensation of movement is congenital in type. Further ophthalmological examination is required to elucidate any associated ocular abnormality.

Nystagmus on lateral gaze may indicate muscle weakness but unsustained nystagmus in extremes of gaze may be seen in otherwise normal individuals. Persistent nystagmus on lateral gaze is always a suspicious sign especially if there are other signs and symptoms of demyelinating disease or other neurological signs of intracranial disease.

Ptosis

Drooping of one or both eyelids (ptosis) is commonly congenital but acquired ptosis is often an important sign of systemic disease. The main causes are summarized in Table 22.4. Damage to the sympathetic supply rarely causes more than slight drooping of the eyelid since only the Müllers muscle is involved.

Pupillary changes

An abnormal pupil reaction is perhaps the most important of all systemic signs in the eye (Fig. 22.6). The normal pupil reaction is present at birth but the small pupils in early infancy make testing difficult.

Table 22.3. Limitation of eye movements (systemic causes)

Muscle disorder
 Thyrotoxic eye disease (ophthalmoplegia — see Fig. 12.6(c))
 Myasthenia gravis — see Fig. 8.10
 Trauma
Nerve lesions
 Vascular — hypertension, diabetes
 Intracranial space-occupying lesion
 Raised intraocular pressure (especially III or VIth — see Figs 8.7 and 8.8)
 Trauma
 Demyelinating disease

Table 22.4. Causes of ptosis

Mechanical ptosis	Inflammation, tumour, redundant skin
Myogenic ptosis	Myasthenia gravis, some myopathies
Neurogenic ptosis	Sympathetic (Horner's syndrome), IIIrd nerve palsy, any lesion in the pathway of these nerves
Drugs	Guanethidine eye-drops
Congenital	
Pseudoptosis	Small eye, atrophic eye, lid retraction on other side

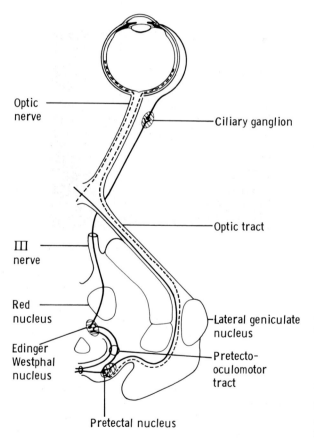

Fig. 22.6 The pupillary reflex pathways. The afferent fibres for the pupillary light reflexes run in the optic nerve and the optic tracts. The fibres then leave the tracts to synapse in the pretectal nucleus where the second neurone fibres arise; these then link with the ipsilateral and contralateral Edinger–Westphal nuclei. The pupilloconstrictor fibres (parasympathetic) arise in the Edinger–Westphal nucleus and pass in the third nerve to the ciliary ganglion.

Older children have larger pupils and the size then diminishes slowly into old age. The pupils dilate with excitement and constrict during sleep or general anaesthesia. Patients being treated for glaucoma with pilocarpine eye-drops have small pupils as do morphine addicts.

When testing the pupils the initial size and any irregularity should be noted. Unequality of the pupils is sometimes called anisocoria. The reaction to direct light and consensual stimulation should also be observed as well as the reaction to accommodation. The pupil reaction gives an important measure of conduction in the optic nerve. A unilateral afferent defect is best detected by swinging the light from normal to affected eye. The pupils will dilate as the light is moved from normal to abnormal eye. This is sometimes called the 'swinging flashlight test'. Since the direct pupil reaction is a response to light rather than one to formed images, it is unimpaired by opaque media in the eye. Localized retinal damage may not impair the pupil reaction but more severe macular disease may do so. Optic nerve damage on the other hand may cause an afferent pupillary defect out of proportion to the loss of vision. It is an important sign in the diagnosis of optic neuritis.

The non-reactive pupil

When a pupil fails to react it is important to test it in the dark; the small pupils of elderly patients may appear to be non-reactive to the naked eye when tested in daylight. The pupils of diabetic patients may be small and show little reaction owing to autonomic degeneration. Patients who have suffered chronic iridocyclitis may have adhesions between iris and lens which prevent the normal movement of the iris. The same may apply in patients who have undergone cataract surgery. The non-reactive pupil may be too large or too small and these situations can be considered separately.

The abnormally dilated pupil

The commonest reason for unilateral mydriasis is drugs in the form of locally administered eye-drops. A less common cause is the Holmes–Adie syndrome, a condition which is most common in young women. The affected pupil is usually dilated and contracts very slowly in response to direct and indirect stimulation. In bright light the pupil may be constricted on the affected side and take up to half an hour to dilate in the dark. This tonic-pupil reaction may be combined with absent tendon-jerks in the limbs. After a delay of months or years the other eye may become affected. The overall disability is minimal and the condition is not related to any other systemic disease.

Acute, narrow-angle glaucoma can occasionally present as a dilated pupil without very much pain in the eye; confusion may arise if the eye is not red. Close examination should make the diagnosis obvious.

Since the nerve fibres which cause constriction of the pupil are conveyed in the oculomotor nerve, oculomotor palsy if complete is associated with mydriasis. For this reason dilatation of the pupil may be a sign of raised intracranial pressure after head injury.

Occasionally one pupil may be larger than the other as a congenital abnormality but both usually react briskly under these circumstances.

The abnormally constricted pupil

Again drugs are a common cause. Miotic drops are still used for the treatment of chronic, simple glaucoma though they are now largely replaced by β-blockers.

When a constricted pupil on one side is observed it is important to note the position of the eyelids. A slight degree of ptosis indicates the possibility of Horner's syndrome. The total syndrome comprises miosis, narrowing of the palpebral fissure owing to paralysis of the smooth muscle in the eyelids, loss of sweating over the affected side of the forehead and a slight reduction of the intraocular pressure. Horner's syndrome may be caused by a wide diversity of lesions anywhere along the sympathetic pathway but quite often it is noted in the elderly as an isolated finding and investigation fails to reveal a cause.

The Argyll–Robertson pupil is a very rare but well-known example of the small pupil which responds to accommodation but not to direct light. This type of pupil reaction was originally described as being due to neurosyphilis but now is much more frequently seen in diabetics.

Iris colour

The normal iris may vary in colour from blue or green to brown and the exact pattern of pigmentation is a subtle facial characteristic. At birth the iris has a slate-grey colour achieving its adult colour after about six months.

Certain disease states can alter the iris colour. Intraocular haemorrhage can give the iris a green tinge and siderosis resulting from a retained intra-ocular foreign body may turn the iris brown. A severely ischaemic eye as seen occasionally in diabetics or following a retinal vein occlusion, may show a pinkish-coloured iris due to the spread of fine new vessels across its anterior surface (rubeosis iridis). Albino subjects have blue eyes but the irides can be shown to transilluminate by shining a torch along the line of view through the pupil.

In Down's syndrome a series of pigmented white nodules are usually seen arranged around the iris. They are known as Brushfield's spots but are not specific for Down's syndrome being seen occasionally in normal subjects. Patients with Von Reckling-hausen's disease (neurofibromatosis) show a number of brown, neurofibromatous nodules on the iris known as Lisch nodules (Fig. 22.7).

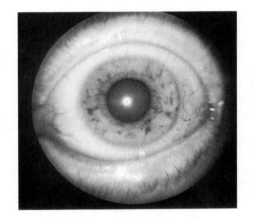

Fig. 22.7 Lisch nodules. These are sometimes helpful in the diagnosis of neurofibromatosis.

Eye signs with basic instruments

Visual acuity measurement

This simple and basic test of vision is sometimes overlooked by the non-specialist and yet eye signs can be crudely classified into serious or non-serious depending on whether or not they are linked with normal visual acuity. Furthermore, the patient's reports of visual status may be proved to be quite erroneous once the visual acuity has been tested.

A series of different sized letters are presented at six metres on a chart. Under each letter is usually printed a small number indicating the distance in metres at which the letter would be just visible to a normal-sighted person. Thus the big letter at the top should be seen at 60 metres by a normally sighted person. If the patient can only just see the top letter at six metres the visual acuity is said to be 6/60. Normal subjects have a visual acuity of 6/6 or often 6/5 or 6/4. It is obviously important to quantify a patient's visual symptoms in this way but when systemic disease threatens the eyesight it may have caused considerable damage to the peripheral field of vision before the visual acuity is affected. This is because the physiological process of seeing fine detail such as small letters on a chart or reading a book is performed by the central 5° representing a small but vitally important area of retina at the fovea. Extensive damage to the peripheral retina may go unnoticed by the patient.

Visual field testing

The simplest method of visual field testing is by confrontation (see Chapter 8). The patient is instructed to cover one eye with a hand and the observer also covers one eye so that the patient's field can be compared with that of the observer. The patient is then asked to say 'Yes' if he can see fine movements of the observer's fingers. The test can be made more accurate by using a pin with a red head on it as a target. By convention the target is moved from non-seeing to seeing parts of the field. However, none of the confrontation methods can match the accuracy of formal perimetry. A number of specialized instruments of varying complexity are available. Using such equipment the patient is presented with a number of different-sized targets in different parts of the visual field and a map of the field of vision is charted. The Goldman perimeter is commonly employed in eye clinics.

The pattern of a visual field defect gives useful localizing information for lesions in the visual pathway and retina. Because the right half of each retina is linked by nerves to the right occipital cortex and because splitting of nerve fibres from each optic nerve occurs at the chiasm, lesions in the optic nerve anterior to the chiasm cause unilateral defects whereas those posterior to the chiasm produce hemianopic or quadrantinopic defects.

Lesions of the occipital cortex tend to be more congruous (i.e. similar on each side). Cortical lesions also show better preservation of central vision (macular sparing).

A special type of field loss is seen with expanding pituitary tumours, the resulting pressure on the centre of the chiasm producing a bitemporal defect.

Localized defects in the retina produce equivalent localized defects in the visual field. Defects due to retinal disease are relatively common, for example due to glaucoma in the elderly, and care must be taken to interpret field defects with this possibility in mind. It is surprising how patients fail to notice quite extensive field loss; hemianopic patients may like to continue to drive in spite of the risks to life and limb and the doctor should be on his guard against such hazardous behaviour.

Ophthalmoscopy

The study of eye disease was revolutionized by the invention of the ophthalmoscope in 1850 by Herman Von Helmholtz. The problem may seem simple enough to us today; it is that of trying to look into a dark cupboard through the keyhole. As soon as one's eye is placed against the keyhole no light enters the

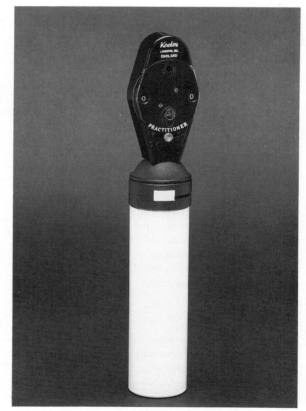

Fig. 22.8 The ophthalmoscope. When learning, familiarize yourself with a basic instrument.

cupboard. The secret is to look down a beam of light. This can be achieved by looking through a hole in a tilted mirror. The modern instrument (Fig. 22.8) incorporates a battery, preferably rechargeable; a bulb, preferably halogen; a light path with small mirror and a set of minute lenses which can be interposed to allow for the spectacle correction of patient and observer. This is achieved by rotating the knurled rim of a disc in which the lenses are fitted.

The technique of ophthalmoscopy is as follows: ask the patient to sit in a chair and to look straight forward. Hold the instrument vertically, close to the patient's eye (Fig. 22.9). The instrument is held in the right hand to view the right eye and the observer uses the right eye. The left hand and left eye are used to view the patient's left eye. Learn to do it this way; otherwise noses come into contact in an embarrassing way.

It is useful to have a routine method of examination:

- *Look for the optic disc* This is situated slightly medial (nasal) to the posterior pole of the eye and slightly above the horizontal meridian. The various features of a normal optic disc should be noted
- *Follow the vessels* Upper and lower branches of the central retinal vessels divide into nasal and temporal so that each of the four branches should be followed out to the periphery in turn
- *Look at the fovea* Simply ask the patient to look at the light. The fovea can only be properly seen with the pupil dilated. It appears as a minute dot representing the reflection from the foveal pit. Careful inspection reveals the yellowish surrounding pigment
- *Look at the background* Scan the optic fundus between the vessels noting any abnormalities such as haemorrhages, exudates or abnormal pigmentation. The choroidal vascularization outside and beyond the retinal vessels can be seen in many normal fundi

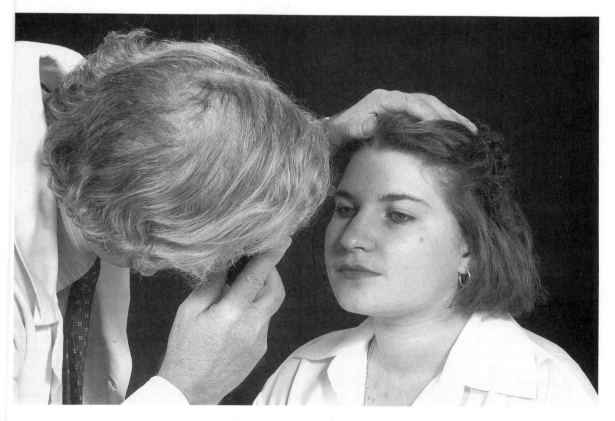

Fig. 22.9 The technique of ophthalmoscopy. Examine the patient in a darkened environment. Learn to use right eye to patient's right eye and left eye to patient's left eye.

- *Look at the periphery* Ask the patient to look to the extremes of gaze and dial a 'plus lens' on the ophthalmoscope. The examination of the peripheral fundus is critical in routine ophthalmoscopy but demands more time and skill than the examination of the posterior pole

When learning ophthalmoscopy there are two main problems. First, the field of view is quite small and serial pictures of the fundus must be put together in one's mind. Secondly, reflections of light from the cornea can seem a nuisance and at first interfere with the view. Practice and proper co-ordination of hand and eye gradually eliminate these difficulties.

There are other ways of looking at the optic fundus. The above technique is known as direct ophthalmoscopy whereas the fundus may also be viewed from 60 or 90 cm away by interposing a convex lens. This technique of indirect ophthalmoscopy is more difficult to master but gives an excellent wide-field view of the fundus.

The laser scanning ophthalmoscope is now available. This instrument gives a television picture of the fundus of the eye which can be stored on disc and visualized on a VDU; the student of the future may not even need to learn ophthalmoscopy once such instruments become readily available.

Ophthalmoscopic signs of systemic disease

Cardiovascular system

Changes in the retinal vessels reflect the rate of progression and severity of systemic hypertension (Fig. 22.10). Irregularity of arteriolar calibre and tortuosity of the perimacular arterioles is an early sign. The light reflex from the walls of the arterioles is heightened giving the description of 'silver wiring'. Nipping of the veins at the point of crossover of an arteriole is also an important early sign. In patients with accelerated hypertension the retinal arterioles become more markedly narrowed and irregular and hard exudates may appear radiating from the macula to give the appearance of a macular star. Soft exudates (cotton wool spots) indicate the presence of infarcts in the nerve fibre layer. Papilloedema is present in severe cases.

Central retinal artery occlusion (Fig. 22.11) presents as sudden loss of vision in one eye and the retina looks pale and oedematous with grossly narrowed arterioles. The macula region may stand out as a normal red colour against the surrounding oedema-

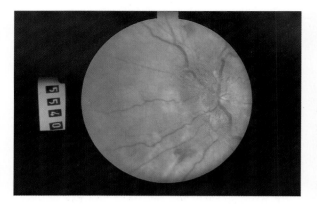

Fig. 22.10 The fundus in severe systemic hypertension with papilloedema, haemorrhages and exudates. When hypertension is associated with these vascular changes it is termed 'accelerated hypertension'.

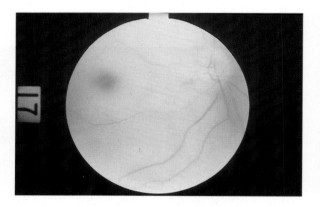

Fig. 22.11 Central retinal artery occlusion showing grossly narrowed arteries.

tous retina. The condition may be secondary to vascular disease and hypertension or may be due to emboli from the heart or internal carotid arteries.

Central retinal vein occlusion (Fig. 22.12) presents as blurred vision rather than loss of vision and the most striking feature of the fundus is the multiplicity of haemorrhages with engorgement of the veins. The condition may be associated with hypertension or hyperviscosity of the blood; however, in many instances the underlying cause cannot be demonstrated. There is an association between central retinal vein occlusion and chronic open-angle glaucoma.

Cranial (or temporal) arteritis is a cause of sudden loss of vision in the elderly; the second eye may subsequently be involved, causing complete blind-

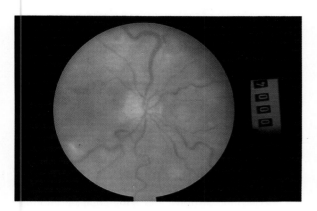

Fig. 22.12 Central retinal vein thrombosis. In more severe cases there may be very large haemorrhages round the disc.

ness. This not uncommon disease of the elderly usually presents with severe headache and tenderness over the extracranial arteries which become inflamed, tender and often occluded. The temporal arteries are frequently affected. The visual loss which may occur at any stage in the untreated disease is due to arterial insufficiency and inspection of the fundi may reveal papilloedema and marked narrowing of the arterioles. The picture of central retinal artery occlusion is also seen in some cases.

Inflammatory changes in the retina and retinal vessels are seen in a wide variety of systemic diseases. They may take the form of venous engorgement and sheathing with leakage of blood into the vitreous or arterial narrowing with consequent retinal ischaemia. Systemic lupus erythematosus may produce multiple cotton wool spots in the fundi and Behçet's syndrome similarly may be associated with retinal ischaemia although here the presence of recurrent hypopyon (pus in the anterior chamber) may obscure a view of the fundus.

Respiratory system

In cases of severe respiratory insufficiency papilloedema may be present due to hypercapnia and consequent increased cerebral and retinal blood-flow. The retinal veins may be engorged and central cyanosis may be evident on ophthalmoscopic examination. Specific chest diseases which manifest themselves with important ophthalmoscopic signs are tuberculosis and sarcoidosis. Miliary tuberculosis can sometimes be diagnosed by discovering the miliary tubercles in the choroid. They are seen as whitish-yellow, slightly raised lesions at the posterior

pole of the fundus which fade and become pigmented. Sarcoidosis may present as acute iridocyclitis or as lacrimal insufficiency causing a dry eye. The fundoscopic changes include retinal periphlebitis. The retinal veins become sheathed and careful examination may reveal small, white patches in the internal limiting membrane of the retina known as candle-wax patches. Horner's syndrome may result from infiltration of the cervical sympathetic ganglion by bronchial carcinoma.

Haemopoietic system

Severe anaemia from whatever cause may be associated with presence of scattered haemorrhages some of which have a white centre to them. Soft exudates may also be present. These changes are most marked in pernicious anaemia and the acute leukaemias.

Sickle-cell disease causes quite specific eye changes which can often be diagnosed simply by ophthalmoscopy. Eye changes which are due to vascular occlusion rather than anaemia are seen most often in sickle-cell haemoglobin C disease (SC) but also in homozygous sickle-cell (SS) disease and in sickle-cell thalassaemia. Vascular occlusions are seen in the peripheral retina with unusual-looking haemorrhages and subsequent tendency to peripheral neovascularization.

Central nervous system

Papilloedema is an important ophthalmic sign in central nervous system disease which has already been discussed in Chapter 8. It is essential to distinguish true swelling of the optic disc (Fig. 22.13) from apparent swelling as is sometimes seen in hypermetropic eyes or when there are 'drusen' of the optic nerve head.

The main causes of papilloedema are listed in Table 22.5.

Optic atrophy (Fig. 22.14)

When nerve fibres in the optic nerve become atrophic

Table 22.5. Causes of papilloedema

Raised intracranial pressure
Severe hypertension (accelerated)
Central retinal vein thrombosis
Temporal arteritis
Respiratory insufficiency (hypercapnia)

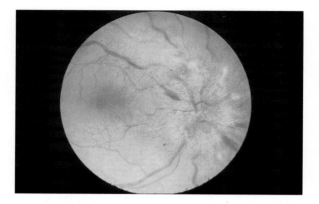

Fig. 22.13 Papilloedema. In the early stages of papilloedema there is filling in of the physiological cup with blurring of the edges. Radial haemorrhages are frequently present around the swollen optic disc.

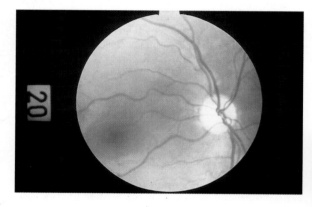

Fig. 22.14 Optic atrophy. This patient had a pituitary tumour.

the optic disc becomes abnormally pale and black dots are seen on the disc. These are the openings in the sclera through which nerve fibres have passed; the so called cribriform markings. They are seen in the elderly with otherwise normal eyes. The following may cause optic atrophy:

- previous obstruction of the central retinal artery or veins
- compression of the nerve by an aneurysm or tumour
- retrobulbar neuritis: rapid progressive loss of central vision in a young person with pain on eye movement is characteristic of retrobulbar neuritis. The fundus at this stage is usually normal but optic atrophy may begin to appear after two or three weeks. An afferent pupillary

defect is present. About half of the patients with retrobulbar neuritis subsequently develop demyelinating disease in other parts of the body after a delay of some years

- resolution of papilloedema
- congenital causes, e.g. retinitis pigmentosa which is an inherited retinal degeneration in which there is a progressive night-blindness, constriction of the visual fields and scattered pigmentation in the fundus. As the disease advances towards blindness the discs become atrophic (Fig 20.15). Optic atrophy may also appear in certain families without any other apparent pathology, for example Leber's optic atrophy and congenital or infantile optic atrophy. It is also seen in the rare cerebromacular degeneration which presents with progressive blindness, epilepsy and dementia
- toxins: a number of poisons can specifically damage the optic nerve. Methanol is the classical example
- trauma
- glaucoma

Diabetes

See Chapter 12.

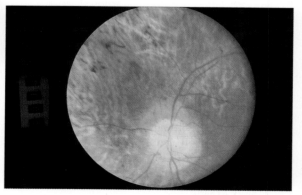

Fig. 22.15 Retinitis pigmentosa. There is scattered pigmentation of the fundus. As the disease progresses the disc becomes atrophic.

Generalized infections manifesting themselves ophthalmoscopically

Bacterial infections

Bacterial septicaemia can cause metastatic infections in the eye which may take the form of Roth's spots

(Fig. 22.16). These are typically seen in subacute bacterial endocarditis and appear as isolated, oval haemorrhagic lesions with a white centre. Sometimes an endophthalmitis may develop with destruction of the eye. The ocular consequences of tuberculosis have been mentioned but episcleritis, keratitis and uveitis may also appear. Syphilitic eye changes are now largely limited to congenital cases in the Western

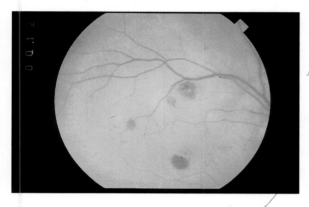

Fig. 22.16 Roth's spots. These appearances are typically seen in subacute bacterial carditis but are by no means as specific as many textbooks would suggest.

world which show evidence of previous interstitial keratitis (a particular kind of corneal scarring) recognizable with the slit-lamp microscope and chorioretinitis producing the 'salt-and-pepper fundus'. These findings are often combined with deafness and Hutchinson's teeth. Acquired syphilis is associated with Argyll—Robertson pupils, anterior uveitis, chorioretinitis and optic neuritis.

Viral infections

The triad of cataract, deafness and congenital heart disease in children born from a mother who suffered rubella infection during the first trimester of pregnancy is well known. Such children also tend to suffer from other abnormalities of the eyes such as microphthalmia, iris hyperplasia or iridocyclitis. Less well-recognized is a characteristic diffuse finding associated with the characteristic x-ray appearance of calcification of the brain and positive serological findings. Acquired toxoplasmosis is rarely associated with ocular disease but there is an abnormally high incidence of positive serology for the infection in patients who present with focal choroiditis and no other apparent systemic upset.

Drugs affecting the eyesight

Many drugs can cause transient blurring of the vision and this effect may be more evident in patients approaching the age when glasses are needed for reading (about 45 years). Any drug which has a potential for dilating the pupil has a theoretical risk of causing narrow-angle glaucoma in a susceptible subject. Narrow-angle glaucoma occurs in middle-aged, hypermetropic individuals. If a patient already has known glaucoma then by and large there is no cause for concern because any treatment that is given will override the slight mydriatic effects of, for example antidepressant drugs.

Some drugs are stored in the pigment epithelium of the retina and if they happen to be toxic they can cause permanent damage to the eye. Chloroquine is the most important example of this effect. Small doses of chloroquine appear to be perfectly safe even when administered over several years but if the dose exceeds the recommended maximum then a specific type of fundus pigmentation can appear with associated permanent loss of vision. Chloroquine is also deposited in the cornea but these deposits disappear when the drug is stopped. Amiodarone is also deposited in the cornea in a similar way and here the level of deposition may sometimes interfere with the vision, even though, like chloroquine, it also disappears when the drug is reduced or stopped.

The effect of local or systemic steroids on the eye should also be borne in mind. Steroids can cause a rise in intraocular pressure in susceptible individuals and a form of secondary glaucoma may result. Steroids administered systemically can also increase the rate of formation of cataracts.

References and further reading

Elkington AR, Khaw PT. *ABC of eyes*. London: British Medical Association, 1993.

Galloway NR. *Common eye diseases and their management*. Berlin: Springer, 1985.

Kritzinger EE, Beaumont HM. *A colour atlas of optic disc abnormalities*. London: Wolfe, 1987.

Miller S. *Clinical ophthalmology*. Bristol: Wright, 1987.

23

Physical signs in otorhinolaryngology for the non-specialist

K. P. Gibbin

Introduction
Examination of the ear
Examination of the nose
Pharyngeal and laryngeal disease
Examination of the neck
References and further reading

Introduction

Students and doctors need to be aware of the basic physical signs in otorhinolaryngology. In this field technique of examination is particularly important and whilst the non-specialist may be unable to visualize the nasopharynx or larynx expertly he should be able to carry out a reasonably thorough examination of ears, nose, pharynx and neck. Although for many parts of the examination an otolaryngologist will use a head mirror and bull's-eye lamp much of the examination can be carried out with a suitable auriscope. As with all medical practice, initial examination starts at the foot of the bed or, as in much of Ear, Nose and Throat (ENT practice), when the patient enters the consulting room.

Examination of the ear

Examination of the ears starts during history-taking when hearing is generally assessed. More formal examination of the patient's ears may then be carried out, starting first with the outer ear.

Major abnormalities of the pinna such as total absence or marked degrees of aplasia will readily be noted. Look for the position of the pinnae, their symmetry, preauricular skin tags, pits and sinuses.

Then deflect the pinna forward to examine the post-aural region for scars, bony depressions and other abnormalities including innocent swellings such as sebaceous cysts, gouty tophi (see Fig. 17.16(b)), wrinkling of the ear-lobe (see Fig. 2.7) or more sinister lesions such as skin carcinomas. A small squamous cell carcinoma such as the one depicted in Fig. 23.1 can easily be missed. Look for enlargement of the preauricular and postauricular lymph nodes.

Swelling of the pinna and exquisite tenderness may be noted as with cellulitis (Fig. 23.2) or following

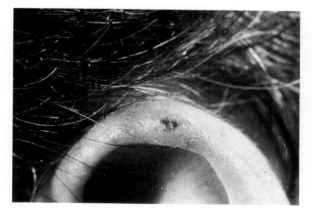

Fig. 23.1 An early squamous cell carcinoma of the pinna.

286

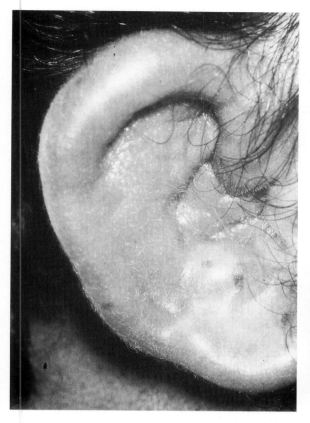

Fig. 23.2 Cellulitis of the external ear. Infection of or trauma to the pinna is often extremely painful.

offensive discharge is frequently the only symptom of atticoantral disease, a more serious type of CSOM in which the main pathological finding is the presence of a cholesteatoma.

The correct way of holding the auriscope will help considerably in enabling a better view to be obtained of the deep ear canal and ear-drum and reducing the risk of hurting and frightening the patient. To examine the left ear the instrument should be held in the left hand, the right hand then being free to retract the pinna, straightening the ear canal and improving visualization of the ear-drum. The ulnar border of the left hand may be rested upon the patient's cheek so that, should the patient move, the examiner's hand holding the auriscope will also move and prevent the speculum impacting in the ear (Fig. 23.3).

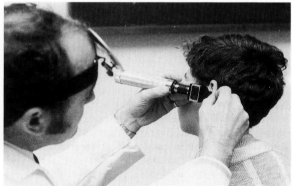

Fig. 23.3 The correct use of the auriscope.

trauma where subperichondral haematomata may cause the so-called cauliflower ear. Discharge from the meatus may cause a secondary eczematous reaction which may extend on to the skin of the neck.

Major abnormalities of size and shape of the pinna may be associated with various syndromes such as the Treacher–Collins syndrome in which there may be severe dysplasia of the pinna and canal as well as other facial features including hypoplastic malae, antimongoloid slant of the eyes and notching of the lower eye-lids. This syndrome may be associated with severe degrees of conductive deafness.

Following external inspection of the ear, the canal should then be examined using a suitable auriscope light. Before inserting the speculum into the canal examine the opening of the ear for discharge and note its nature. It may be thin and watery as seen in some cases of otitis externa; thicker, mucopurulent discharge may indicate tubotympanic or mucosal chronic suppurative otitis media (CSOM). Scanty

Whilst introducing the speculum abnormalities of the ear canal may be seen such as otitis externa, a furuncle (which is extremely tender), a meatal exostosis (bony swellings of the canal frequently found in those who have done a lot of swimming) and rarely, tumours. If wax is present it may need to be carefully syringed away before further examination can take place. Always enquire of a history of discharge or known perforation before syringing an ear. The ear-drum may then be examined. A healthy tympanic membrane has a shallow concavity with an anteroinferior reflection of the examining light, the cone of light, narrowing towards the umbo or middle part of the membrane (Fig. 23.4). The colour is typically a pale grey/pink and the incus–stapes assembly may just be visible posteriorly through the drum. The relationship of the structures in the inner and middle ears can now be demonstrated on CT scanning (23.5(a) and (b)).

If there has been previous infection the ear-drum

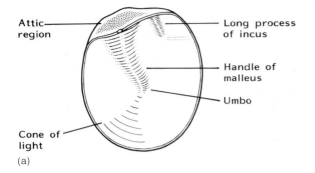

Attic region

Long process of incus

Handle of malleus

Umbo

Cone of light

(a)

Fig. 23.4 Auriscopic appearances of the left tympanic membrane.

may be somewhat dull in appearance and thickened; conversely it may be thinned and retracted onto the medial wall of the middle ear — an atelactic ear. The colour of the drum may be altered; for example, if a middle-ear effusion is present the ear-drum may have a slightly yellow appearance. Very occasionally in this condition a fluid level or air bubbles may be seen. Haemotympanum, a not uncommon sequel to fracture involving the temporal bone, will produce a blue drum; a blue appearance to the drum may also sometimes be seen in cases of secretory otitis.

A central perforation (Fig. 23.6) in the pars tensa will indicate the tubotympanic or relatively safe type of CSOM; an attic defect is indicative of atticoantral disease, typically associated with cholesteatoma. There is a higher incidence of intracranial and other complications such as facial palsy in atticoantral CSOM (Fig. 23.7).

In some cases part of the pars tensa may be severely retracted and give the appearance of a perforation; without the use of a pneumatic otoscope or an operating microscope it may be difficult to interpret this appearance correctly.

Hyaline or chalky patches in the tympanic membrane are relatively common findings and are evidence of previous inflammatory ear disease. They may be found both in intact tympanic membranes and in association with a perforation. Most typically there is a peripheral crescentic white appearance.

Deafness

Most deaf patients have nothing to find on aural examination except an abnormality on tuning-fork testing and, of course, the deafness. When carring out tuning-fork testing, use the 512-Hz tuning-fork as it may be heard rather than experienced through vibration sensation and it has a suitably long decay period.

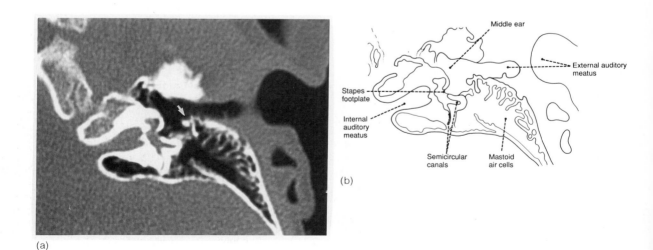

(a)

Stapes footplate

Internal auditory meatus

Middle ear

External auditory meatus

Semicircular canals

Mastoid air cells

(b)

Fig. 23.5 (a) CT scan showing some of the major structures in the temporal bone; the white arrow indicates the position of the ossicles. (b) Explanatory line diagram of scan.

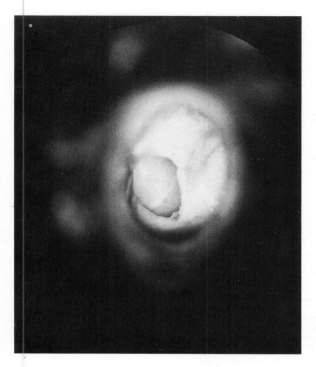

Fig. 23.6 Right tympanic membrane showing posterior central perforation with considerable tympanosclerosis.

CSOM
POINTS

Attico antral (Unsafe)	Tubotympanic (Relatively safe)
Scanty offensive discharge	Discharge profuse and mucopurulent, rarely offensive
Cholesteatoma	Mucosal disease
Perforation/defect in attic region –may be hidden by overlying crust. Membrana tensa may be normal.	Perforation in membrana tensa Attic normal

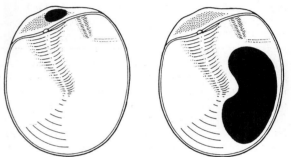

Fig. 23.7 Chronic suppurative otitis media.

In the Rinne test the patient's ability to discriminate between air conduction (through the external meatus) and bone conduction is tested. To test air conduction the tines of the fork are held parallel to the ear canal and about 2.5 cm away (Fig. 23.8(a)); for bone conduction testing the base of the fork is held firmly against the skull adjacent to the ear, typically against the mastoid process (Fig. 23.8(b)). The quickest way to carry out the test is to ask the patient to compare the loudness of bone-conducted and air-conducted sound. A positive Rinne is recorded when air-conducted sound is heard better than that by bone conduction; a negative Rinne when the converse is found.

In the Weber test the tuning-fork is held anywhere on the skull in the midline and the patient asked whether he can hear the sound and if so whether it lateralizes (Fig. 23.8(c)). Finally the absolute bone conduction test may be carried out comparing the patient's bone-conduction threshold with that of the examiner, whose hearing is (it is to be hoped) normal. The results and interpretation of these tests are summarized in Table 23.1.

Table 23.1. Results and interpretation of Rinne's and Weber's tests

Right	Left	Interpretation
Rinne positive Weber central	Rinne positive	Normal, mild, moderate or severe bilateral sensorineural loss
Rinne positive Weber → left	Rinne negative	Left conductive or mixed hearing loss
Rinne negative Weber central	Rinne negative	Bilateral mixed or conductive deafness
Rinne positive Right ← Weber	Rinne negative	Left severe or profound sensorineural loss
(This is referred to as a false-negative Rinne)		

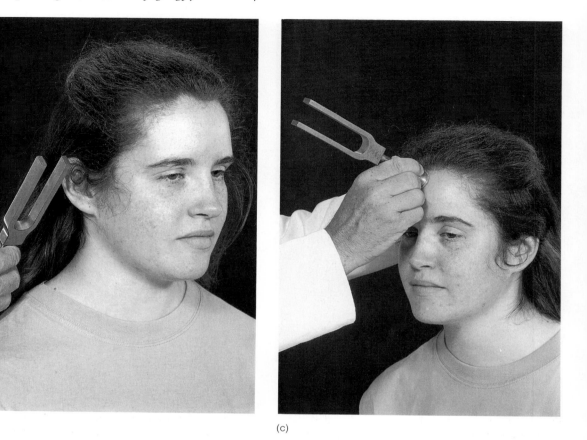

(a)

(c)

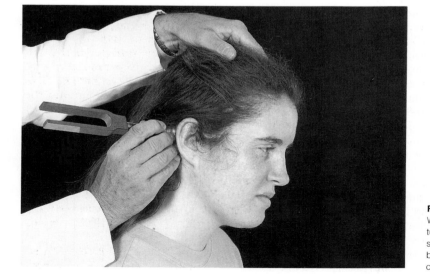

(b)

Fig. 23.8 (a and b). The Rinne test. (c) The Weber test. How to hold and position the tuning-fork; note the examiner's hand supporting the head in order to obtain firm bony pressure when carrying out bone-conduction testing.

Simple voice testing may then be carried out using a quietly spoken voice or a whisper, the examiner covering his mouth to prevent the patient lip-reading. From this the patient's hearing loss may be assessed as mild, moderate, severe or profound. A simple checklist for examination of the ear is shown in Table 23.2.

Table 23.2. Examination of the ear

1. Assess the patient's hearing in conversation
2. Examine position and appearance of the pinnae
3. Examine the postaural region
4. Before examining the tympanic membrane using a speculum, examine the ear canal
5. When using an auriscope or aural speculum be gentle; the ear canal, especially if inflamed, may be very tender
6. Examine the whole tympanic membrane using a good light source
7. Assess deafness

Vertigo

Vertigo presents one of the more challenging diagnostic problems in both otological and general medical practice, the diagnosis resting heavily on thorough history-taking. In many cases of vertigo there may be few, if any, physical signs, their absence often being important in excluding a diagnosis.

In examining a patient with a history of vertigo it is essential to examine the ears for abnormalities including especially an attic perforation which may be associated with a chronic serous labyrinthitis or a labyrinthine fistula. With the latter the patient may volunteer a history of vertigo on pressing the ear to occluding the ear canal. If occlusion of the ear canal with variation in the canal pressure produces vertigo then the fistula sign is said to be positive. This is supported by observing nystagmus which is in the horizontal plane. In the case of a fistula with an infective labyrinthitis persistent horizontal nystagmus may be seen, the rapid phase being variable in its direction. Of course examination of a patient with vertigo is not complete without assessment of the central nervous system and the cardiovascular system. In most cases of vertigo there is no otoscopic abnormality or nystagmus.

Nystagmus may briefly be defined as involuntary eye movements; they may be physiological or pathological; causes are listed in Table 23.3. Examples of physiological nystagmus include end-point nystagmus, elicited in many normal people by taking the direction of gaze more than about 60° either side of the midline position. Other examples include railway nystagmus, a rapid nystagmus produced when watching a scene moving rapidly across the field of vision.

Table 23.3. Causes of nystagmus

Physiological	Spontaneous	Congenital
		Ocular
Pathological	Induced	Vestibular
		Of CNS origin

Vestibular nystagmus typically has two components, a rapid phase and a slow phase, the direction of the rapid phase being used to describe the direction of the nystagmus, i.e. rapid phase to the right = nystagmus to the right. An irritative labyrinthine lesion will produce a nystagmus to the ipsilateral ear, a paralytic nystagmus being to the opposite ear.

Sometimes a vestibular lesion may produce a 'compound' nystagmus with both a horizontal and a rotatory component, an example being the nystagmus elicited in the classic Hallpike positional test for benign paroxysmal positional vertigo. In this the patient is moved from a sitting position to lying with head dependent on one side or the other (Fig. 23.9). In this condition the nystagmus demonstrates the following features: there is a long period in its onset after the head is placed in the appropriate position; it is directed to the undermost ear and the nystagmus rapidly decays. On resuming the sitting position there may again be a brief period of vertigo with nystagmus in the opposite direction. Repetition of the manoeuvre results in a reduced severity of vertigo and shorter duration of nystagmus; indeed both may be absent after the first demonstration. The nystagmus is therefore said to fatigue.

Departure from any of these criteria should alert the examining doctor to the possibility of a non-benign central cause including intracranial space-occupying lesions.

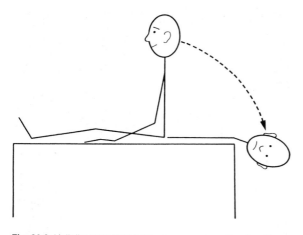

Fig. 23.9 Hallpike tests for benign paroxysmal positional vertigo.

Examination of the nose

As in the case of aural disease, examination starts by observing the patient during the history-taking. Is there obvious rhinorrhoea and if so what is its nature? Are there any obvious abnormalities of the external nose? Does the patient have a blocked nose, the typical hyponasal speech or rhinolalia clausa, or does the patient present with a nasal air leak on talking, rhinolalia aperta, as noted for example in many patients with a cleft palate. Is the patient obviously gasping for breath when talking and does he have dry lips and sit open-mouthed.

More formal examination of the nose starts with observation of the external nose and facial structures looking for displacement of the nose and abnormalities of the skin overlying it such as rhinophyma (Fig. 23.10). Rhinophyma is due to thickening of the skin of the nose and hypertrophy of the sebaceous glands.

Nystagmus may of course arise from disorders of the central nervous system or from ocular disease; congenital forms, producing a pendular motion, also exist and may be familial.

Other tests often helpful in the assessment of the patient with vertigo include the Romberg and the Unterberger test. Both provide non-specific information. In the Romberg test the patient is asked to stand with eyes closed and his ability to maintain balance is noted. The test is said to be positive if the patient sways unduly or is unable to maintain balance at all. A positive Romberg's test usually indicates defective joint-position sense but vestibular impairment may also cause Rhombergism when position sense is normal. Too much significance should not be attached to this sign.

In the Unterberger test the patient is asked to walk on the spot with eyes closed and arms stretched in front; in patients with a unilateral labyrinthine lesion there will be a tendency to rotate towards the side of the lesion.

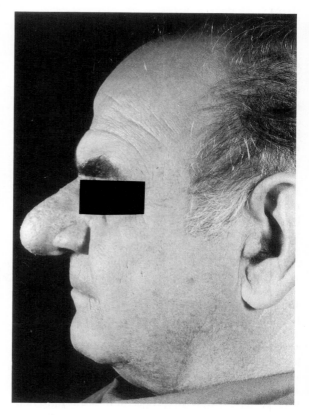

Fig. 23.10 Rhinophyma. Do not assume that this is always caused by alcohol!

Although seen with alcoholism it is not always due to it! The nature of nasal discharge should be noted. Anterior rhinoscopy may then be carried out. In many instances an adequate examination may be carried out simply by lifting the tip of the nose with the thumb and inspecting inside the nose using a good light. As with otoscopy, the hand-held auriscope may often be adequate. After examination of the tip and the anterior part of the nose has been carried out a more detailed intranasal inspection may be performed by using either a thudicum speculum or by utilizing the hand-held auriscope with a suitably large aural speculum which may be introduced into the nostril.

Among points to note on anterior rhinoscopy are the position of the septum, any bleeding points, the nature of the nasal mucosa, and the appearance of the turbinates. In health both the inferior and middle turbinates may be clearly visible within the nose and although there is a superior turbinate this is rarely, if ever, seen. The inferior turbinate is commonly mistaken for a nasal polyp by the inexperienced rhinoscopist!

Posterior rhinoscopy is not always possible even for an experienced ENT surgeon and without the appropriate equipment cannot be tackled. However, examination of the oropharynx may yield important clues to nasal disease, for example a mucopurulent postnasal discharge from infected nasal sinuses, perhaps even with a secondary pharyngitis. Additional information about the nasal airway may be obtained by placing a cold metal tongue depressor under both nostrils and noting the degree of misting on expiration through the nose.

Finally the nose may be palpated noting any structural abnormalities and testing also for tenderness over the maxillary sinuses and medially below the supraorbital ridges for frontal tenderness. Gentle percussion similarly may elicit pain.

Nasal obstruction

One of the commonest nasal symptoms is nasal obstruction and in many instances the non-specialist may make the diagnosis of the underlying cause. Clearly the commonest cause of this symptom is the common cold, producing short-lived symptoms. In adults one of the more common causes of chronic nasal airways obstruction is a deviated nasal septum (Fig. 23.11). It may not always be appreciated that the deflection need not be towards the side that the patient says is most obstructed and indeed the

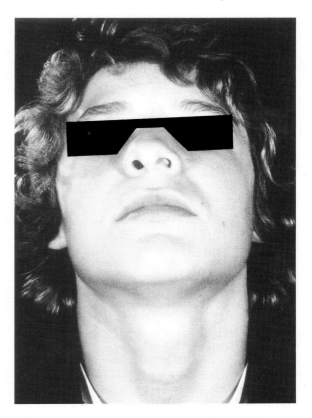

Fig. 23.11 Deviation of the nasal septum. Note the displacement of the nasal pyramid to the side opposite to that of the deflection.

obstruction may fluctuate from one side to the other even in cases of quite marked deflection.

Vasomotor rhinitis (VMR) and allergic rhinitis produce a similar clinical appearance, the distinction being made on the history and on testing for appropriate allergens. The nasal mucosa, especially over the turbinates is usually pale, almost a lilac colour and there is often considerable clear mucus present. Polypi may also be seen. The complex relationships between the various common causes of nasal congestion and sinusitis are indicated in Fig. 23.12.

Many patients with nasal obstruction resort to the use of topical decongestant drops, easily available from retail pharmacists. Whilst useful for short-term use chronic usage produces a chemical rhinitis (vasomotor rhinitis medicamentosa) with its characteristic appearance of a florid red mucosa and engorged turbinates.

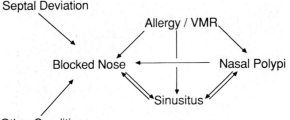

Fig. 23.12 Some of the interrelated factors causing a blocked nose.

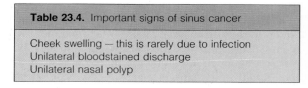

Table 23.4. Important signs of sinus cancer
Cheek swelling — this is rarely due to infection Unilateral bloodstained discharge Unilateral nasal polyp

Nasal discharge

Nasal discharge is similarly a frequent symptom and the appearance of the discharge may give a clue to the underlying pathology; a clear, often profuse, watery discharge is most commonly seen in allergic and vasomotor rhinitis; clear rhinorrhoea is not uncommon in the elderly. After head injury of course, the appearance of clear rhinorrhoea points to a CSF leak, usually from a fracture through the cribriform plate. Purulent discharge typically is associated with sinusitis, although if the discharge is unilateral the most likely cause, particularly in the very young and the mentally infirm, is a foreign body in the nose. In an older patient a unilateral bloodstained discharge may be the first sign of a malignant tumour in the nose or paranasal sinuses.

Cheek swelling and proptosis

Maxillary sinus tumours may also present with cheek swelling (Fig. 23.13(a)–(d)) and frontoethmoid tumours may be associated with proptosis of the eye (Fig. 23.14) (Table 23.4). However, not all such swellings are neoplasms and mucoceles of the frontal sinuses typically may present with proptosis. The presence of orbital cellulitis (Fig. 23.15) should prompt full investigation to exclude an underlying sinusitis, typically of the frontal sinuses in adults, of the ethmoidal sinuses in younger children.

Nose bleeds

Nose bleeds (epistaxes) are common, especially in children, the majority arising from Little's area — the anterior part of the nasal septum — the area most easily reached by the patient's probing finger! Contrary to popular belief, nose bleeds in adults are not usually due to high blood pressure. Hypertension in a patient suffering a torrential nose bleed is much more likely to be due to fright than to pre-existing

disease. Do not forget the possibility of a bleeding disorder in a patient with recurrent epistaxis; look for evidence elsewhere such as skin purpura and bleeding gums. Blue spots on the lips may betray the cause in hereditary haemorrhagic telangiectasia (see Fig. 5.4). Finally remember that nose bleeds may be a sign of serious intranasal pathology (Fig. 23.16).

Pharyngeal and laryngeal disease

The voice

The quality and timbre of the patient's voice may give a clue to underlying disease both in the larynx and pharynx and also more general disease such as the hoarseness in patients with myxoedema. The weak, 'breathy' voice of a patient with a paralysed vocal cord indicates the possibility of an underlying bronchial neoplasm affecting the left recurrent laryngeal nerve. Noisy breathing on inspiration, inspiratory stridor, usually indicates glottic or supraglottic airway obstruction and if the stridor is biphasic, both inspiratory and expiratory, the possibility arises of tracheal airway narrowing. Stridor should not be confused with the wheezing sound of a patient with lower airway obstruction, nor with the sound produced by pharyngeal and nasopharyngeal obstruction, stertor. In patients with hoarseness, the examiner should look for other evidence of central nervous system disease such as palatal or tongue paralysis.

The mouth

Although this has been described in Chapter 5 it is worth re-emphasizing the importance of thorough examination of the whole buccal mucosa using adequate lighting and also, where appropriate, a tongue depressor or depressors. Intraoral examination is not complete without asking the patient to remove his or her dentures. It is essential to ask the patient to lift the tongue to inspect the floor of the mouth otherwise lesions such as a carcinoma of the

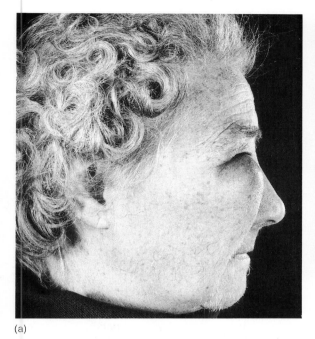

(a)

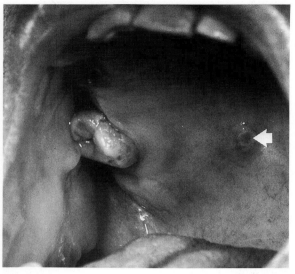

(b)

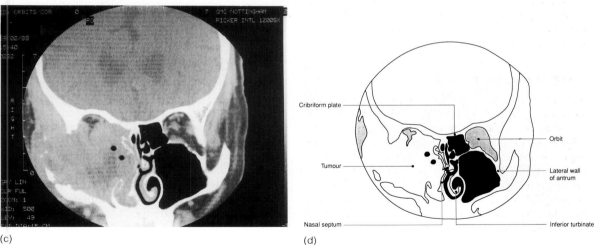

(c)

(d)

Fig. 23.13 (a) A maxillary sinus tumour presenting with swelling of the right cheek. (b) Oral examination reveals the same tumour (arrowed) invading the hard palate. (c) CT scan of tumour which has replaced the whole of the sinus and has invaded the orbit. (d) Identification of structures shown on the scan.

tongue may be missed. Many young and middle-aged women may complain of feeling a lump in the throat for which no cause is ever found. This is often termed 'globus'. Such symptoms should not be dismissed without inspection of the throat (Fig. 23.17).

Sore throats

Sore throats may be due to primary pharyngeal disease or as part of a systemic illness. Patients may present with an acute sore throat and malaise and it

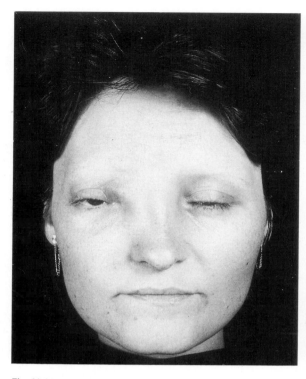

Fig. 23.14 A frontoethmoid tumour causing displacement of the globe.

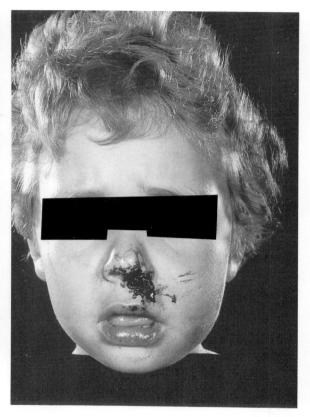

Fig. 23.16 Epistaxes may have a serious cause; recurrent unilateral nose bleeds in this child were due to an intranasal rhabdomyosarcoma.

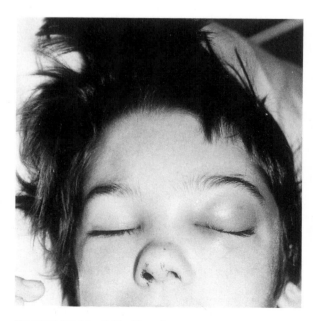

Fig. 23.15 Orbital cellulitis; this serious condition demands urgent investigation (see text).

is often extremely difficult to differentiate on clinical grounds alone between a patient with an acute parenchymal tonsillitis and a patient with glandular fever (Fig. 23.18). In the latter disease the lymphadenopathy is, of course, much more generalized but the final diagnosis rests on the peripheral blood film and the positive Paul Bunnell test.

The appearance of the pharynx in patients with a recurrent tonsillitis may seldom give an indication as to whether surgery is indicated. The tonsils may appear to be large, or small, but their true size is not reflected in their clinical appearance; the tonsils may be superficially placed within the tonsillar fossae or may be very deeply recessed within them.

The tonsils drain to the upper deep cervical nodes which quickly enlarge in acute tonsillar infections. The node below the angle of the mandible and deep to the upper portion of the sternomastoid muscle is termed the tonsillar node; this is often the first to

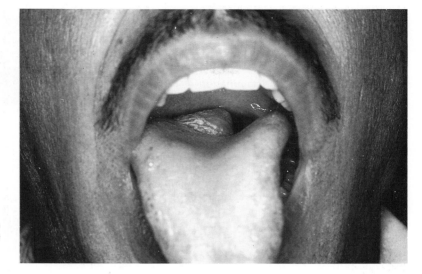

Fig. 23.17 This man complained of a lump in the throat which he surely had! Inspection revealed a tumour at the base of the tongue and excision later showed it to be a neurofibroma.

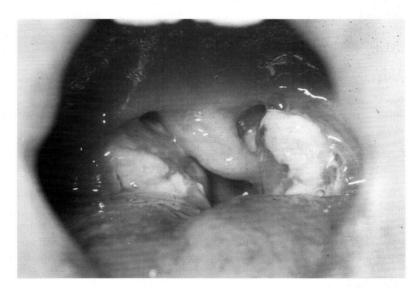

Fig. 23.18 The throat in glandular fever. In addition to lymphadenopathy a white membrane on the tonsils often gives a clue as to the diagnosis.

become tender and enlarged with a sore throat. Recurrent throat infections may cause chronic firm enlargement of this node up to 2 cm in diameter Larger glands than this should be regarded with suspicion and tuberculosis should be considered.

The presence of thrush produces a very typical appearance (see Fig. 5.11). Its significance depends on the age and clinical status of the patient. It is common at the two extremes of life, in babies and in debilitated old folk. In middle life it commonly complicates antibiotic and immunosuppressive therapy.

Do not forget the possibility of AIDS when thrush appears unexpectedly.

Sometimes the tonsillar crypts may be seen to contain debris which in rare instances may accumulate and produce a large mass — a tonsillolith. Finally the physician should be alert to the possibility of a tonsillar neoplasm — any irregularity in appearance or marked asymmetry in size of the tonsils needs further investigation to exclude either a carcinoma or a lymphoma.

Examination of the neck

Examination of the neck is an essential part of a full examination of the ears, nose and throat. It may be required to complete the examination of the patient who presents, for example, with hoarseness or dysphagia to exclude metastatic disease; alternatively the patient may present with a neck swelling. In both instances it is important to have a thorough method of palpation of the neck and to be aware of the underlying anatomy. With the patient sitting upright and the head flexed slightly forward, palpate in turn the submental region, the submandibular region extending back to the angle of the mandible, the jugular chain to the clavicles, and then laterally into the posterior triangle of the neck. The anterior triangle may then be examined more thoroughly, not forgetting the midline. Do not omit to examine the sub-occipital region and the posterior aspect of the neck. In some instances as with a thyroid swelling or carotid body tumour it may be appropriate to carry out auscultation over the swelling for a bruit.

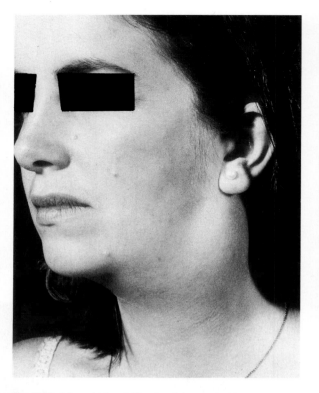

Fig. 23.19 A branchial cyst. The site of the cyst in this patient is typical; it was smooth and fluctuation could be elicited. If such cysts are aspirated the fluid is yellow and contains fat and cholesterol crystals.

Neck swellings

Neck swellings can be notoriously difficult to diagnose. The majority are likely to be lymph nodes which are enlarged either as a result of primary disease such as lymphoma or of secondary disease such as metastatic carcinoma. Primary diseases of the lymph nodes are dealt with in Chapter 9.

Branchial cysts

Branchial cysts are derived from remnants of a branchial cleft, usually the second. Although present at birth they may not necessarily distend and become palpable until adult life. Most present during early adult life and are sited deep to the sternomastoid muscle at the junction of its upper and middle thirds (Fig. 23.19). Because they are cystic, fluctuation can be elicited but if the cyst is very tense the lesion may feel solid.

Most branchial cysts are painless but they may become infected when they enlarge rapidly and are associated with regional lymphadenopathy. Under these circumstances they may simulate a tuberculous abscess. Branchial cysts are not associated with other congenital abnormalities.

Salivary gland swellings

Disorders of the salivary glands have been considered in Chapter 5. They consist of three pairs of glands: the parotids, submandibulars and sublinguals. Broadly speaking, unilateral disease is of a surgical nature, i.e. abscess, stone or tumour whereas bilateral disease is medical, i.e. sarcoidosis or Sjögren's disease. Some of the major causes of swelling of the glands are listed in Table 23.5.

Of the surgical diseases the commonest tumour is the pleomorphic adenoma which affects mainly the parotid gland. Approximately 30 per cent of all salivary tumours are malignant, being carcinomas. Some of these arise in pre-existing pleomorphic adenomas. The carcinoma is differentiated from the adenoma in that it is painful, it grows quickly and invades skin and surrounding structures including the facial nerve.

Acute infection of the salivary glands (almost always the parotid) occurs in debilitated, dehydrated,

Table 23.5. Salivary gland swellings		
Unilateral		
Tumours	Pleomorphic (mixed parotid tumour) Carcinoma	Mainly parotid gland
Abscess Stones in duct		Mainly submandibular
Bilateral		
Mumps Alcoholism Sarcoidosis Sjögren's disease Lymphoma		Both glands affected

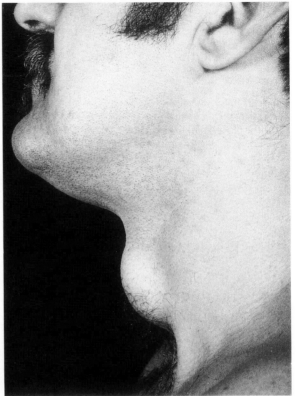

Fig. 23.21 A thyroglossal cyst.

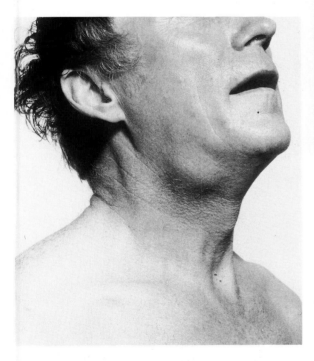

Fig. 23.20 Swelling of the right submandibular gland secondary to a calculus in the submandibular duct. The gland can be distinguished from upper cervical lymph nodes in that it lies beneath the ramus of the mandible 2 cm in front of the sternomastoid muscle.

seriously ill patients almost always suffering from another grave illness.

The characteristic feature of stone in the salivary duct is that pain and swelling in the gland come on just before and during eating and subside afterwards.

Because of the increased viscosity of submandibular salivary juice and the more dependent position of the gland in relation to its duct, calculi are more common in the submandibular duct (Fig. 23.20). Sometimes the calculus can be seen impacted at the end of the submandibular duct at the side of the frenulum of the tongue.

Bilateral (and usually generalized) enlargement of the salivary glands may be secondary to a wide variety of systemic disorders. The term Mikulicz syndrome is a purely descriptive one and refers to combined enlargement of the salivary and lachrymal glands. It is best avoided as it includes a mish-mash of unrelated conditions. Sjögren's syndrome is an autoimmune disorder characterized by enlargement of the lachrymal and salivary glands, with arthritis, dry eyes and dry mouth. The 'sicca' syndrome of dry eyes and dry mouth in primary biliary cirrhosis is probably a variant of this. Sarcoidosis can also cause salivary gland swelling; West Indians and American Negroes seem particularly vulnerable to a florid form of the disease. Occasionally lymphoma and chronic lymphatic leukaemia cause swelling of the salivary glands. Chronic enlargement of the parotids may be seen in the alcoholic.

Thyroglossal cysts

Anterior neck swellings most typically arise in the thyroid gland or along its developmental tract and in the case of thyroglossal cysts the cystic nature may be elicited and displacement upwards of the swelling may be seen on asking the patient to protrude his tongue (Fig. 23.21).

References and further reading

Hall IS, Colman BH. *Diseases of the nose, throat and ear. A handbook for students and practitioners*. Edinburgh: Churchill Livingstone, 1987.

O'Donoghue GH, Bates G and Narula A. *Clinical ENT. An illustrated textbook*. Oxford: Oxford University Press, 1992.

Stafford ND, Youngs R. *ENT Colour aids*. Edinburgh: Churchill Livingstone, 1988.

24

Fever and hypothermia

I. W. Fellows

> Fever
> Physical signs of fever
> Hypothermia
> References and further reading

Fever is a common feature of many illnesses and clues to the diagnosis are often provided by concurrent symptoms such as cough or dysuria. Nevertheless, fever is sometimes the principal or only symptom, in which case a carefully taken history and meticulous physical examination is essential. 'Running a temperature' or 'having a chill' are common complaints by patients that sometimes conceal sinister or serious diseases. Traditionally the term 'pyrexia of unknown origin' (PUO) is used to described a persistent fever, usually of at least two weeks' duration, that is not associated with abnormal, physical signs.

Body temperature in normal subjects

Man is homeothermic, tending to maintain deep-body (core) temperature within narrow limits despite marked changes in environmental temperature. However, core temperature shows diurnal variation of approximately 1 °C with lower waking values and a rise during the hours of consciousness. The body temperature of infants and children can be more labile. The site of measurement also affects the temperature recorded, with rectal temperatures being up to 0.5 °C higher than sublingual temperatures. Conventionally, 37 °C is accepted as the upper limit of normal sublingual temperature.

Core temperature depends upon behavioural changes and the physiological mechanisms of heat production (resting energy expenditure, thermic effort of feeding, exercise, shivering thermogenesis and the more controversial non-shivering thermo-genesis) and heat loss (by radiation, convection, conduction and evaporation). Central control of these mechanisms resides in the hypothalamus.

Physiological causes of an increase in temperature

Severe exertion or exercise such as marathon running may produce significant rises in body temperature to 39 °C; sometimes when the normal body compensatory mechanisms fail levels of 41 °C may be reached (hyperpyrexia). Hot, humid climatic conditions may cause small increases in body temperature. The mean body temperature in women is higher in the second half of the menstrual cycle than it is in the first.

Fever

Fever occurs when the regulatory 'set-point' of the hypothalamus is increased. The precise mechanisms involved remain unclear but involve 'endogenous pyrogens' such as interleukin-1, tumour-necrosis factor and interferon, as well as elevations in hypothalamic prostaglandin E2 levels.

Non-infective causes of fever

It is essential to realize that not all fevers are due to infective conditions. Tissue necrosis such as in myocardial infarction or pulmonary infarction commonly causes fever as does profound anaemia (characteristically as in pernicious anaemia) and the connective tissue diseases. Malignant disease, particularly the lymphomas and carcinoma of the kidney, may also be associated with fever. The intermittent, relapsing, so-called Pel–Ebstein fever is rarely seen in Hodgkin's disease and it remains controversial to what extent patterns of fever are of diagnostic assistance.

A wide range of drugs may cause fever either in therapeutic doses or in overdose, e.g. salicylate. The most dramatic and dangerous examples are malignant hyperpyrexia (an autosomal dominantly inherited disorder) provoked by inhalational anaesthetics, and the malignant neuroleptic syndrome induced by drugs such as haloperidol. Some of the commoner causes of non-infective fevers are shown in Table 24.1.

Table 24.1. Non-infective causes of fever
Malignancy
Particularly the lymphomas
Note carcinoma of the kidney as a cause of PUO
Tissue necrosis
Myocardial infarction
Pulmonary infarction
Trauma
Connective tissue disease
SLE
PAN
Polymyalgia arteritica
Severe anaemia
Particularly pernicious anaemia
Granulomatous disease
Sarcoidosis
Pontine haemorrhage
Drugs
Malignant neuroleptic syndrome
Malignant hyperpyrexia
Factitious

Fever due to infections

Here, of course, the list covers the whole field of microbial disease; however, some basic features are worth remembering. Rigors or shivering attacks commonly occur at the onset of acute infections usually of bacterial aetiology. In the Western world rigors are often due to cholangitis, ascending urinary tract infections or pneumonia. The shivering or shaking phase corresponds to the rise in core temperature with cool vasoconstricted skin; this is associated with a sensation of coldness. Following the rigor there is a hot, drenching sweat. In certain diseases of the tropics, particularly malaria, the remitting character of the fever may help with the diagnosis of the

type of infection (see Chapter 19 and Fig. 19.1). Undulent or relapsing fevers may be seen in such chronic infections as brucellosis. A biphasic, 'saddle-back' type of fever is sometimes, but not typically, seen in dengue fever.

Recovery of untreated lobar pneumonia may be by crisis. This implies a sudden fall in temperature associated with clinical improvement. Such reactions are now rarely seen because of antibiotic therapeutic regimens. More usually a steady fall (lysis) indicates clinical response to treatment.

Earlier reference has been made to the perplexing problem of a PUO — that is a persisting fever without obvious cause and without associated physical signs. Some of the causes of PUO are shown in Table 24.2. In patients presenting ostensibly with a PUO it is important to look for clues as to the cause (Fig. 24.1).

Table 24.2. Causes of PUO
Infections (40%)
Subacute infective endocarditis
Liver abscess
Perinephric abscess
Tuberculosis
Neoplastic disease (20%)
Lymphomas
Carcinoma of the kidney
Connective tissue disease (20%)
SLE
PAN
Other unusual causes (20%)
Familial Mediterranean fever
Crohn's disease

Physical signs of fever

These are of course influenced greatly by the basic cause of the fever. The skin is flushed and much sweating, particularly at night, is a feature of tuberculosis, sepsis, rheumatic fever and lymphoma. The patient may describe how he has to change his pyjamas and bedding having awakened in a drenching sweat. The heart rate is often increased in febrile patients, though in some infections such as typhoid the pulse may be relatively slow. Herpes labialis may complicate fever of any cause but particularly in the immunosuppressed. In severe infections with high fever, (over 39 °C in children and over 40 °C in adults), mild confusion progressing to delirium and convulsions may dominate the picture.

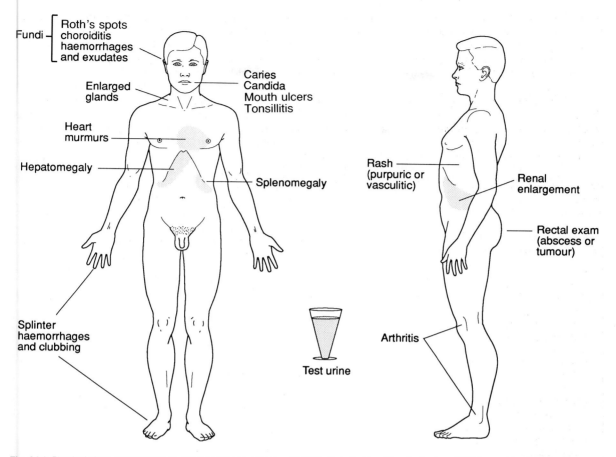

Fig. 24.1 Physical signs that need to be searched for in patients with PUO. Note that traditionally the term PUO is used to describe fevers without signs. This does not excuse the doctor from examining such a patient regularly as the illness progresses; the signs highlighted in the diagram may appear at any time.

Core temperatures over 42 °C may cause rhabdomyolysis, coma and death.

Hypothermia

A core temperature of less than 35 °C denotes hypothermia. In hypothermic patients, it is not possible to record core temperature in the oral cavity or axilla. A low-reading thermometer inserted 15 cm into the rectum provides an accurate measurement of core temperature.

The causes of hypothermia are:

- exposure to cold, which may affect fit, young people as well as the vulnerable elderly. Immersion in cold water causes hypothermia more rapidly because of the higher thermal conductivity of water compared with air

- impaired thermoregulation in infants and the elderly
- pathological conditions:
  - (a) myxoedema — many of the effects of myxoedematous hypothermia are similar to those of simple hypothermia so that this diagnosis can be difficult
  - (b) hypoglycaemia and hypopituitarism — hypoglycaemia causes abolition of shivering by a central effect
  - (c) undernutrition — this results in defective thermogenesis in response to a cold environment
  - (d) any severe illness, e.g. stroke, septicaemia, diabetic ketoacidosis and coma, can result in hypothermia

(e) drugs — alcohol can impair protective behaviour as well as induce hypoglycaemia; barbiturates, phenothiazines and narcotics can also induce hypothermia

(f) injury — accidental and surgical

Physical examination may reveal impaired consciousness or coma. The skin feels cold but at core temperatures of 32–30 °C, vasodilatation may result in a pink colour. At lower temperatures, cyanosis is present. The heart rate slows and at temperatures below 29 °C, cardiac arrhythmias are common, e.g. atrial fibrillation. Ventricular fibrillation can result and attempts at resuscitation should not be abandoned until core temperature has been restored to normal. Falls in arterial blood pressure and respiratory rate, muscular rigidity and diminution or loss of tendon reflexes, and sluggish or absent pupillary reflexes can be seen. Acute pancreatitis and acute tubular necrosis may be induced.

References and further reading

Dinarello CA, Cannon JG, Wolff SM. New concepts on the pathogenesis of fever. *Review of Infectious Diseases (Chicago)*. 1988; **10**: 168–9.

Kluger MJ. Fever: role of pyrogens and cryogens. *Physiological Reviews*. 1991; **71**: 93–127.

Lonning PE, Skulberg A, Abyholm F. Accidental hypothermia. *Acta Anaesthiologica Scandinavica*. 1986; **30**: 601–13.

Moss J. Accidental severe hypothermia. *Surgery, Gynaecology and Obstetrics*. 1986; **162**: 501–13.

Glossary

A Glossary of terms which have not necessarily been defined in the text

Abduction	Movement away from the midline of body or limb.
Adduction	Movement towards the midline of body or limb.
−algia	A suffix meaning 'pain arising in or from'.
Amnesia	Loss of memory.
Aneurysm	Dilatation of an artery.
Anorexia	Loss of appetite.
Anosognosia	Lack of awareness or acceptance of severe disability, usually a left hemiplegia.
Anuria	Failure of secretion of urine.
Aplasia	Lack of development or growth.
Ascites	Fluid in the peritoneal cavity.
Blepharitis	Inflammation or redness of the eyelid margins.
Brady−	A prefix meaning slow.
Bruit	A noise due to turbulent flow in a blood vessel.
Bulla (pl. ae)	Large blisters in the skin.
Cachexia	Wasting.
Chemosis	Oedema of the conjunctiva.
Cholestasis	Stagnation of bile.
Circadian	A description of a rhythm recurring on a daily basis.
Coarctation	A narrowing of a blood vessel.
Crepitus	Grating or creaking with joint or bone movement.
Cyanosis	Blue colour of the skin due to deoxygenation of the blood.
−cytopenia	A suffix meaning a reduced number of cells.
Diverticulum (pl. a)	A blind sac.
Dys−	A prefix meaning pain or difficulty with certain activities.
Dysarthria	Difficulty in articulation.
Dysphagia	Difficulty or pain on swallowing.
Dysphasia	A language defect in putting thoughts into words (expressive) or understanding the spoken word (receptive).
Dysphonia	Difficulty in phonation.
Dysplasia	Abnormal development of growth.
Dyspnoea	Breathlessness or difficulty in breathing.
Dyspraxia	Difficulty in formulating and synthesizing movement patterns.
Dysuria	Scalding or pain on micturition.
Ecchymosis (pl. es)	Bruise.
Effusion	A collection of fluid in a potential space.
Embolus (pl. i)	Substance carried in the blood stream and large enough to occlude a vessel.

Epigastrium	Upper abdomen.
Erythema	Redness or flushing of the skin due to dilatation of superficial blood vessels.
Erythrodermia	Red skin.
Exophthalmos	Protrusion of the globe of the eye in thyroid disease.
Fistula (pl. ae)	An abnormal track between two hollow organs or between an organ and the skin surface.
Fossa (pl. ae)	A hollow.
Frequency	Frequent passage of small volumes of urine.
Gangrene	Death and infective necrosis of tissue.
Gingivitis	Inflammation of the gums.
Haematemesis (pl. es)	Vomiting of blood.
Haematuria	Blood in the urine.
Haemolysis	Breakdown or destruction of erythrocytes.
Haemoptysis (pl. es)	Coughing up blood.
Hallucinations	Abnormal perceptions of objects.
Hemianopia	Half of the visual field on one side.
Homonymous	On the same side, as in vision.
Hyper—	A prefix meaning overactivity or more than normal.
Hyperacusis	Sounds seeming to be unduly loud.
Hyperaemia	Increased blood flow.
Hyperhidrosis	Excess sweating.
Hyperphagia	Increased eating.
Hypo—	A prefix implying underactivity or less than normal.
Iatrogenic	Caused by doctors or as a result of treatment.
Ichthyosis	Scaly, fish-like skin.
Idiopathic	Cause unknown.
—itis	A suffix implying 'inflammation of'.
Illusions	Misinterpretations of stimuli.
Intertrigo	Eczema at skin flexures.
Koilonychia	Spoon shaped nails.
Kyphos	An increase in the forward flexion of the thoracic spine by sharp angulation at one point.
Kyphosis	An increase in the anteroposterior curvature of the spine.
Lanugo	Soft fine hair as in the newborn.
Macro—	Large.
Macule	A small, visible but non-palpable skin lesion.
Mydriasis	Dilatation of the pupil.
Naevus (pl. i)	A skin blemish, not necessarily vascular in origin.
Nocturia	Passing urine at night.
—nychia	A suffix meaning 'of the nail'.
Oedema	Fluid in tissues.
Oligo—	Prefix meaning reduced or little.
Oligomenorrhoea	Scanty periods.
Oliguria	Secretion of small volumes of urine.
Onycholysis	Separation of the distal nail from the nail bed.
—orrhoea	A suffix meaning 'discharge from'.
Orthopnoea	Breathlessness on lying flat.
Osteomalacia	Failure of calcification of new osteoid.
Osteoporosis	Reduction in bone mass.
Phlebitis	Inflammation of a vein.
—plasty	A suffix denoting repair or correction by surgery.
Pleurisy	Pain arising from the pleura.
Pneumo—	Prefix meaning air in an organ or cavity.

−**pnoea**	A suffix meaning 'related to breathing'.
Polycythaemia	Excess of erythrocytes in the blood.
Polyphagia	Increased appetite.
Polyuria	Passing large volumes of urine.
Prognathos	Protrusion of the lower jaw.
Proptosis	Protrusion of the globe.
Pruritus	Skin itching.
Ptosis	Drooping of the eyelid.
Scoliosis	A lateral curvature of the spine.
Stenosis (pl. es)	A narrowing.
Stigma (pl. ata)	A characteristic sign.
Sulcus (pl. i)	A groove or furrow.
Tachy−	A prefix meaning fast.
Telangiectasia	Enduring dilatation of blood vessels in skin.
−**uria**	A suffix used relating to the urine.
Vesicles	Small blisters in the skin.
Viscus (pl. era)	Hollow internal organ.
Xanthoma (pl. s)	Deposits of lipids in the skin.
Xanthelasma (pl. s)	Plaques of lipids in the skin of the eyelids.

Subject Index